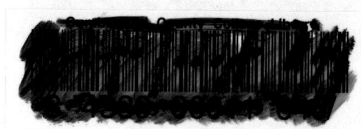

EKG for Nursing

DeMYSTiFieD

Notice

Medicine is an ever-changing science. As new research and clinical experience broaden our knowledge, changes in treatment and drug therapy are required. The authors and the publisher of this work have checked with sources believed to be reliable in their efforts to provide information that is complete and generally in accord with the standards accepted at the time of publication. However, in view of the possibility of human error or changes in medical sciences, neither the authors nor the publisher nor any other party who has been involved in the preparation or publication of this work warrants that the information contained herein is in every respect accurate or complete, and they disclaim all responsibility for any errors or omissions or for the results obtained from use of the information contained in this work. Readers are encouraged to confirm the information contained herein with other sources. For example and in particular, readers are advised to check the product information sheet included in the package of each drug they plan to administer to be certain that the information contained in this work is accurate and that changes have not been made in the recommended dose or in the contraindications for administration. This recommendation is of particular importance in connection with new or infrequently used drugs.

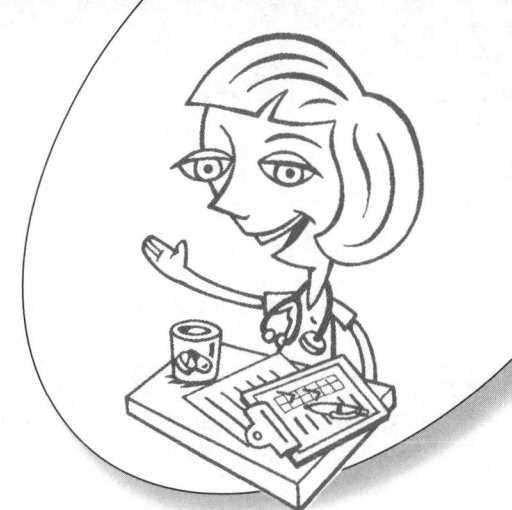

EKG for Nursing
DeMYSTiFieD

Patricia Clutter, RN, MEd, CEN, FAEN

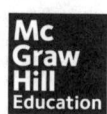

New York   Chicago   San Francisco   Athens   London   Madrid
Mexico City   Milan   New Delhi   Singapore   Sydney   Toronto

EKG for Nursing Demystified

2 3 4 5 6 7 8 9 0   DOC/DOC   19 18 17 16

MHID 0-07-180169-3
ISBN 978-0-07-180169-0

This book was set in Berling by Cenveo® Publisher Services.
The editors were Michael Weitz and Regina Y. Brown.
The production supervisor was Richard Ruzycka.
Production management was provided by Anupriya Tyagi, Cenveo Publisher Services.
RR Donnelley was printer and binder.

This book is printed on acid-free paper.

Library of Congress Cataloging-in-Publication Data

Clutter, Patricia, author.
    EKG for nursing demystified / Patricia Clutter.—First edition.
        p.; cm.
    Includes index.
    ISBN 978-0-07-180169-0 (pbk. : alk. paper)—ISBN 0-07-180169-3 (pbk. : alk. paper)
    I. Title.
    [DNLM: 1. Electrocardiography—methods—Nurses' Instruction. WG 140]
    RC683.5.E5
    616.1'207547—dc23
                                                            2014020120

McGraw-Hill Education books are available at special quantity discounts to use as premiums and sales promotions, or for use in corporate training programs. To contact a representative please e-mail us at bulksales@mcgraw-hill.com.

This book is dedicated to the myriad of patients and their loved ones that I have had the joy to work with throughout my 40 plus years in the profession of emergency nursing. Through each of them, I have learned a little bit more each time and hopefully have provided the excellent care that I desired to provide. For each of my colleagues who have worked and continue to work beside me, I tip my nurses' hat and breathe a sigh of "thank you" for each time you offered your support and knowledge.

This book is also dedicated to my children, Justace and Ben, and the women in their lives, Huan and Melanie, my mother, Celia, and my sisters and brothers, who listened endlessly to the phrase, "I'm working on the book." They were awesome in their conversations with me and held me up when the strains of working on multiple projects and jobs attempted to overcome me.

And, of course, my husband, Randy, who has been my constant cheerleader and shoulder to cry upon when things didn't always go right at work and who was a saint during the writing of this book. He heard "just a minute" a million times and supported me during every written word. Thank you for always letting me "be me."

—Pat Clutter

Contents

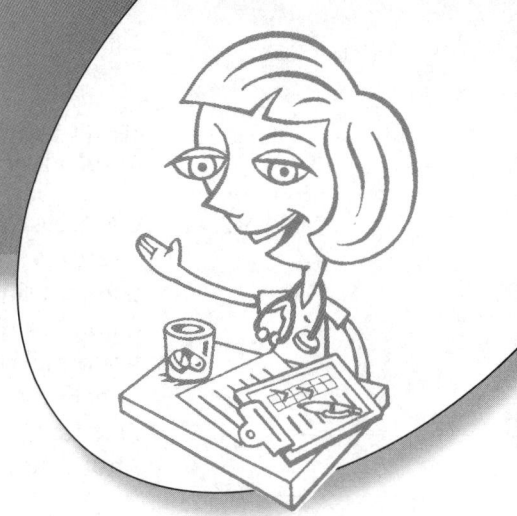

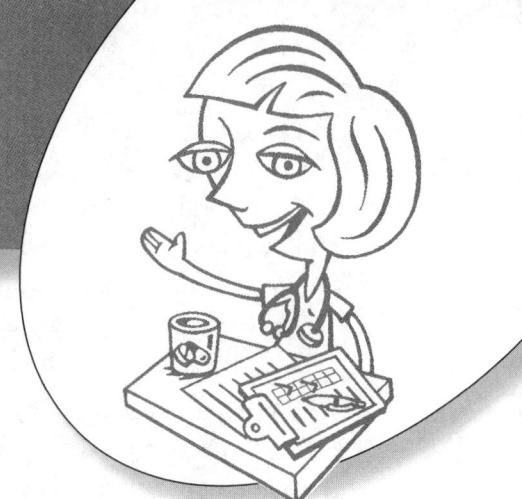

Preface

Understanding and interpreting EKGs and dysrhythmias can be a daunting task for nurses everywhere. Creating a knowledge base and incorporating tools that can help make this charge of our profession easier is the mission of this book. Once general rules are understood, the undertaking of this chore can be a positive addition to our roles of caring for our patients and their loved ones; for it is not only the patient who has multiple questions about the things that we do and the machines that we use to help us attain optimal care. Students who are studying to achieve an understanding of this aspect of care, new nurses who are building confidence in their skills, and the experienced nurse who desires to resharpen their knowledge can all benefit from the contents of this book.

We have worked hard to "demystify" this difficult facet of nursing by starting at the beginning and building upon the blocks of learning as each chapter takes on a different aspect of the world of electrocardiography. Through this book, we provide background physiology and pathophysiology, appreciation for concepts, and highlighted "clinical alerts" in order to provide a thorough comprehension of not only the science of this subject, but also the art that must be incorporated so that our patients feel comfortable with the process and with us.

Each chapter is built around the following tools that contribute to the reader's ability to grasp the intent and purpose of each topic:

Objectives and key terms that are used within that particular chapter
An overview to highlight the target goals of each chapter
Clinical alerts to bring out important components of subject matter
Tables to provide information in an easy to understand format

Boxes that highlight significant factors
Figures to visualize essential portions of information
Real world practical wisdom that has stood the test of time
Key points highlighted in the conclusion
Practice questions to explore the reader's comprehension
Answer keys with rationales and reiteration of concepts
A final exam to test the learner's knowledge level

We hope that you enjoy your journey through this part of the prism that extends to so many facets of care. Each of us must continue the learning process throughout our careers in our chosen specialties so that we may provide excellent attention to the details of our patient care. May you attain and maintain wisdom and knowledge, clarity of thought, skillful hands, and a compassionate heart as we all work towards the highest level of protection for those entrusted to our care.

Patricia Clutter, RN, MEd, CEN, FAEN

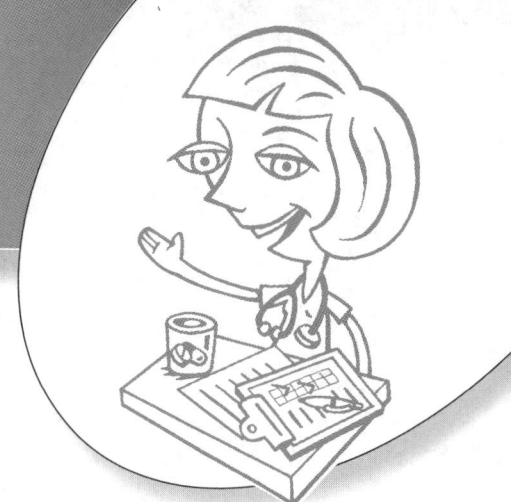

Acknowledgments

My sincerest gratitude and appreciation to the individuals at McGraw-Hill—Michael Weitz, and Regina Brown; and Anupriya Tyagi (Cenveo Publisher Services)—who kept me on track and helped me understand this process. Their patience was overwhelming! Also, much thanks to Joanna Cain who believed in me and approached me regarding taking on this project. I owe each of these individuals a great deal.

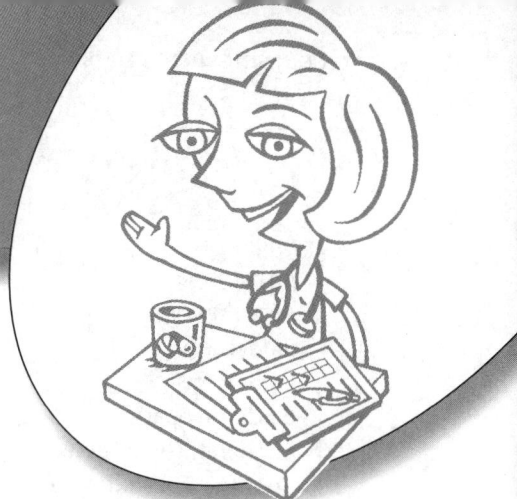

chapter **1**

Introduction

At the end of this chapter, the student will be able to:

❶ Describe an electrocardiogram (EKG) and the equipment needed to perform this diagnostic test.

❷ Detail the history of EKG and related advances in today's technology.

❸ List the clinical uses for EKG.

❹ Distinguish the health care personnel who may conduct EKG and the certification opportunities available in the discipline.

KEY WORDS

Angina	Endocarditis
Arrhythmia	Heart failure
Auscultation	Heart valve disease
Bradycardia	Holter monitor
Cardiologist	Ischemia
Cardiomyopathy	Myocardial infarction
Congenital heart defects	Pacemaker
Coronary heart disease	Pericarditis
Dysrhythmia	Physiologist
Electrocardiogram	Stress test
Electrodes	Tachycardia

Overview

Electrocardiogram, or EKG—also referred to as ECG—is a diagnostic test, performed at the bedside, that assists in the assessment of problems or disturbances with the electrical activity of the heart. This electrical activity within the heart is observed by means of an external EKG machine that connects via cables to **electrodes**. These electrodes are placed on the patient's skin where they detect the heart's electrical impulses. These electrical impulses are then "translated" by the EKG machine and recorded as line tracings on paper. The tracings on the special paper are referred to as a "12 lead." A "rhythm strip" is different than an EKG. An EKG looks at all angles of the electrical conduction system providing 12 views. (There are also 15- and 18-lead EKGs that are performed to diagnose specific **myocardial infarction** processes.) A "rhythm strip" shows one lead. This is useful to determine rate and rhythm and as an ongoing tool during patient observation. Today's cardiac monitors have many tools built into them to assist health care personnel to screen for patient problems. A rhythm strip can also be produced by an EKG machine.

Figure 1–1 shows a normal EKG strip and Fig. 1–2 shows a 12-lead EKG. By the time you finish this book, you will be able to recognize a normal EKG rhythm strip that can be obtained from an EKG tracing or a cardiac monitor, identify all the common electrical cardiac abnormalities, and understand common concepts relative to the EKG and disease processes.

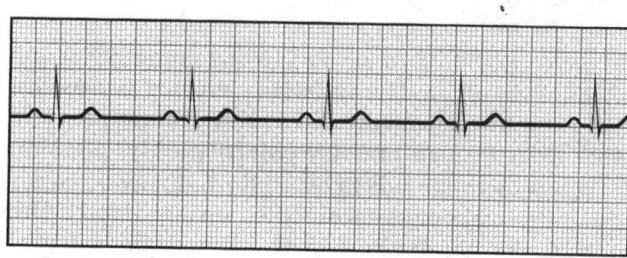

FIGURE 1–1 • **Normal EKG strip.** Strip shows normal sinus rhythm. [*From Saladin KS. (2012). Anatomy & Physiology: The Unity of Form and Function, 6e. McGraw-Hill.*]

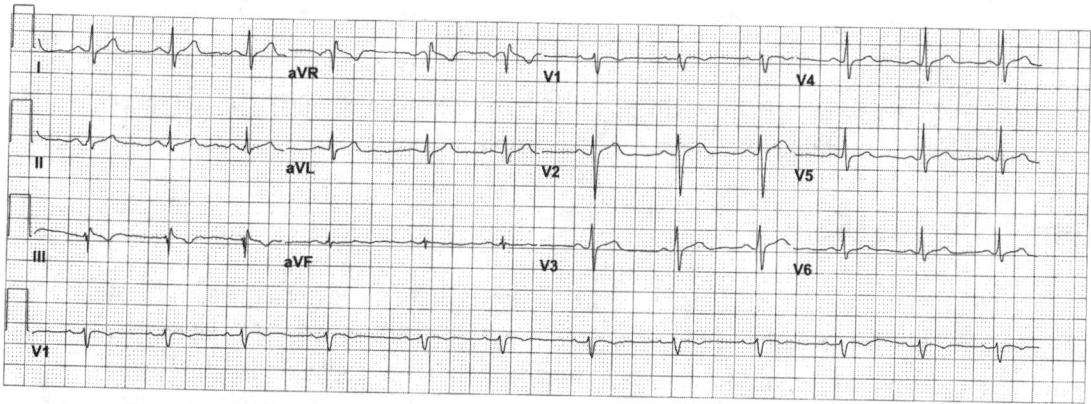

FIGURE 1–2 • **12-lead electrocardiogram.** A standard 12-lead electrocardiogram showing a rhythm strip taken from lead V_1. [*From Raff, Hershel and Levitzky, Michael, (2011). Medical Physiology A Systems Approach, McGraw-Hill.*]

History of EKG

Willem Einthoven, a Dutch **physiologist**, introduced the EKG in 1903. Although Carl Ludwig and his student Augustus Waller are credited with initially tracing the heartbeat onto a phonographic plate fixed to a toy train that allowed the heartbeat to be recorded in real time in 1887, Einthoven perfected this system in 1903 to create a much more sensitive device. Einthoven's participants would immerse each of their limbs into containers of salt solution from which the EKG was recorded as opposed to today's method of using self-adhesive electrodes. This original machine weighed 500 pounds and required multiple people to function.

Einthoven assigned the letters P, Q, R, S, and T, still used today, to the waves and segments found in the EKG (Fig. 1–3). This earned him the Nobel Prize in Medicine in 1924.

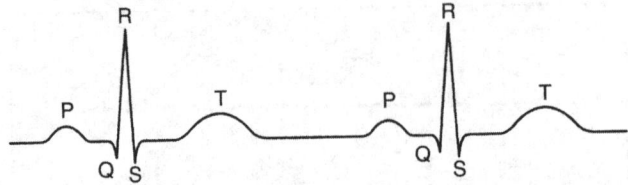

FIGURE 1–3 • Normal electrocardiogram showing the P, Q, R, S, T waves. [*From Huff, Jane.(2012). ECG Workout Exercises in Arrhythmia Interpretation 6e.*]

Many advances have been made in electrocardiography through the decades. Once cumbersome laboratory machines, today's EKG devices are compact electronic systems that offer computerized interpretation of EKG. In keeping with the future's mobile trends, a sleek, low-power wireless case can be attached to a smartphone to transform the phone to a clinical-quality cardiac event recorder with the help of a smartphone application.

Clinical Uses of EKG

The clinical uses of EKG are vast. EKGs are utilized in every aspect of health care. They can be used in physician's or provider's offices or in any department in the hospital environment including (but not limited to) the emergency department, medical/surgical departments, intensive care units, labor and delivery, surgery, postanesthesia care unit, and pediatrics. EKGs are also used routinely in the prehospital setting, often being electronically transmitted to the emergency department physician prior to arrival. They can also be completed in a patient's home by home health care agency personnel or individuals who work for insurance companies. EKGs may be performed at health screenings, routine physical examinations, or presurgical workups in a planned elective situation. They are also an emergent diagnostic tool in potentially life-threatening situations. The individual receiving an EKG ranges from someone who is initiating a new exercise regimen to a person who is having chest pain. The use of the EKG is cross-generational, providing clues to care for all age groups from the infant with congenital heart disease to the centenarian with shortness of breath.

EKGs are also performed to determine heart rhythms that are different than the normal rhythm when abnormal electrical impulses disturb the cardiac cycle. These are called **arrhythmias** or **dysrhythmias** (Fig. 1–4). These terms are usually used interchangeably; however, "dysrhythmia" is more accurate since the term "arrhythmia" can officially mean an absence of heart rhythm. In this book, the term dysrhythmia will be utilized to differentiate an abnormal rhythm. These dysrhythmias will be explored in detail later in this book.

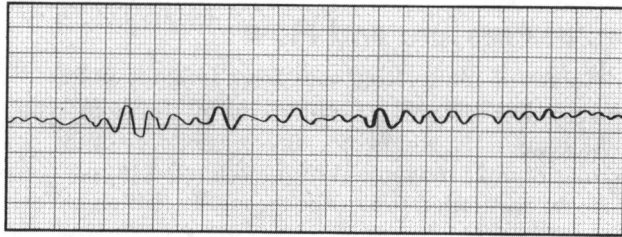

FIGURE 1−4 • EKG strip showing dysrhythmia. Ventricular Fibrillation, a type of dysrhythmia, can be seen in myocardial infarction (heart attack). [*From Saladin KS. (2012). Anatomy & Physiology: The Unity of Form and Function, 6e. McGraw-Hill.*]

CLINICAL ALERT

During dysrhythmia, the heart can beat too fast (**tachycardia**), too slow (**bradycardia**), or with an irregular rhythm.

EKG is used to

- Assess heart rhythm (rate and regularity of heartbeats)
- Diagnose poor blood flow to the heart muscle (**ischemia**)
- Diagnose a heart attack (myocardial infarction)
- Diagnose abnormal electrical conduction of the heart
- Diagnose heart chamber enlargement
- Measure the effects of drugs or devices used to regulate the heart (such as a **pacemaker** or cardiac medications)

An EKG may be recommended for patients who experience the following signs and symptoms:

- Chest pain (**angina**)
- Breathing problems
- Tiredness and weakness
- Unusual heart sounds found upon **auscultation**
- Unusual heartbeat, fluttering, racing, or pounding

An EKG can show

- Dysrhythmia
- Birth defects in the heart (**congenital heart defects**)
- Problems with the heart valves (**endocarditis**)
- A heart that does not pump blood forcefully enough (**heart failure**)

- Lack of blood flow to the heart muscle (**coronary heart disease**)
- Inflammation of the sac that surrounds the heart (**pericarditis**)
- Heart muscle that is too thick or parts of the heart that are too big (**cardiomyopathy**)

Who Can Perform an EKG?

An EKG may be performed by health care workers who have received specific EKG training, such as physicians, physician assistants, nurse practitioners, nurses, certified nursing assistants, medical assistants, paramedics, emergency medical technicians, cardiac technicians, and specifically EKG technicians. Training includes EKG operation and troubleshooting, electrode placement, use of EKG grid paper, and the recognition of normal and abnormal EKG patterns.

Health care workers can obtain this training from their educational institutions. However, most EKG technicians are trained on the job in a facility by an EKG supervisor or a **cardiologist**. On-the-job training usually lasts 8 to 16 weeks. Certification programs that can last up to 1 year are also available and offer programs for basic EKG, **Holter monitoring**, and **stress testing**. Holter monitoring involves equipping the patient with a portable EKG monitor that attaches to the patient's belt and electrodes that reside on the patient's chest. The patient's normal activity is monitored for 24 or 48 hours in order to detect any abnormal heart rhythms. The test results are printed out and interpreted by a specialist to diagnose heart conditions such as dysrhythmias and pacemaker problems.

A stress test involves recording a patient's base EKG reading while the patient stands still. Then the patient is asked to first walk and then run on a treadmill as the technician increases the treadmill's speed. The specialist then interprets the test results to determine the effect this increased exertion has on a patient's heart. Stress tests can also be performed with medications that speed up the heart for those patients who cannot walk on a treadmill.

CLINICAL ALERT

State laws vary as to which medical professionals can legally interpret EKG results for diagnostic purposes. In all states, physicians can interpret EKG results. Do not provide a patient with an interpretation of EKG results unless it is within your scope of practice to do so.

Conclusion

Electrocardiogram is a diagnostic test that checks for problems with the electrical activity of the heart. EKG is used to identify and diagnose a wide range of heart problems. Note these key points:

- An EKG machine is an external device that uses electrodes attached to the patient's skin to detect the heart's electrical impulses.
- Special paper records the EKG tracings.
- Willem Einthoven created the EKG in 1903 and won a Nobel Prize in Medicine for its creation in 1924.
- EKG is used to assess heart rhythm; diagnose poor blood flow to the heart muscle; diagnose a heart attack; diagnose abnormal electrical conduction of the heart; diagnose heart chamber enlargement; and measure the effects of drugs or devices used to regulate the heart.
- EKG may be recommended for patients who experience angina; breathing problems; tiredness and weakness; unusual heart sounds; and unusual heartbeat, fluttering, racing, or pounding.
- EKG can provide evidence for dysrhythmias, congenital heart defects, **heart valve disease**, heart failure, coronary heart disease, pericarditis, and cardiomyopathy.
- EKG may be performed by health care workers who have received specific EKG training, such as physicians, physician assistants, nurse practitioners, nurses, certified nursing assistants, medical assistants, paramedics, emergency medical technicians, cardiac technicians, and specifically EKG technicians.
- EKG is performed in the clinical setting such as a physician's office, health clinic or hospital, and in other areas such as the patient's home.

PRACTICE QUESTIONS

1. **Electrocardiogram is a diagnostic test that checks for**
   A. fluid overload in the circulatory system.
   B. electrical conduction problems of the heart.
   C. carotid artery plaque.
   D. heart chamber atrophy.

2. **Einthoven had his participants immerse their limbs into which solution to help record the heart's impulses?**

   A. Hydrogen peroxide

   B. Betadine

   C. Salt solution

   D. Tap water

3. **The letters assigned to the waves and segments as determined by Einthoven and still used in EKG today are**

   A. A, B, C, D, E

   B. M, N, O, P, Q

   C. P, Q, R, S, T

   D. S, T, U, V, W

4. **The term *dysrhythmia* refers to**

   A. abnormal electrical impulses of the heart.

   B. any cardiac disease or condition.

   C. a pacemaker device.

   D. a device that measures heart activity.

5. **EKG is used to diagnose**

   A. Ludwig angina.

   B. Jugular venous distention.

   C. Compartment syndrome.

   D. Pericarditis.

ANSWER KEY

1. **B.** Electrocardiogram is a diagnostic test that checks for electrical conduction problems of the heart.

2. **C.** Einthoven had his participants place their limbs in salt solution to help record the heart's impulses.

3. **C.** P, Q, R, S, and T are the letters assigned to the waves and segments by Einthoven that are still used today.

4. **A.** *Dysrhythmia* refers to abnormal electrical impulses of the heart.

5. **D.** EKG is used to diagnose pericarditis, which is an inflammation of the sac that surrounds the heart.

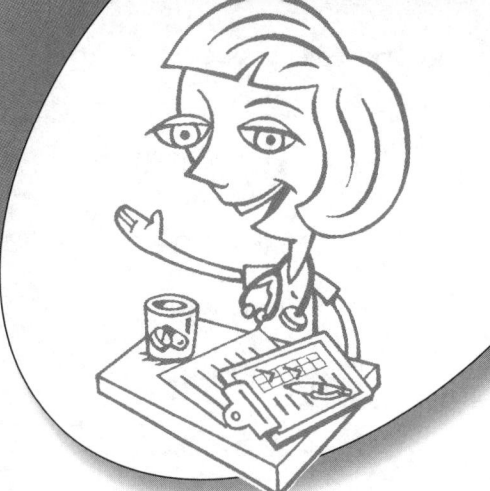

chapter **2**

Heart Anatomy and Physiology

LEARNING OBJECTIVES

At the end of this chapter, the student will be able to:

1 Describe the anatomy of the heart including the layers of the heart, the pericardial space, and coronary circulation.

2 Detail the structure and function of the heart's chambers.

3 List the heart's four valves including their anatomical location and purpose.

4 Describe the sympathetic and parasympathetic nervous systems in relation to heart function.

5 Compare the differences among the four major heart sounds.

6 Explain the flow of the blood through the heart and how this impacts the cardiac cycle.

7 Describe the components of cardiac output and its relationship to blood pressure.

KEY WORDS

Acute myocardial infarction
Afterload
Aortic valve
Apex
Atrial gallop
Atrial kick
Atrioventricular (AV) valves
Atrium
Autonomic nervous system
Base
Blood pressure
Cardiac output
Cardiac tamponade
Carotid sinus massage
Chronotropic
Chordae tendineae
Contractility
Coronary artery disease (CAD)
Depolarization
Diastasis
Diastole
Ejection fraction
End-diastolic volume
Endocardium
End-systolic volume
Epicardium
Exudate
Fibrous pericardium
Gallop rhythm
Hypertension
Hypertrophy
Hypotension

Inotropic
Ischemia
Mediastinum
Mitral valve
Murmur
Myocardial vortex
Myocardium
Ostium
Parasympathetic nervous system
Pericardial fluid
Pericarditis
Pericardial effusion
Pericardiocentesis
Pericardium
Peripheral vascular resistance
Preload
Pulmonic valve
Purulent
Regurgitation
Semilunar (SL) valves
Serous pericardium
Sternum
Stroke volume
Subendocardial area
Subepicardial area
Sympathetic nervous system
Systole
Tachycardia
Tricuspid valve
Valvular prolapse
Ventricle

Overview

The human heart is a hollow, cone-shaped, muscular organ roughly the size of its owner's fist that weighs approximately 9 to 12 oz (250-350 g) (Fig. 2–1). The heart measures about 5 in (13 cm) long from base to apex, 3.5 in (9 cm)

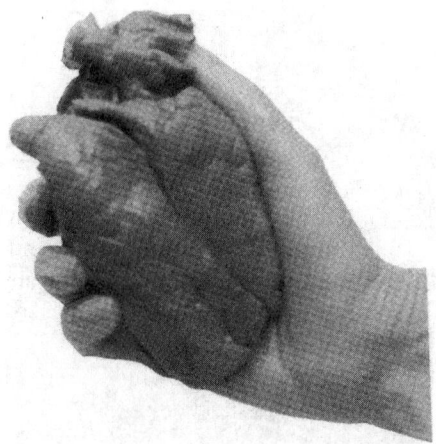

FIGURE 2–1 • Size of the human heart. The heart is approximately the same size as the individual's fist. [*Modified from Aehlert, Barbara (2011). ECG's Made Easy, 4e. Mosby Elsevier.*]

wide (at the base or top of the heart), and 2.5 in (6 cm) thick. It comprises approximately 0.45% of a man's and about 0.40% of a woman's body weight. Variances that can be noted would be an athlete whose heart would most likely weigh more than someone who does not exercise regularly, a person with heart disease whose heart has increased in size and mass (**hypertrophy**), and an elderly individual whose heart would weigh less than someone in early adulthood. A person's heart size and weight are influenced by body weight, physical build, exercise regimen, age, sex, and illnesses such as heart disease, scoliosis, and diabetes.

The heart is located in the chest slightly to the left of the breastbone. The heart resides in a space behind the **sternum** and in front of the spine between the lungs called the **mediastinum**. It sits above the diaphragm and tilts like an inverted triangle with two thirds of the heart lying to the left of the sternum. The remaining third of this organ extends into the right side of the sternum.

The top of the heart (the part closest to the head) is the **base**. The major portion of the base, which lies below the second rib, is established by the left **atrium**. The right atrium contributes a smaller portion of this base. The base is where the great vessels, including the aorta and the pulmonary artery, are attached to the heart. The heart lies in front of the esophagus and the trachea and the descending portion of the aorta lies behind this portion of the heart. The lower portion of the heart (the point of the triangle) is the **apex** and consists of the left **ventricle** which tilts down and forward, toward the left side of the body. It is positioned between the fifth and sixth ribs in the left midclavicular line and rests superior to or above the diaphragm (Fig. 2–2).

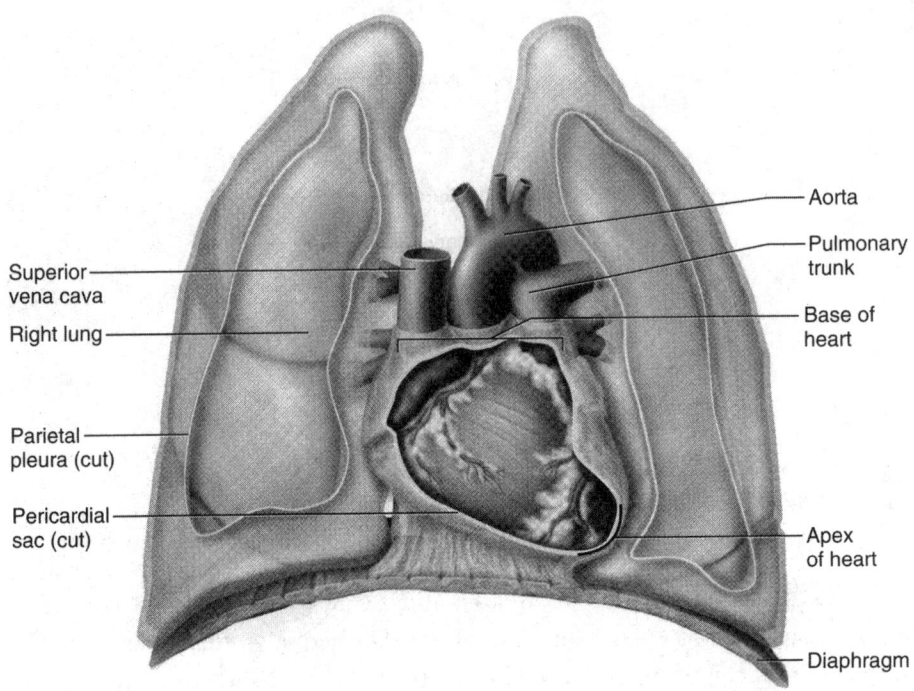

FIGURE 2–2 • Position of the heart in the chest. Frontal view of the chest showing the position of the heart. [*Modified From Saladin KS. (2011). Human Anatomy, 3e. McGraw-Hill.*]

The position of the heart can vary considerably depending on body build, size and shape of the chest, and the level of the diaphragm. The heart of tall, slender people tends to hang vertically and be positioned centrally. Short, stocky people tend to have hearts that lie more left and horizontally. The infant heart lies in a more horizontal position until the age of approximately 7. The apex of the heart in the infant population is positioned at the fourth intercostal space.

CLINICAL ALERT

The function of the heart is to pump blood through the network of arteries and veins called the cardiovascular system.

Heart Layers

The heart's wall is made up of three tissue layers: **endocardium**, **myocardium**, and **epicardium** (Table 2–1).

TABLE 2–1 Layers of the Heart Wall		
Endocardium	**Myocardium**	**Epicardium**
• Innermost layer • Thin, smooth • Consists of endocardial cells and connective tissue • Lines heart's inner chambers, valves, muscles • Continuous with vessel system • Capillaries made up of one thin layer of endothelial cells	• Middle layer • Thick, muscular • Consists of cardiac muscle fibers • Largest portion of heart's wall • Contracts with each heartbeat and pumps blood • Subdivided into subendocardial and subepicardial areas • Left ventricle is thickest due to the function of this portion of the heart	• Outermost layer • Continuous with inner lining of pericardium • Consists of squamous epithelial cells overlying connective tissue • Contains nerve fibers, blood vessels, lymph capillaries, and fat • Main coronary arteries lie on epicardial surface

- **Endocardium:** Innermost layer of the heart wall made up of a thin layer of endothelial cells and connective tissues. This smooth endocardium lines the heart's inner chambers and valves and is continuous with the interior layer of the arteries and veins. Capillaries, the connection between the arteries and veins in the body, are made up of one thin layer of endothelial cells. This allows for ease of movement of oxygen and other crucial elements to move across the membrane to nourish the cells and for waste products such as carbon dioxide to pass into the vascular space to be carried to their exit points.

- **Myocardium:** Thick, muscular, middle layer of the heart wall consisting of cardiac muscle fibers which are found only in the heart. The myocardium is the largest portion of the heart's wall and is responsible for the pumping action of the heart because this layer of muscle tissue contracts with each heartbeat. The muscle fibers in this layer are laid out in a spiral fashion which assists in the work of this muscle by creating a twisting or spiral motion that enhances each contraction. This is called the **myocardial vortex**. The myocardium is subdivided into two areas: the **subendocardial area** and the **subepicardial area**.

  - **Subendocardial area:** Innermost section of the myocardium

  - **Subepicardial area:** Outermost section of the myocardium

CLINICAL ALERT

The myocardial layer of the ventricles is much thicker than that of the atria because the ventricles pump blood to the lungs and the rest of the body whereas the atria encounter little resistance when pumping blood through the valves to the ventricles. The left myocardium, which pumps blood against greater resistance to feed the arteries of the body as it exits the aorta, is also thicker than the right ventricle which propels blood into the nearby pulmonary system presenting a lesser degree of resistance.

- **Epicardium:** Outermost layer of the heart wall formed by squamous epithelial cells and connective tissue containing nerve fibers, blood vessels, lymph capillaries, and fat. This is also the visceral layer of the serous pericardium, establishing a continuum with the inner lining of the pericardial sac. The main coronary arteries are located on this layer. These arteries receive oxygenated blood first prior to entering the myocardium itself which then supplies the inner layers with oxygen rich blood.

CLINICAL ALERT

The heart's endocardial area is at the greatest risk for **ischemia** (decreased supply of oxygenated blood to an organ or body part). This area is fed by the distal branches of the coronary arteries that lie on the epicardial surface of the heart. It has excessive requirements for oxygen.

A layer of connective tissue called the **pericardium**, which is a tough, double-walled sac that protects the heart from injury and infection, encloses the heart. The pericardium consists of the outer **fibrous pericardium** and the inner **serous pericardium**.

- **Fibrous pericardium:** Tough fibrous tissue that serves as the outer, protective layer. This layer fits around the heart in a loose fashion which allows the heart to expand with each heartbeat, but contains it within a specific area preventing expansion beyond acceptable limits. The fibrous pericardium anchors the heart to surrounding structures, such as the diaphragm and sternum with ligaments and prevents the heart from moving around excessively in the chest.

- **Serous pericardium:** Thin, smooth, inner portion of the pericardium that has two layers. The inner layer is called the parietal layer. This layer lines the inner portion of the fibrous pericardium described above. The visceral layer lies on the outermost portion of the heart itself and is contiguous with the epicardium (Fig. 2–3).

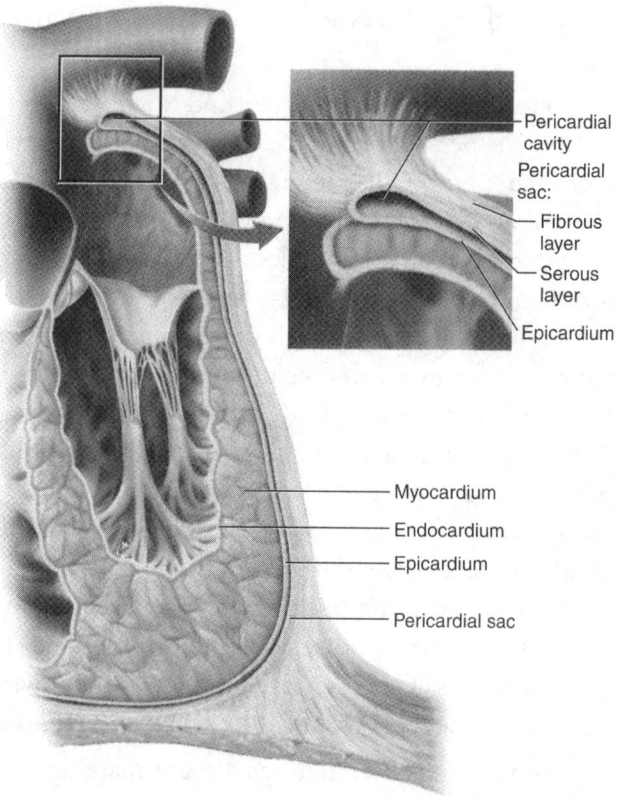

Pericardial cavity

Pericardial sac:

Fibrous layer

Serous layer

Epicardium

Myocardium

Endocardium

Epicardium

Pericardial sac

FIGURE 2–3 • **Layers of the heart's wall.** Layers of the heart wall include the epicardium, endocardium, and myocardium. The pericardial sac is made up of fibrous and serous layers. [*From Saladin KS. (2011). Human Anatomy, 3e. McGraw-Hill.*]

Pericardial Space

Between the parietal and visceral layers of the serous pericardium is an area called the pericardial space. This space contains roughly 20 mL of thin, clear fluid secreted by the serous layers—called **pericardial fluid**—that acts as lubricant and cushion to prevent friction each time the heartbeats.

Situations can occur in which too much pericardial fluid is present, blood is present within the space, or an **exudate** exists within the space leading to disruptions to the heart's function.

- **Pericarditis**: Inflammation of the pericardium that results in an excess of pericardial fluid production. This can occur due to rheumatoid arthritis, systemic lupus, a heart attack that destroys the heart muscle, viral or bacterial infection, or heart surgery.

- **Pericardial effusion**: A condition where blood, a **purulent** exudate, and/or pericardial fluid builds up in the pericardial space compressing the heart and interfering with the heart's ability to relax and fill with blood between heartbeats.

- **Cardiac tamponade**: A life-threatening condition in which the extra fluid or blood within the pericardial space creates a situation in which the heart is restricted and cannot fill adequately with blood. This results in a decreased amount of blood which the ventricles are able to pump out to the body. If a decreased amount of blood is forced out through the arterial system (**cardiac output**), this will in turn lead to a decreased amount which can return to the heart through the venous system. This obstruction of blood flow results in an emergent condition which must be treated immediately. This can occur quickly from a traumatic event or can be produced over a longer period of time from disease processes such as malignancies or kidney disease. A pericardial tamponade associated with trauma can produce a life threat with as little as 100 mL of blood in the pericardial sac while a chronic situation can increase the fluid content to as much as 1000 mL with no significant consequences due to the ability of the pericardium to stretch over a period of time. The risk of death is dependent on the rate of the increase in fluid or blood within the space and the capacity of the sac to adjust to the increasing fluid buildup.

Pericardial effusion and cardiac tamponade are managed by a procedure called **pericardiocentesis** where a needle is inserted into the pericardial space and the excess fluid is removed (aspirated) through the needle. Pericarditis is treated with medications.

> ### CLINICAL ALERT
>
> Pericardiocentesis is performed by a physician or mid-level provider who has specialized training, but, requires the entire team who is responsible for, among other things, watching the electrocardiogram during the process for both rhythm and EKG changes. In the emergent situation of trauma, removal of as little as 5 mL of blood can save the patient's life.

Heart Chambers

The heart consists of four major chambers—two atria and two ventricles—that are made of cardiac muscle. The right and left atria are receiving cavities that function as reservoirs prior to blood being pumped into the ventricles. The right **atrium** receives deoxygenated blood that has already traveled around the body and is returning to the heart via the inferior and superior vena cavae. This deoxygenated blood also returns from the heart itself through the coronary sinus. Four pulmonary veins direct newly oxygenated blood into the left atrium. These two atria are separated by the interatrial septum which assists in the force of contraction of the atria as they pump blood into the ventricles.

Cardiac cells that make up the heart muscle communicate with each other through the exchange of nutrients and other substances such as anions, cations, and metabolites. The cardiac muscle contracts as a result of calcium that travels from the interstitial fluid surrounding the heart's cells into the heart's muscle fibers, thus creating an electrical impulse that is quickly conducted throughout the wall of a heart chamber. Because of this, calcium plays an important role in the force of contraction. Without available calcium, the heart muscle remains in a relaxed state.

The "pumps" of the heart are the right and left ventricles and aid in blood flow through the heart. The right ventricle receives deoxygenated blood from the right atrium and pumps it into the pulmonary system by way of the pulmonary artery which branches into the right and left lungs, where it exchanges carbon dioxide for oxygen. This is the only time that an artery carries unoxygenated blood. The left atrium sends oxygenated blood to the left ventricle. The left ventricle pumps the now oxygenated blood out through the aorta to nourish the body. The ventricles are aided in their pumping action by the interventricular septum that separates the two distinct ventricles (Fig. 2–4).

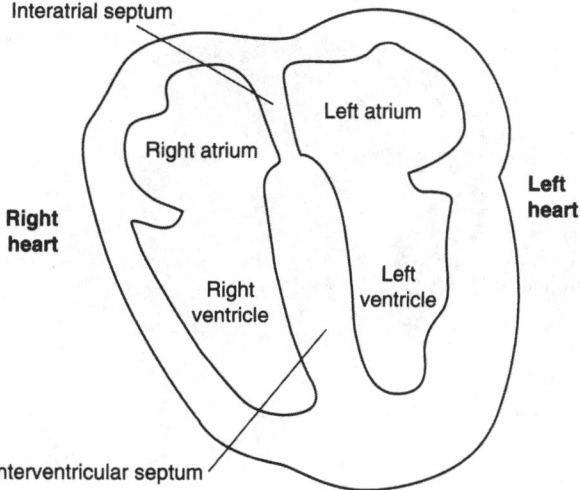

FIGURE 2–4 • The four chambers of the heart. [*From Huff Jane. (2012). ECG Workout Exercises in Arrhythmia Interpretation, 6e.*]

> **CLINICAL ALERT**
>
> The pumping action of the heart can be affected by many things including disease processes of the heart muscle, valves, or conduction system.

Heart Valves

The heart has four valves: two **atrioventricular (AV) valves** and two **semilunar (SL) valves** (Fig. 2–5). The AV valves are the **tricuspid valve** on the right side of the heart and the **mitral or bicuspid valve** on the left side. The SL valves are the **pulmonic** and **aortic valve** located in each of these great vessels of the heart (the pulmonary artery and the aorta). Valves ensure that blood flows in a forward direction through the heart's chambers, therefore, no backflow occurs. The valves open and close in response to the pressure in the corresponding heart's chambers to which they connect. When the valves close, they prevent the blood from flowing backwards (called **regurgitation**) into the chamber. The heart sounds ("lub-dub" sounds) that are heard through a stethoscope are created by the closing of the heart valves.

- **Atrioventricular valves:** Controls flow of blood between the atria and their corresponding ventricles. These valves consist of tough, fibrous rings, cusps (also called leaflets or flaps) of endocardium, **chordae tendineae**, and papillary muscles. Pressure gradients control the opening and closing of these valves, propelling blood in a forward direction creating the opening and

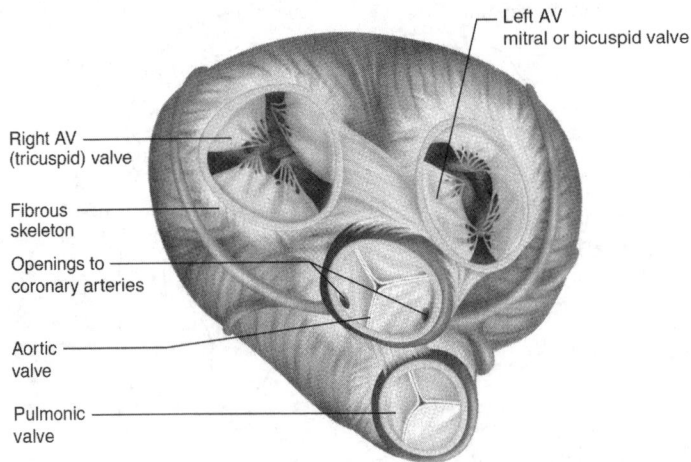

FIGURE 2–5 • **Heart valves.** Two atrioventricular valves (tricuspid valve and mitral valve) and the two semilunar valves (aortic valve and pulmonic valve). [*Modified From Saladin KS. (2011). Human Anatomy, 3e. McGraw-Hill.*]

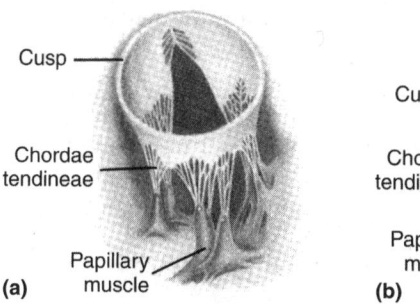
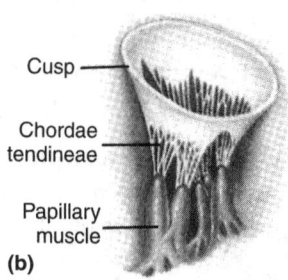

FIGURE 2−6 • **(a) The tricuspid and (b) mitral (bicuspid) valves.** The tricuspid valve has three cusps or flaps and has associated chordae tendinae and papillary muscle tissue. The mitral (bicuspid) valve has two cusps or flaps and associated chordae tendinae and papillary muscle tissue. [*Modified From Aehlert, Barbara (2011). ECG's Made Easy, 4e, Elsevier.*]

closing when then gradient pushes backward. The backward pressure gradient does not have to be great in order for the valves to close. A fibrous skeleton is present in the heart that includes thick connective tissue at the valves and also helps to shape and separate the atria from the ventricles. The AV valves have associated chordae tendineae, strands of connective tissue, which have the appearance of parachute lines. These strands are then attached to myocardial tissue called papillary muscles that extend into the ventricular floors. When the ventricle contracts the papillary muscles pull on the chordae tendineae which keep the valvular flaps from pulling back into the atrial chamber. Due to the appearance of the chordae tendineae, they are sometimes referred to as "heart strings" (Fig. 2–6).

- **Tricuspid valve:** Lies between the right atrium and right ventricle. The tricuspid valve consists of three separate cusps and is thinner than the **mitral valve**.

- **Mitral valve:** Lies between the left atrium and left ventricle. The mitral valve (also called bicuspid valve) has two cusps and takes its name from the fact that it bears the shape of a bishop's hat called a mitre when it is open.

- **Semilunar valves:** Located in the aorta and pulmonary artery to avoid backflow of blood back into the ventricles. These valves are shaped like half-moons (therefore the name "semilunar"), have smaller openings than the AV valves, and have smaller, thicker cusps than the AV valves. The SL valves have three cusps. These valves do not have associated chordae tendinae or papillary muscles. As ventricular contraction occurs, these valves open allowing blood to flow out of the ventricle into the connecting vessel. The SL valves close at the end of ventricular contraction when the pressure in the pulmonary artery and aorta exceeds that of the ventricles and pushes the cusps closed.

- **Pulmonic valve:** Located where the pulmonary artery and right ventricle meet. The **pulmonic valve** allows deoxygenated blood to flow from the right ventricle into the pulmonary arteries without allowing blood to flow backwards into the right ventricle.

- **Aortic valve:** Located where the left ventricle and aorta meet. The aortic valve allows freshly oxygenated blood to flow into the aorta and out to the remainder of the body without backflow of blood into the left ventricle.

A malfunctioning heart valve can disrupt the flow of blood through the heart. When this happens a **murmur** can be heard. Types of valvular heart disease as a result of a malfunctioning of heart valve include:

- **Valvular regurgitation:** Blood flows back into the heart chambers when a heart valve does not close properly. For instance, blood would flow back into the right atrium from the right ventricle if the tricuspid valve did not have complete closure. Other terms for this problem are valvular incompetence or valvular insufficiency.

- **Valvular stenosis:** A stenosed valve occurs when a valve thickens, constricts, or for some reason becomes rigid. This can cause the heart to work harder to pump blood through the narrower or less flexible valve.

- **Valvular prolapse:** A **valvular prolapse** occurs when a valve cusp inverts. This typically occurs when one valve cusp is larger than the other(s). Elongated or ruptured chordae tendineae can also cause valvular prolapse.

CLINICAL ALERT

Rupture of papillary muscles, which can be caused by an **acute myocardial infarction**, can cause incomplete closure of the valves resulting in regurgitation or prolapse of the valve. When rupture of the papillary muscles occurs, **cardiac output** can be decreased and place the patient into potentially fatal complications. Emergency surgery may be necessary.

Heart Sounds

As the heart contracts and relaxes and blood flow increases and decreases within the chambers and the valves open and close, vibrations are created. These vibrations that occur in the heart tissue as the valves close create heart sounds.

- During one heartbeat cycle ("lub-dub"), the heart's ventricles contract (called ventricular **systole**) and relax (called ventricular **diastole**). More specifically, during ventricular systole, the atria relax (atrial diastole) and fill with blood while the mitral and tricuspid valves close. This closure of the mitral and tricuspid valves causes the first heart sound ("lub"). This first heart sound is referred to as S_1. The aortic and pulmonic valves are then forced open by a rise in ventricular pressure. This rise in ventricular pressure causes the ventricles to contract, and blood flows through the circulatory and pulmonic systems. During diastole, the ventricles relax while the atria contract, which forces blood through the open tricuspid and mitral valves. The aortic and pulmonic valves close during this time causing the second heart sound—S_2—"dub" (Fig. 2–7). It is thought that the actual creation of the sounds occurs due to turbulence of the blood flow and heart wall motion.

Extra Heart Sounds

A third heart sound (S_3), occurs at the beginning of diastole after S_2 (ventricular filling). S_3 is not caused by valve closure, but instead is caused by blood moving quickly back and forth between the walls of the ventricles due to blood rushing in from the atria. S_3 is lower in pitch than S_1 or S_2. A third heart sound occurring in youth is benign, but is considered abnormal in persons older than 30 to 40 years of age and is frequently associated with heart failure or a mitral valve regurgitation. An S_1-S_2-S_3 sequence sounds like "lub-dub-ta", "slosh-ing-in" or "Ken-tuck-y" and is referred to as a ventricular gallop or **gallop rhythm**.

A fourth heart sound (S_4) is rare but when heard in an adult is referred to as a presystolic gallop or **atrial gallop**. S_4 sounds like "ta-lub-dub", "Ten-es-see", or "a-stiff-wall" and is a sign of a failing left ventricle possibly due to a stiffening or enlargement of the wall. The sound occurs after atrial contraction at the end of diastole and immediately before S_1. The sequence with this gallop rhythm is S_4-S_1-S_2.

CLINICAL ALERT

The combination of an S_3 and S_4 is called a "Hello-Goodbye" gallop.

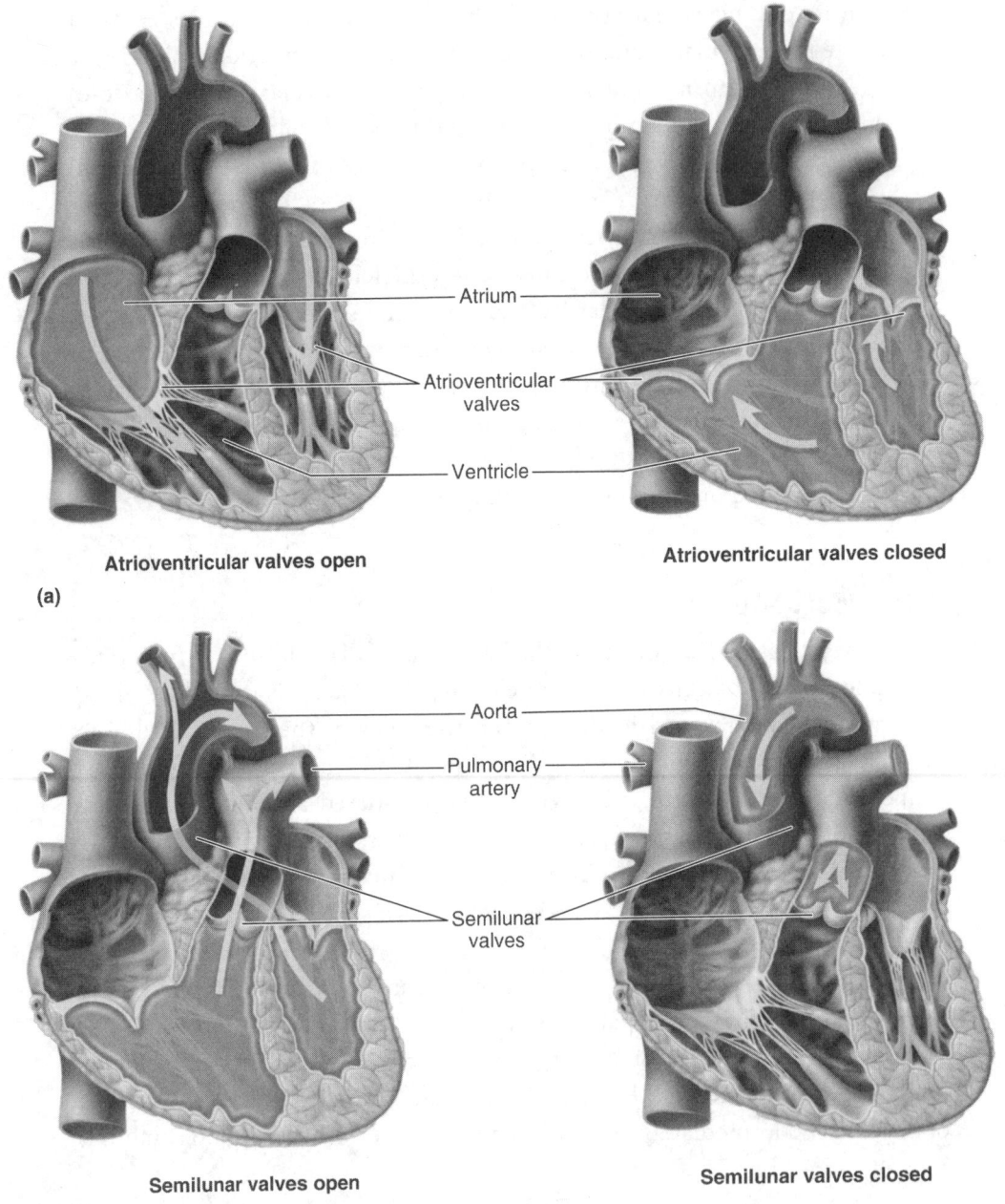

Atrioventricular valves open

Atrioventricular valves closed

(a)

Atrium

Atrioventricular valves

Ventricle

Aorta

Pulmonary artery

Semilunar valves

Semilunar valves open

Semilunar valves closed

(b)

FIGURE 2–7 • Opening and closing of the heart valves creating heart sounds. (a) Atrioventricular valves. These valves open and blood flow is directed into the ventricles when atrial pressure is greater than ventricular pressure (atrial systole). Blood in the ventricle then pushes the valve closed, creating S_1 or "lub", when the ventricular pressure becomes higher than the pressure in the atria (ventricular systole). (b) Semilunar valves. When pressure within the ventricles increases and contraction of the ventricles occurs (ventricular systole), these valves are forced open and blood enters the pulmonic and aortic vessels. When ventricular pressure is lower than arterial pressure (ventricular diastole), the valves close and the second heart sound, S_2, or "dub" is heard. [*From Saladin KS. (2011). Human Anatomy, 3e. McGraw-Hill.*]

Heart Nerves

The sympathetic and parasympathetic nervous systems that make up the **autonomic nervous system** are part of the heart's physiology. This system does not cause the initiation of the electrical impulses within the cardiac tissue, but, can strongly impact the overall function. The **sympathetic nervous system** (also called the adrenergic nervous system) supplies norepinephrine and epinephrine which prepares the body to function under stress ("fight-or-flight" response).

When this system is activated, the following results can be expected related to heart function:

- Increase in heart rate (**chronotropic** response)
- Increase in **contractility** (**inotropic** response)
- Increase in blood pressure through constriction of the blood vessels
- Increase in cardiac output
- Increase in speed of conduction
- Increase in blood flow to the tissues
- Increase in blood flow to organs necessary for survival (heart, lungs, brain)

Other systems throughout the body are also impacted when the sympathetic nervous system is stimulated. Some of these are:

- Increase in size of the bronchi to enhance oxygenation
- Increase in release of stored energy to supply the brain with glucose and muscles with fatty acids
- Increase in sweating
- Increase in size of pupils

The **parasympathetic nervous system** (also called the cholinergic nervous system) releases the chemical acetylcholine that slows heart rate, decreases automaticity of the AV node, decreases conduction of impulses through the AV node, decreases the force of contraction of the atria, and can mildly decrease the strength of ventricular contractions. The parasympathetic nerve that influences the heart is the vagus nerve. Baroreceptors, specialized nerve cells located in the aortic arch and the carotid arteries, also stimulate the vagus nerve, which then activates the parasympathetic response. These baroreceptors are sensitive to changes in vascular tone and blood pressure. As with the sympathetic nervous system, other organs in the body are also affected by the parasympathetic system including vascular dilation and pupillary constriction. The parasympathetic nervous system conserves and restores body resources ("feed-and-breed" or "rest and digest" response).

> **CLINICAL ALERT**
>
> A maneuver called **carotid sinus massage** is sometimes performed in situations of rapid heartbeat in an intentional attempt to stimulate the baroreceptors, activate the vagus nerve, and slow the heart. This is known as a vagal maneuver and is performed by the physician or provider.

Blood Flow Through the Heart

The right atrium receives deoxygenated blood (low in oxygen and high in carbon dioxide) from the superior (from the head, neck and, upper extremities) and inferior (from the lower body) vena cavae and the coronary sinus, the largest vein that drains the heart. Blood flows through the tricuspid valve from the right atrium into the right ventricle. The right ventricle then contracts causing the tricuspid valve to close. The right ventricle propels blood through the pulmonic valve into the main pulmonary artery which then branches off to become the right and left pulmonary arteries. The deoxygenated blood reaches the lungs where oxygen and carbon dioxide are exchanged. The now oxygen-rich blood flows from the lungs through the four pulmonary veins into the left atrium. This completes the circuit called pulmonary circulation. Blood flows from the left atrium through the mitral valve (bicuspid) into the left ventricle. The left ventricle contracts and the mitral valve closes. Blood travels through the aortic valve from the left ventricle to the aorta. The aorta and its branches deliver blood throughout the body (systemic circulation) (Box 2–1). Blood also flows through the **ostium**, located near the aortic valve, into the coronary circulation. This occurs mainly during ventricular diastole when the aortic valve is closed and the ostium is more pronounced as it is partially hidden when the valve is in an open position (Fig. 2–8).

> **CLINICAL ALERT**
>
> In rapid heartbeat (**tachycardia**) situations, the resting period (**diastole**) for the ventricle is shortened. This can create a problem with a decrease in coronary blood flow as less oxygenated blood is allowed to enter these arteries. Also, the increase in contractions causes the vessels on the heart to be compressed adding to the decrease in coronary blood flow.

BOX 2-1   Blood Flow Through the Heart

- Blood low in oxygen and high in carbon dioxide travels from the body to the superior and inferior vena cavae and the coronary sinus into the right atrium.
- Blood flows from the right atrium through the tricuspid valve into the right ventricle.
- The right ventricle contracts and the tricuspid valve closes.
- The right ventricle expels the deoxygenated blood through the pulmonic valve into the right and left pulmonary arteries.
- Blood travels to the lungs via the pulmonary arteries.
- Oxygen and carbon dioxide are exchanged in the lungs.
- The oxygenated blood travels from the lungs to the left atrium via four pulmonary veins (two from the right lung and two from the left lung).
- Blood flows from the left atrium through the mitral (bicuspid) valve into the left ventricle.
- The left ventricle contracts and the mitral valve closes.
- Blood leaves the left ventricle through the aortic valve and travels to the aorta.
- Blood reaches the body through the aorta and the coronary arteries via the ostium.

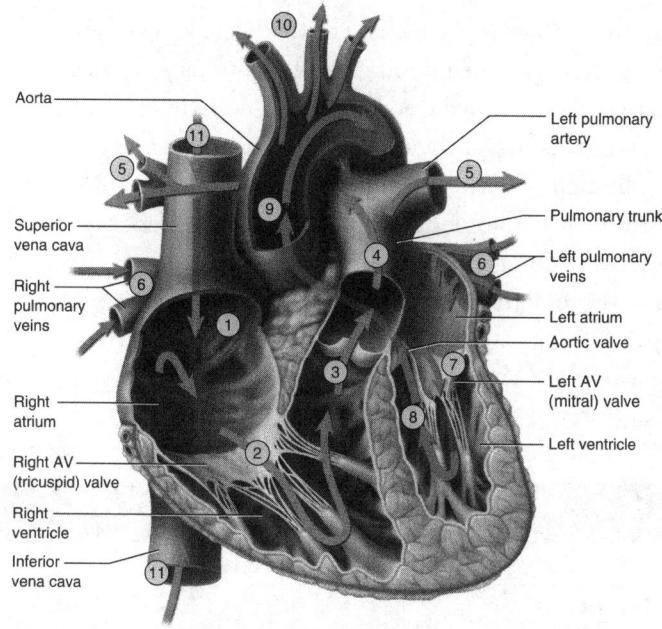

1. Blood enters right atrium from superior and inferior venae cavae. (Coronary circulation is also emptied into the right atrium through the coronary sinus.)
2. Blood in right atrium flows through right AV valve into right ventricle.
3. Contraction of right ventricle forces pulmonary valve open.
4. Blood flows through pulmonary valve into pulmonary trunk.
5. Blood is distributed by right and left pulmonary arteries to the lungs, where it unloads carbon dioxide and loads oxygen.
6. Blood returns from lungs via pulmonary veins to left atrium.
7. Blood in left atrium flows through left AV valve into left ventricle.
8. Contraction of left ventricle (simultaneous with step 3) forces aortic valve open.
9. Blood flows through aortic valve into ascending aorta. (Blood is also pushed into the coronary arteries through the ostium as the ventricle relaxes.)
10. Blood in aorta is distributed to every organ in the body, where it unloads oxygen and loads carbon dioxide.
11. Blood returns to heart via venae cavae.

FIGURE 2-8 · **Blood flow through the heart.** 4 through 6 represents the pulmonary circuit, and 9 through 11 represents the systemic circuit. Steps 1-5 carry deoxygenated blood and steps 6-10 carry oxygenated blood. [*Modified From Saladin KS. (2011). Human Anatomy, 3e. McGraw-Hill.*]

Coronary Circulation

The heart itself must also be nourished with oxygen rich blood and have an avenue available to remove waste products such as carbon dioxide. This is performed through the coronary circulation. As oxygenated blood passes through this system, approximately 60% to 75% of the oxygen within the blood stream is extracted as it passes through the heart. This is the highest amount of extracted oxygen for any organ and demonstrates the extreme importance of oxygen to cardiac tissue. When the demand for oxygen increases, there must be an increase in coronary artery blood flow in order to meet the needs of the myocardium. This coronary blood flow accounts for 4% to 5% of the total cardiac output or about 250 mL/min. The rate of blood flow through the entire cardiovascular system is about 5000 mL/min.

CLINICAL ALERT

Coronary artery disease (CAD) occurs when there is a greater than 50% narrowing of the diameter in any of these major coronary arteries.

The coronary arteries lie on the surface (epicardium) of the heart and supply the heart muscle with blood and oxygen. The opening for the coronary arteries is known as the coronary ostium located near the aortic valve. The right and left coronary arteries branch off from this initial opening at the base of the aorta. From here these arteries then branch off into smaller arteries that extend into the heart's muscle mass and supply it with blood. This network of smaller arteries is called collateral circulation. Even when the major coronary arteries become clogged with plaque, the collateral circulation continues to supply blood to the heart. The major coronary arteries are the right coronary artery (RCA) and the left coronary artery (LCA) which divides into the left anterior descending (LAD) artery and the circumflex (CX) artery (Table 2–2).

TABLE 2–2 Major Coronary Arteries

Right Coronary Artery	Left Coronary Artery	
	Left Anterior Descending	**Circumflex**
Supplies the right atrium, right ventricle, portions of the back of left ventricle	Supplies the anterior (front) of the left ventricle	Supplies left atrium, lateral (sides) of left ventricle, posterior portion (back) of left ventricle

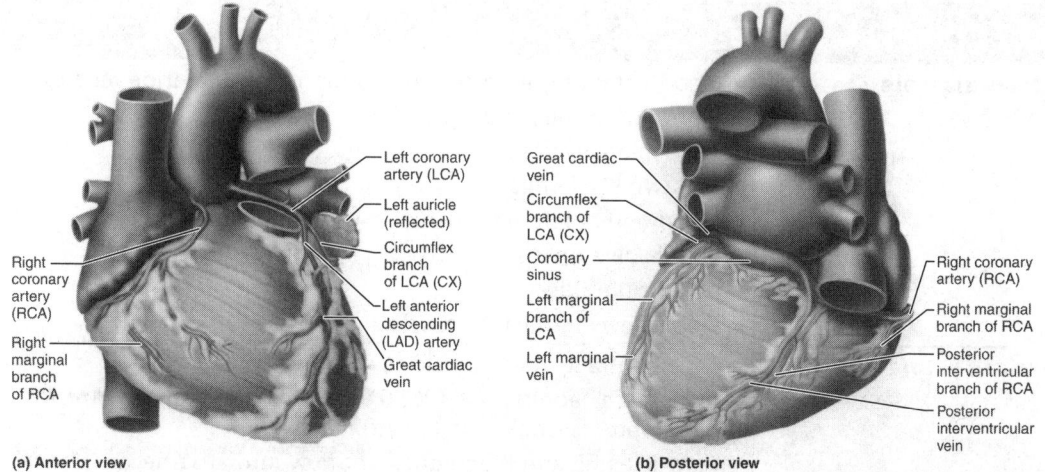

(a) Anterior view

(b) Posterior view

FIGURE 2–9 • **The coronary arteries and veins.** The major coronary arteries (a) anterior or front view; (b) posterior or back view : Vessels of the heart including the left coronary artery (LCA), left anterior descending (LAD) artery, circumflex (CX) artery, and the right coronary artery (RCA). [*Modified From Saladin KS. (2011). Human Anatomy, 3e. McGraw-Hill.*]

These arteries also supply various portions of the conduction system which will be discussed in Chapter 3.

The coronary veins travel alongside the arteries. Cardiac veins collect deoxygenated blood from the capillaries of the myocardium. This venous system includes the great cardiac vein, the middle cardiac vein, and the left marginal vein which empties into the coronary sinus. Eighty percent of returning deoxygenated blood returns through the coronary sinus. This large coronary sinus lies in the area between the atria and the ventricles and drains directly into the right atrium. The other 20% of blood returning to the circulation empties by way of multiple smaller veins that have direct pathways to the right atrium and ventricle (Fig. 2–9).

Cardiac Cycle

The cardiac cycle that is responsible for the blood flow through the heart consists of the systolic and diastolic phases (Table 2–3). Systole occurs in both the atria and ventricles and is the period during which the chambers are contracting and projecting blood. Diastole also occurs in both the atria and the ventricles and is the phase of relaxation when the heart's chambers fill with blood. Ventricular diastole is the phase when the myocardium receives its fresh supply of oxygenated blood from the coronary arteries.

The cardiac cycle is propelled by a pressure relationship where blood flows from one heart chamber to another from higher to lower pressure. In diastole, the pressure in the heart chambers decreases while it increases in systole. The

TABLE 2-3 Cardiac Cycle	
Atrial diastole	• Blood enters right atrium from superior and inferior vena cavae • Right atrium fills and distends • Tricuspid valve opens • Right ventricle fills • Blood enters left atrium from four pulmonary veins • Mitral valve opens • Left atrium fills • Blood flows into left ventricle
Atrial systole	• Atria contract when ventricles are filled to 70% • Atria forces additional 10%-30% of ventricular capacity worth of blood into ventricles (called atrial kick) • Ventricles fill and blood does not flow into atria because atrial pressure exceeds venous pressure
Ventricular systole	• Occurs as atrial diastole begins • Ventricles contract • Blood moves through systemic and pulmonary circulations • SL valves close; ventricular diastole begins
Ventricular diastole	• Ventricles passively fill with blood • Both atria and ventricles relax

heart's valves keep the blood moving forward. Precise timing of the contractions is an important aspect regarding the pressure relationships. The timing of atrial and ventricular systole is dependent upon the heart's conduction system that controls the nerve pathways and electrical impulses.

The atria work in concert with each other and the ventricles also are working synchronously during the cardiac cycle. Each cardiac cycle takes about 1 second to complete. The four stages (Fig. 2–10) of the cardiac cycle are:

1. **Ventricular Filling:** During ventricular filling, two activities occur. First, the pressure in the ventricles becomes less than the atria and the AV valves (tricuspid and mitral) open to allow blood to enter the ventricles. Initially there is a rapid filling followed by a slower period of movement of blood volume from the atria into the ventricles. This second slower filling period is known as **diastasis**. At the end of diastasis, the atria contract (atrial systole) providing "**atrial kick**" which propels an extra 10% to 30% of blood into the ventricles. This amount of blood that is now in the ventricles is known as the **end-diastolic volume** (EDV). This is different in individuals but is usually approximately 130 mL.

2. **Isovolumetric ventricular contraction:** Pressure in the ventricles increases due to ventricular depolarization and causes the mitral and tricuspid

valves to close. During this phase the pulmonic and aortic valves remain closed due to a higher amount of pressure in the aorta and pulmonary vessels, therefore, no blood is being ejected into the systems at this time. The term isovolumetric is used to help describe this phase because no change in ventricular volume occurs. During this phase, the atria are in a relaxed state (atrial diastole).

3. **Ventricular ejection:** The aortic and pulmonic valves open in response to ventricular pressure that exceeds that of the aortic and pulmonary arterial pressure. The SV valves (aortic and pulmonic) open and the ventricles eject blood at this stage (ventricular systole). The entire **end-diastolic volume** (approximately 130 mL) is not expelled. About 70 mL is ejected during this phase and is known as the **stroke volume**. The percentage of the amount of ejected blood is known as the **ejection fraction** which should be at least 55%. The blood that remains in the ventricle at the end of this phase is known as the **end-systolic volume** (ESV).

CLINICAL ALERT

An echocardiogram is one way to assess cardiac contractile functionality. This testing modality provides information regarding performance of the cardiac valves, levels of different chamber volumes, and contractile malfunctions. A clinical measurement obtained from this piece of equipment is called the ejection fraction as listed above. Ejection fractions (EF) can range from 55% to 80%. This is calculated from the stroke volume (SV) and end-diastolic volume (EDV)(EF = SV divided by EDV). Exercise can increase ejection fraction up to 90% in some individuals. Cardiac disease will produce a decreased ejection fraction. EF measuring less than 55% indicate a decline in the contractile strength of the myocardium.

---

4. **Isovolumetric relaxation:** The aortic and pulmonic valves close in response to a decrease in ventricular pressure below that of the aorta and pulmonary artery (ventricular diastole). All valves are closed at this stage, atrial diastole takes place, and blood fills the atria. This phase is also known as isovolumetric since no blood is passing through any valves again.

CLINICAL ALERT

Loss of atrial kick can seriously diminish the amount of blood pumped out into the vascular system with each cardiac cycle (cardiac output). If less blood is pumped into the ventricles, less blood will be available to be ejected into the systemic circulation. This can occur with certain heart rhythms such as atrial fibrillation.

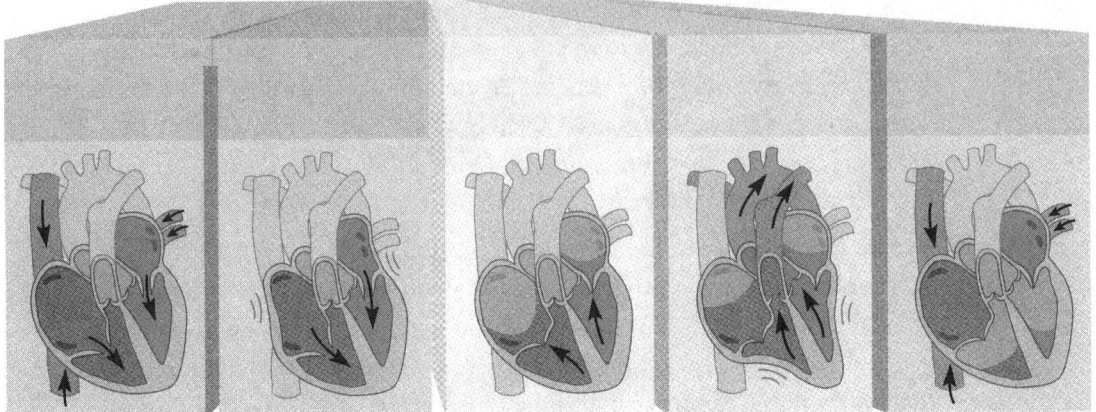

FIGURE 2−10 • Phases of the cardiac cycle. The first phase, ventricular filling, includes two activities. The cardiac cycle completes in one second and includes ventricular fillling, contraction, ejection, and relaxation. [*Modified From Saladin KS. (2010). Anatomy and Physiology - The Unity of Form and Function, 6e. McGraw-Hill.*]

Cardiac Output

The term cardiac output is used to describe the amount of blood pumped into the systemic circulation through the aorta each minute. This is measured by multiplying the stroke volume (SV) (amount of blood ejected from a ventricle with each contraction) times the heart rate. Cardiac output in most adults is between 4 and 8 L/min. Decreased cardiac output can place individuals at risk for life threatening problems and can occur for a variety of reasons. Symptoms that can be noted are listed in Box 2–2.

Stroke Volume

Preload, **afterload**, and myocardial contractility affect stroke volume and must be in balance for optimal cardiac output to occur.

- **Preload:** The amount of force placed on the walls of the ventricles causing the cardiac muscle to stretch. This is established by the pressure exerted and the volume of blood present within the left ventricle at the end of its resting phase (diastole). It is affected by the amount of blood returning to the right atrium; therefore, an increase or decrease in preload can be appreciated with increases and decreases in blood volume. Larger volumes will stretch the cardiac fibers prior to contraction allowing the ventricles to eject the increased volume through an increase in the force of contraction. In a normal heart, the greater the preload, the greater the force of ventricular contraction and the greater the stroke volume, resulting in increased cardiac output. The heart adjusts its pumping capacity in

BOX 2–2   Manifestations of Decreased Cardiac Output

- Fatigue
- Shortness of breath
- Difficulty breathing while lying flat (orthopnea)
- Increased respiratory rate
- Cough
- Blood pressure alterations
- Restlessness
- Changes in mentation
- Cold extremities
- Dizziness
- Fainting or near fainting
- Pallor
- Cyanosis (bluish discoloration to skin)
- Edema
- Clammy skin
- Dysrhythmias
- Abnormal breath sounds such as crackles or wheezing

response to venous return. This is important when individuals are exercising because it allows the fibers to stretch before contracting. It can also be stretched beyond normal limits at which time it could produce a decrease in cardiac output. This could occur with an overload of volume causing a failing of the work of the heart.

- **Afterload:** The pressure against which the ventricles must work to pump blood. Three factors affect afterload—arterial blood pressure, arterial resistance, and the ability of the arteries to stretch. Lower resistance means that blood flow is more easily ejected. When resistance is increased, the heart must work harder to eject blood. This increase in resistance can occur with increased viscosity (thickness) of the blood, increased blood pressure, or a rigid (stenosed) aortic valve. Pulmonary disorders such as chronic obstructive pulmonary disease can cause scarring within the lung fields that can increase the resistance against which the right ventricle must work. This causes an increased afterload for the right side of the heart as well.

- **Contractility:** The ability of cardiac muscle cells to respond to stimulation causing contraction. This is not the tension itself, but, rather the responsiveness that occurs within the cardiocytes (heart cells). This occurs after **depolarization** (response of a myocardial cell to an electrical impulse that triggers myocardial contraction). The amount the muscle fibers are stretched at the end of diastole affects contractility and the volume of blood pumped out of the ventricles. Too much or too little stretch affects the actual SV that is delivered. A term used when discussing contractility is "inotropic". Positive inotropes will increase contractile strength and negative inotropes will decrease contractility. Calcium is a positive inotropic agent. It increases the strength of contraction. Patients with a low calcium level will not have good contractile strength. However, in extremely high levels of calcium, cardiac arrest can occur. Negative inotropic effects can occur with many things including high levels of potassium.

Heart Rate

The second piece of the formula for cardiac output is heart rate. This is the chronotropic response. Things that increase heart rate have positive chronotropic responses and those that decrease heart rate have negative chronotropic reactions. Both high and low pulse rates will have a strong bearing on cardiac output. Sympathetic stimulation, low levels of calcium, and increased levels of thyroid hormone or caffeine will produce positive chronotropic effects (fast heart rate). Parasympathetic stimulation, high levels of calcium and potassium as well as decreased levels of potassium will cause negative chronotropic effects (slow heart rate). Infants respond to a decrease in cardiac output with fast heart rates (tachycardia) because they have fixed stroke volumes. Therefore, the only way for them to attempt to increase their cardiac output is to increase their heart rates.

Blood Pressure

Blood pressure is the pressure of circulating blood that is exerted on the walls of the arteries and is a principal vital sign. Blood pressure refers to the arterial pressure of the systemic circulation. At each heartbeat, blood pressure changes due to varying systolic and diastolic pressures that is maintained by the pumping action of the heart. It is equal to cardiac output multiplied by peripheral vascular resistance. **Peripheral vascular resistance** is the resistance to the flow of blood. Two factors influence this resistance—blood vessel diameter and the tone (balanced tension) of the vascular musculature. Therefore, any condition that changes either cardiac output or peripheral vascular resistance affects blood pressure. An increase in blood pressure is due to an increase in cardiac output or peripheral vascular resistance, whereas a decrease in blood pressure is due to a decrease in cardiac output or peripheral vascular resistance.

> ### CLINICAL ALERT
>
> When blood pressure drops below 80 mm Hg (systolic), decreased cardiac output can cause a deficiency in the coronary artery blood flow. This can produce a lack of oxygenated blood to cardiac tissue and dysrhythmias may occur.

Blood pressure is expressed in terms of the systolic pressure over diastolic pressure and is measured in millimeters of mercury (mm Hg), for example, 118/68 mm Hg. Ideal blood pressure for adults is 90 to 119 mm Hg systolic and 60 to 79 mm Hg diastolic. Blood pressure may be affected by a person's age, weight, medications, life-style choices, medical conditions, nutrition, exercise habits, and environmental factors, such as responses to stress. **Hypertension** refers to arterial pressure that is abnormally high, as opposed to **hypotension**, which is abnormally low blood pressure.

> ### CLINICAL ALERT
>
> Risk factors for developing high blood pressure are family history, advanced age, gender-related risk patterns, lack of physical activity, poor diet (especially one that includes too much salt), overweight and obesity, and consumption of too much alcohol. Possible contributing factors include stress, smoking and second-hand smoke, and sleep apnea.

Conclusion

The heart acts as a pump that moves blood through the circulatory system. Note these key points about the heart:

- The human heart is a hollow, cone-shaped, muscular organ, roughly the size of its owner's fist that weighs between 250 and 350 g (roughly 9-11 oz).
- The heart is located in the chest slightly left of the breastbone in a space called the mediastinum.
- The heart's wall is made up of three tissue layers: endocardium, myocardium, and epicardium.
- Between the parietal and visceral layers of the serous pericardium is an area called the pericardial space. This space contains roughly 20 mL of

thin, clear serous fluid—called pericardial fluid—that acts like a lubricant and cushion to prevent friction as the heartbeats.

- The heart contains four chambers—two atria and two ventricles—that are made of cardiac muscle and act as two separate pumps that work in concert with each other.

- The heart has four valves: two atrioventricular valves (tricuspid valve and mitral valve) and two semilunar valves (aortic valve and pulmonic valve). These valves ensure that blood flows in a forward direction through the heart's chambers without creating a backflow of blood.

- The heart has two normal heart sounds (S_1 and S_2) that can be heard as the heart valves close, and they sound like "lub-dub." Extra heart sounds are S_3 and S_4.

- The sympathetic and parasympathetic nervous systems that make up the autonomic nervous system contribute to the heart's function.

- Blood flow through the heart consists of pulmonary and systemic circulations.

- The cardiac cycle that is responsible for the blood flow through the heart consists of the systolic and diastolic phases that occur in four stages.

- Cardiac output is equal to stroke volume times the heart rate.

- Three factors affect stroke volume—preload, afterload, and contractility.

- The heart has its own vascular system which provides oxygenated blood to the coronary arteries.

- An echocardiogram provides information related to contraction of the heart muscle.

- Blood pressure is equal to cardiac output multiplied by peripheral vascular resistance and is affected by any condition that increases cardiac output or peripheral vascular resistance.

PRACTICE QUESTIONS

1. **The apex of the heart is formed by the tip of the _____ _____.**
   A. right atrium
   B. left atrium
   C. right ventricle
   D. left ventricle

2. The middle layer of the heart wall that is thick and muscular and consists of cardiac muscle fibers is the

   A. endocardium.

   B. myocardium.

   C. epicardium.

   D. subendocardium.

3. The tricuspid valve

   A. is shaped like a bishop's hat.

   B. directs freshly oxygenated blood to the aorta.

   C. lies between the right atrium and ventricle.

   D. lies between the left atrium and ventricle.

4. In systemic circulation, blood from the upper extremities empties into the

   A. superior vena cava.

   B. inferior vena cava.

   C. aorta.

   D. left atrium.

5. In which stage of the cardiac cycle does the mitral and tricuspid valves open in response to atrial pressure?

   A. Ventricular filling

   B. Isovolumetric ventricular contraction

   C. Isovolumetric relaxation

   D. Ventricular ejection

6. Cardiac output is the measurement of

   A. peripheral vascular resistance × blood pressure

   B. stroke volume × heart rate

   C. stroke volume × blood pressure

   D. blood vessel diameter × vascular tone

7. Afterload is the

   A. force exerted on the walls of the ventricles causing the muscle to stretch.

   B. pressure against which the atria must work to pump blood.

   C. force within the atria that creates the atrial kick.

   D. pressure against which the ventricles must work to pump blood.

8. **Blood pressure is the**

   A. venous pressure of the pulmonary circulation.
   B. venous pressure of the systemic circulation.
   C. arterial pressure of the systemic circulation.
   D. arterial pressure of the pulmonary circulation.

9. **A positive inotropic response would increase**

   A. contractility.
   B. heart rate.
   C. automaticity.
   D. blood vessel diameter.

10. **Which of the following would cause a decrease in heart rate?**

    A. Activation of the sympathetic nervous system
    B. Stimulation of the vagus nerve
    C. Ingestion of caffeine
    D. Increased exercise

ANSWER KEY

1. **D.** The lower portion of the heart, the apex, is formed by the tip of the left ventricle and tilts down and forward, toward the left side of the body.

2. **B.** The myocardium is the thick, muscular middle layer of the heart wall that consists of cardiac muscle fibers.

3. **C.** The tricuspid valve lies between the right atrium and right ventricle.

4. **A.** Blood from the head, neck, and upper extremities empties into the superior vena cava while blood from the lower body returns to the inferior vena cava.

5. **A.** In ventricular filling, the mitral and tricuspid valves open in response to atrial pressure which causes blood to flow passively into the ventricles.

6. **B.** Cardiac output is measured by multiplying the stroke volume by the heart rate.

7. **D.** Afterload is the pressure against which the ventricles must work to pump blood into the circulation.

8. **C.** Blood pressure refers to the arterial pressure of the systemic circulation.

9. **B.** Positive inotropic responses increase contractility which would increase cardiac output.

10. **A.** A decreased heart rate would be caused by stimulation of the vagus nerve which is part of the parasympathetic system.

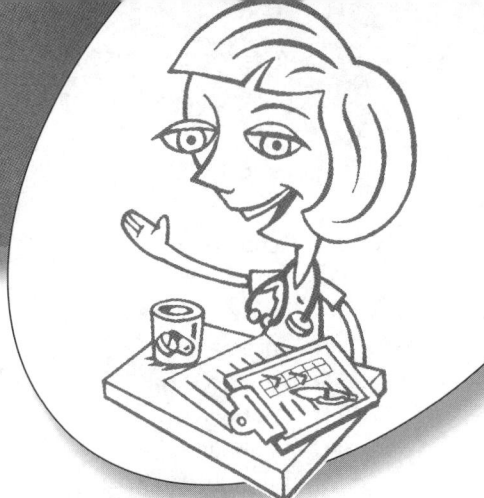

chapter **3**

Cardiac Electrical Conduction System

LEARNING OBJECTIVES

At the end of this chapter, the student will be able to:

1 List the functionality differences between myocardial and pacemaker cells.

2 Identify the differences between acting and resting potential.

3 Define depolarization, repolarization, and refractoriness.

4 Explain the process of the cardiac conduction system.

5 Explain ways in which abnormal heart impulses are generated.

Key Words

Action potential	Inotropic
Atrial fibrillation	Ischemia
Atrioventricular (AV) node	Isoelectric line
Automaticity	Membrane potential
Conductivity	Myocardial cells
Contractility	Myocytes
Defibrillation	Pacemaker cells
Depolarization	Refractoriness
Ectopic	Repolarization
Enhanced automaticity	Resting potential
Excitability	Sinus node
His-Purkinje system	Ventricular fibrillation

Overview

As discussed in the prior chapter, the heart works as a pump to circulate blood throughout the body. However, without the specialized cells that make up the heart, it would not be able to function. The heart is able to maintain this pumping function through electrical impulses that spread from one cell to the next. This electrical system is also known as the cardiac conduction system. The electrical impulses of the heart are independent from the nervous system. This means that the heart can beat independently even if ties to the nervous system have been severed.

Cardiac Conduction

Cardiac Cells

The heart's cardiac cells (**myocytes**) have one of two functions: mechanical (contractile) or electrical (pacemaker). The mechanical cells, also called **myocardial cells**, create the contractile strength of the myocardium. These contractile cells form the muscular layers of the atrial and ventricular walls and rely on the pacemaker cells to generate the impulse to contract.

Pacemaker cells, also called conducting cells or automatic cells, spontaneously produce and conduct electrical impulses without stimulation by a nerve.

Cardiac cells have four characteristics that make them conducive to generating and transmitting electrical impulses (Box 3–1).

BOX 3–1   The Characteristics of Heart Cells

Automaticity is the ability of cardiac pacemaker cells to create an electrical impulse without stimulation by a nerve. Automaticity is maintained by normal concentrations of sodium (Na^+), potassium (K^+), and calcium (Ca^{++}); increased amounts of these cations can produce a decrease in automaticity; however, decreased amounts of potassium and calcium can increase automaticity. The SA node is the normal pacemaker of the heart. Only pacemaker cells have this property.

Excitability, or irritability, is the ability of cardiac muscle cells to respond to chemical, mechanical, or electrical stimuli. Cardiac muscle remains electrically excitable because of an ionic imbalance across the cells. All cardiac cells have the ability to respond in this way.

Conductivity is the cardiac cell's ability to receive an electrical impulse and transmit it to another cardiac cell. This characteristic allows a generated impulse from any part of the myocardium to be distributed throughout the heart muscle. The speed of conductivity can be influenced by medications as well as stimulation from both the sympathetic and parasympathetic nervous systems. All cardiac cells are capable of conductivity.

Contractility refers to the cell's ability to contract after receiving an impulse. Normally the SA node sends an impulse that causes the heart to contract. Only myocardial cells have the ability to perform this function.

CLINICAL ALERT

Medications such as digitalis, dopamine, and epinephrine can improve the heart's ability to contract. This would be considered to be an **inotropic** response. (Chronotropic responses have to do with heart rate.)

Action and Resting Potential

Ions move across cell membranes causing a slight difference in the concentration of charged particles. This imbalance in the charged particles creates energy and makes the cells excitable. The inside of cardiac cells has a negative charge due to the larger amount of negatively charged molecules in the cell. When this intracellular negativity exists, the cell is considered to be polarized or in a resting state (**resting potential**). The difference in the electrical charges across the cell membrane is the **membrane potential**. The movement of the electrolytes across the cell membrane requires energy in the form of ATP (adenosine triphosphate) to create a flow of current that is then expressed in volts. This voltage produces waveforms and spikes on the EKG recording. When the cell is in the resting state (polarized), it produces a straight line on the EKG known as the **isoelectric line**.

Action potential describes the electrolyte exchanges that occur across the cardiac cell membranes during **depolarization**. This action potential occurs in five stages and these stages are described in Table 3–1.

TABLE 3−1 Phases of the Cardiac Action Potential

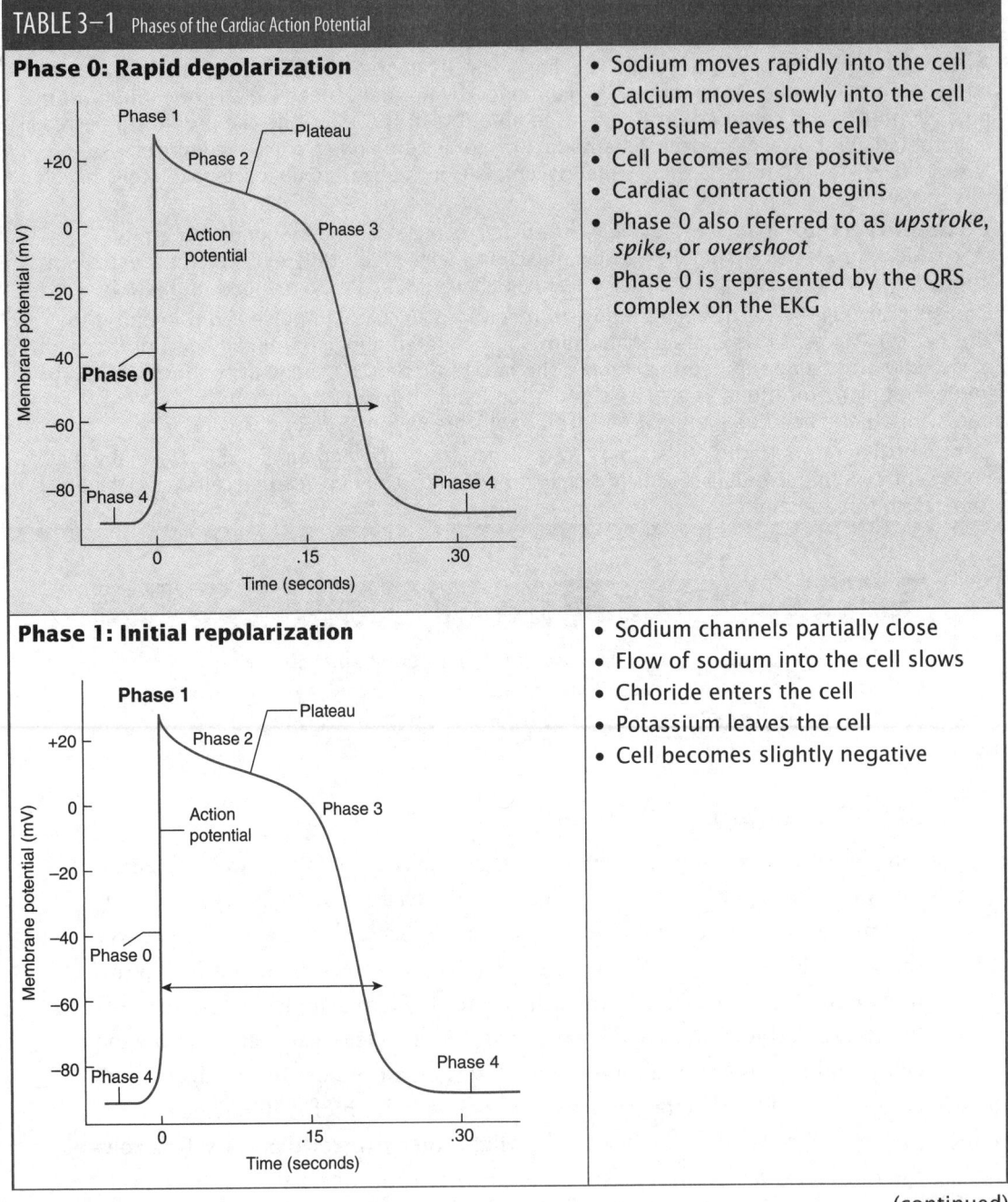

Phase 0: Rapid depolarization

- Sodium moves rapidly into the cell
- Calcium moves slowly into the cell
- Potassium leaves the cell
- Cell becomes more positive
- Cardiac contraction begins
- Phase 0 also referred to as *upstroke*, *spike*, or *overshoot*
- Phase 0 is represented by the QRS complex on the EKG

Phase 1: Initial repolarization

- Sodium channels partially close
- Flow of sodium into the cell slows
- Chloride enters the cell
- Potassium leaves the cell
- Cell becomes slightly negative

(continued)

TABLE 3–1 Phases of the Cardiac Action Potential (continued)

Phase 2: Plateau	
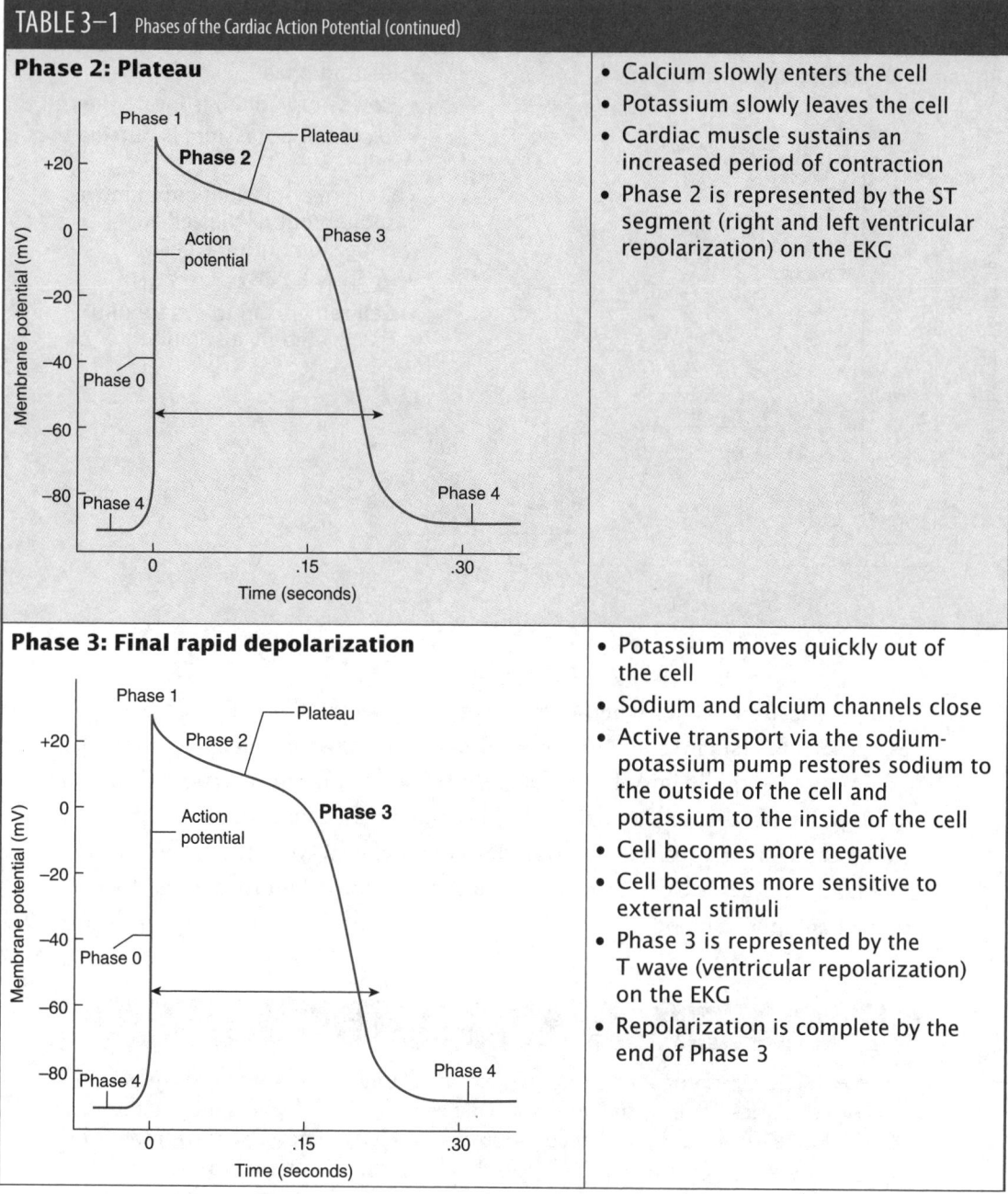	• Calcium slowly enters the cell • Potassium slowly leaves the cell • Cardiac muscle sustains an increased period of contraction • Phase 2 is represented by the ST segment (right and left ventricular repolarization) on the EKG
Phase 3: Final rapid depolarization	
	• Potassium moves quickly out of the cell • Sodium and calcium channels close • Active transport via the sodium-potassium pump restores sodium to the outside of the cell and potassium to the inside of the cell • Cell becomes more negative • Cell becomes more sensitive to external stimuli • Phase 3 is represented by the T wave (ventricular repolarization) on the EKG • Repolarization is complete by the end of Phase 3

(continued)

TABLE 3–1 Phases of the Cardiac Action Potential (continued)

Phase 4: Diastolic depolarization	
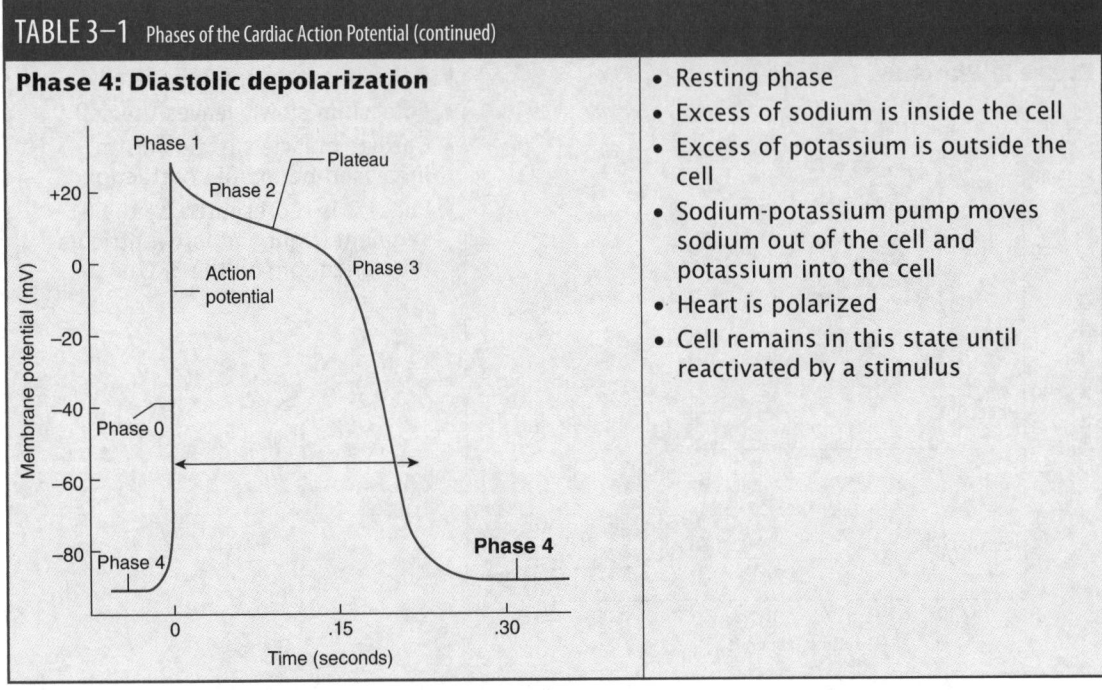	• Resting phase • Excess of sodium is inside the cell • Excess of potassium is outside the cell • Sodium-potassium pump moves sodium out of the cell and potassium into the cell • Heart is polarized • Cell remains in this state until reactivated by a stimulus

Depolarization occurs when cardiac cells are electrically activated by the passage of ions (such as sodium and potassium) across the cell membrane. Sodium moves rapidly into the cardiac cells while calcium moves more slowly. At this point, potassium leaves the cell. This movement causes the inside of the cell to become more positive that translates to a spike (waveform) on the EKG. Depolarization is a very active process and must occur before the heart can contract and pump blood.

CLINICAL ALERT

Some medications impact the movement of calcium in the channels. One of these categories of drugs is known as calcium channel blockers and would slow the heart rate due to a decrease in conductivity. They also have other properties such as opening up (vasodilation) the coronary arteries and decreasing contractility. Examples of this type of medication would be diltiazem (Cardizem) and verapamil (Calan). Other medications that can be used to treat irregular heart rhythms disrupt the sodium (Na^+) and potassium (K^+) channels. When any of these medications are utilized, particular EKG changes can be noted for each type.

An impulse begins in the pacemaker cells of the sinoatrial (SA) node of the heart and moves through each heart cell until all the cells have been depolarized. This chain reaction is a wave of depolarization. The impulse spreads from the pacemaker cells to the myocardial cells that contract when stimulated. A P wave is recorded on the EKG when the atria are stimulated, representing atrial depolarization. A QRS complex represents ventricular depolarization and is recorded on the EKG when the ventricles are stimulated. Figure 3–1 displays the cardiac cycle and its relationship to the depolarization and repolarization that is occurring within the heart.

Conversely, the resting potential occurs when a fully depolarized cell returns to its resting state and restores its electrical charges to normal in a process called **repolarization**. The electrical charges in depolarization reverse and return to normal leaving negatively charged particles inside the cell. Repolarization moves from the epicardium to the endocardium and occurs rapidly at first, then plateaus, and surges again until the resting state is achieved. This ventricular repolarization presents as an ST segment and T wave on the EKG.

It is important to remember that while these electrical events are taking place, they correlate with the mechanical action of the heart muscle as well. During the depolarization of the atria (the P wave), atrial systole is occurring.

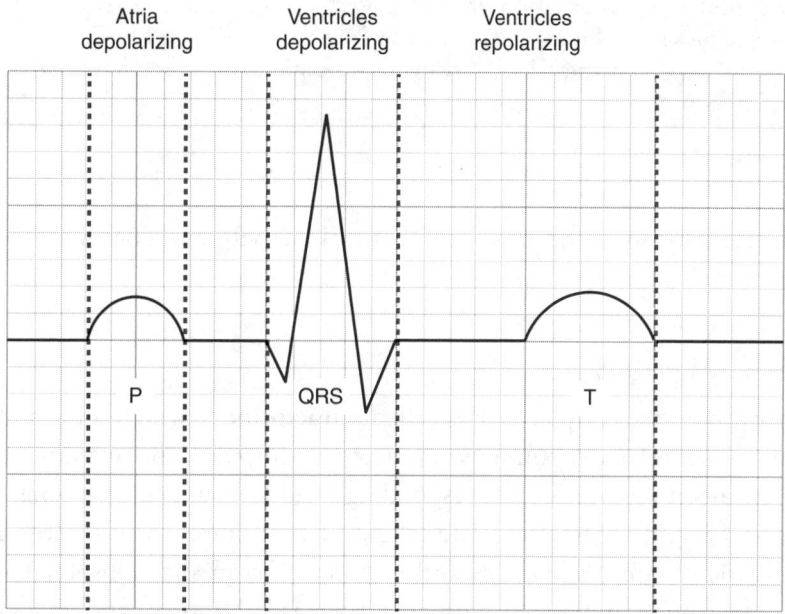

FIGURE 3–1 • The cardiac cycle and the EKG. Correlation of cardiac cycle and EKG waveforms.

As stated in Chapter 2, this is when active contraction is taking place. Ventricular depolarization (the QRS wave) causes ventricular systole. Atrial diastole or repolarization actually occurs at the same time that the ventricles begin their depolarization process however the strength of its signal is not as strong as the ventricular signal and therefore is "lost" within the QRS waves. The progression of the depolarization through the ventricles begins at the Q wave and continues through to the beginning of the T wave. The mass of the contraction essentially takes place at the end of the QRS during the plateau phase depicted on the EKG as the ST segment. Cardiac cells respond differently than skeletal muscle to stimuli. Skeletal muscles react with a short twinge type response, whereas, cardiac cells act with a longer, sustained type of contraction due to the necessity of pumping blood through the heart chambers. Repolarization of the ventricles, ventricular diastole, is identified on the EKG recording as the T wave.

CLINICAL ALERT

When the Electrical Activity (depolarization) of the heart occurs, it does not necessarily mean that the mechanical portion of the heart's contraction will occur as well. In order for the heart to function it must have both electrical and mechanical activity. If Electrical Activity occurs without the mechanics of a contraction, a condition known as PEA or pulseless Electrical Activity occurs. This is a serious situation which is not easily resolved. Electrical Activity is seen on the EKG; however, the patient does not have pulses or blood pressure.

The relationship of the EKG to Electrical Activity and contraction of the myocardium is found in Fig. 3–2.

Refractory Periods

Another property of cardiac cells is called **refractoriness**, which is the ability to remain unresponsive to a stimulus or to reject an impulse. The refractory period where the heart recovers before responding to additional stimuli is longer than the heart's actual contraction. The length of time for each of the refractory phases varies among individuals and is affected by medications, recreational drugs, electrolyte imbalance, disease, myocardial injury, and myocardial ischemia.

Figure 3–3 depicts the timing of refractoriness.

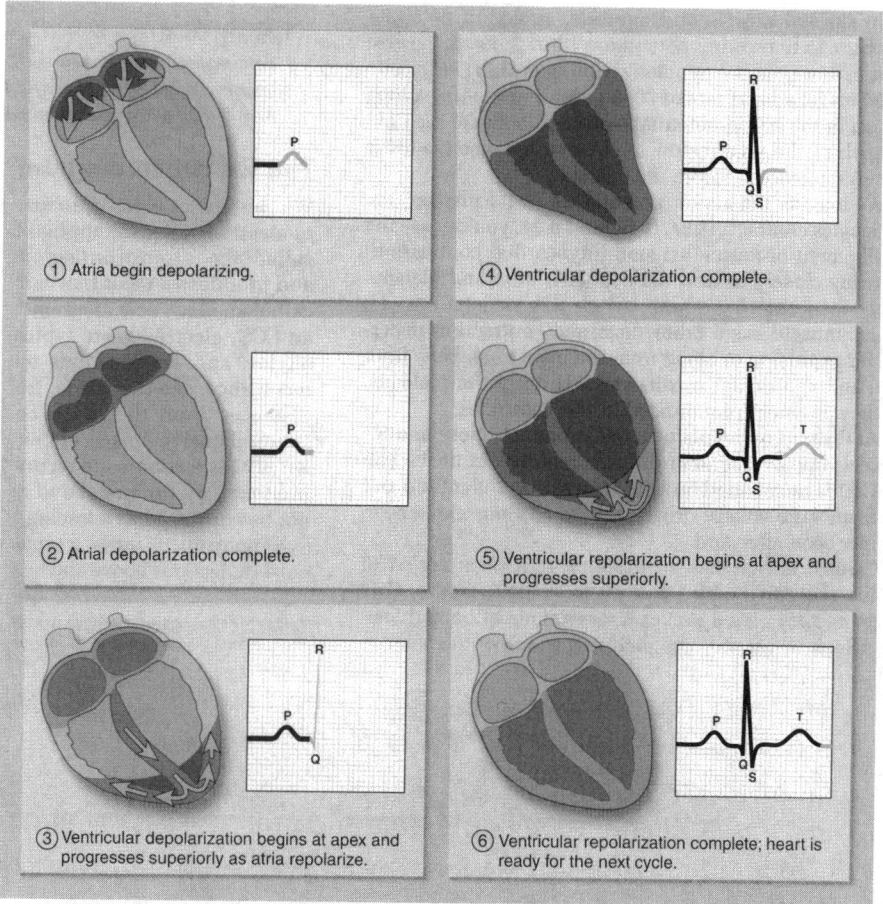

① Atria begin depolarizing.

② Atrial depolarization complete.

③ Ventricular depolarization begins at apex and progresses superiorly as atria repolarize.

④ Ventricular depolarization complete.

⑤ Ventricular repolarization begins at apex and progresses superiorly.

⑥ Ventricular repolarization complete; heart is ready for the next cycle.

FIGURE 3–2 • **Relationship of the EKG to electrical activity and contraction of the myocardium.** Each heart diagram indicates the events occurring as the waves of depolarization and repolarization progress through the heart. Arrows indicate the direction in which a wave or depolarization or repolarization is traveling. [*From Saladin, KS (2012). Anatomy Physiology. McGraw-Hill.*]

Refractoriness occurs in three periods:

- **Absolute refractory period:** This period occurs when the cardiac cells cannot respond to stimuli. The myocardial cells do not contract and electrical impulses are not generated by the electrical conduction system despite the strength of the stimulus. This period is synonymous with depolarization and the beginning of repolarization and corresponds with the onset of the QRS complex to the peak of the T wave on the EKG. Phases 0, 1, 2, and part of phase 3 of the cardiac action potential are included in this period.

- **Relative refractory period:** This period is also called the *vulnerable period*, a time when only a strong stimulus can cause depolarization. During this

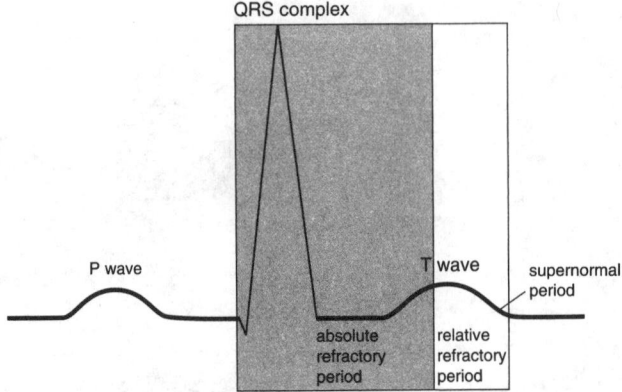

FIGURE 3—3 • **Relationship of refractory periods and the EKG tracing.** Refractory periods occur during the depolarization and repolarization of the ventricles. [*From Huff, Jane (2012). ECG Workout Exercises in Arrhythmia Interpretation.*]

period, repolarization is almost complete and some cells may respond to stimuli, some cells may respond in an unusual fashion, and some cells may not respond at all. Cardiac cells are extremely vulnerable during this period and may respond in a disorganized manner resulting in a life-threatening dysrhythmia. The downslope of the T wave, during the period of ventricular repolarization, relates to this refractory period.

- **Supernormal period:** This period occurs at the very end of the T wave. This corresponds to the completion of Phase 3 and the beginning of Phase 4. Cardiac cells can respond to weaker stimuli at this time and is therefore, also a very vulnerable period of time for the development of dysrhythmias.

CLINICAL ALERT

One situation that can occur during the final upswing of the T wave is known as commotio cordis. This most commonly occurs in young mid teenage boys who are hit in the chest at exactly the right time in the cardiac cycle. It can also occur in other individuals, as well, who are in some way administered a blow to the heart during the period of time of 10 to 30 ms before the peak of the T wave. This is in the final stages of depolarization and the beginning of repolarization. This causes instantaneous **ventricular fibrillation** and must be treated immediately with **defibrillation**.

Cardiac Conduction System

The cardiac conduction system is comprised of an electrical system of pathways among the sinus node (SA node), atrial tissue, the atrio-ventricular (AV) junction, the bundle of His, the right and left bundle branches, and the Purkinje

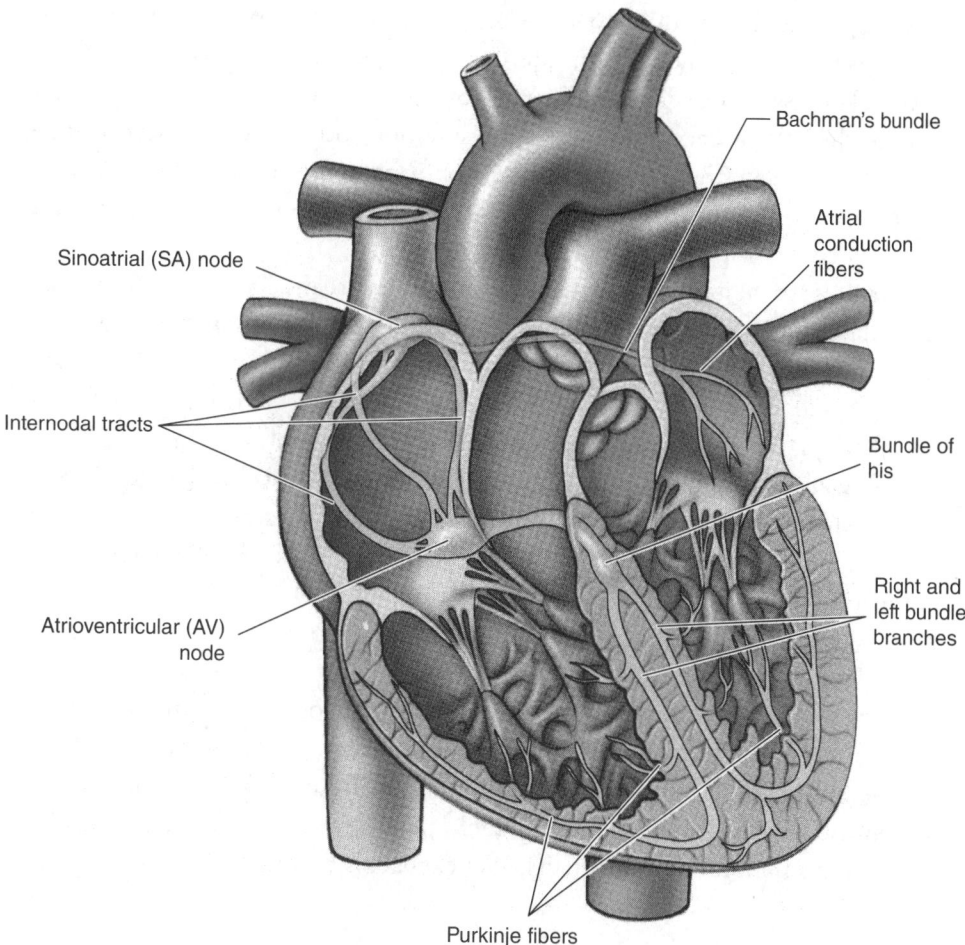

FIGURE 3–4 • **Cardiac conduction system.** Electrical signals travel from the SA node through the system to the Purkinje fibers to create each heartbeat. [*Modified From Aehlert. B (2011) ECG's Made Easy 4e. Mosby Elsevier.*]

fibers (Fig. 3–4). When impulses originating in the SA node are conducted through this system in a normal fashion, the heart chambers will contract in the proper manner to produce each heartbeat.

Sinus Node

The **sinus node** (also called the sinoatrial node or SA node) is located in the upper right corner of the right atrium where the right atrium and superior vena cava join. The SA node is 10 to 20 mm long and 2 to 3 mm wide in the adult and is made up of different types of cells, including pacemaker cells. The SA node is dense with sympathetic and parasympathetic nerve fibers and receives its blood supply from the SA node artery that runs lengthwise through the center of the node. The sinus node is referred to as the *pacemaker* because it reaches potential more quickly than the rest of the cardiac tissue and generates impulses 60 to 100 times per minute. This is the fastest of the intrinsic rates of pacemaker tissue found in the heart. However, other areas of the heart can assume the role of pacemaker if certain situations occur such as the SA node failing to stimulate the atria to contract, not firing at the correct rate, a block in the conduction of the impulse, or inability of the SA node to produce an adequate electrical impulse at all.

As an electrical impulse leaves the SA node, it spreads across the atrial muscle and produces contraction of the right atrium, travels through the interatrial septum through Bachman's Bundle, and then enters the left atrium. This causes the right and left atria to contract at the same time. The ventricles do not contract because fibrous tissue separates the atrial and ventricular myocardium that only allows the atria to contract. This impulse doesn't flow backward, but instead only in a forward motion, because the cardiac cells are unable to respond to a stimulus immediately after the process of depolarization. The contraction of the atria is the P wave. Since the right atrium is depolarized first, this is indicated by the upswing of the P wave and the left atrium is then the downstroke of the P wave (Fig. 3–5).

The impulse travels from the SA node, to the AV node. This impulse reaches the atrioventricular junction through three passages known as the internodal pathways. This is a group of fibers that contain both functional myocardial cells and impulse transmission fibers. Each pathway has a particular name: Bachmann's bundle (anterior tract), Wenckebach's bundle (middle tract), and

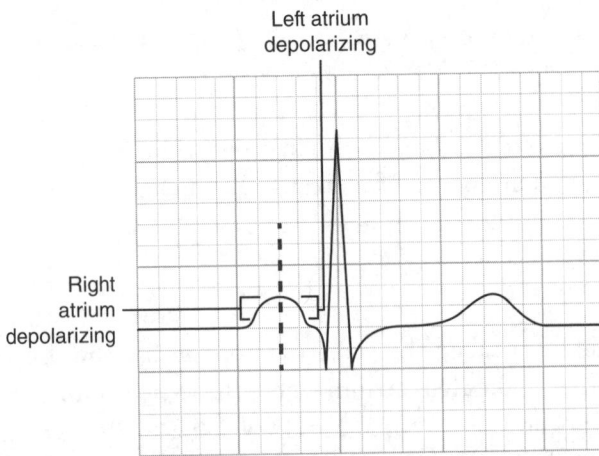

FIGURE 3–5 • Contraction of the right and left atria on EKG tracing. The right atrial contraction is seen on the EKG as the initial upswing of the P wave. The left atrial contraction is indicated by the downstroke of the P wave. [*Modified From Thaler (2010). The Only EKG Book You Will Ever Need 6e.*]

Thorel's pathway (posterior tract). As described above, Bachmann's bundle is also the transmission pathway for the left atrium.

> **CLINICAL ALERT**
>
> The sympathetic nervous system will cause an increase in heart rate ("fight or flight" response) and the parasympathetic nervous system will cause a decrease in heart rate when stimulated.

Atrioventricular Node

The **atrioventricular (AV) node** is located in the inferior right atrium. It is an essential piece of the picture as the fibrous skeleton that is present between the atria and ventricles prevents electrical currents from crossing this barrier otherwise. It sits in close proximity to the opening of the coronary sinus and behind the tricuspid valve. The metrics of this node include a length of 22 mm, a width of 10 mm, and a thickness of 3 mm in the normal adult. This node is also supplied by both sympathetic and parasympathetic nervous system fibers. The AV node is a pathway for the conduction of the impulse and actually has no pacemaker cells. The surrounding junctional tissue does contain pacemaker cells that have the ability to fire at a backup rate of 40 to 60 times per minute if necessary. This is known as an escape pacemaker. For the pediatric patient under the age of three, this AV nodal back up can fire at a rate of 50 to 80 times per minute. The impulse travels from the atria to the AV node, but its course is delayed 0.04 seconds in order to allow the ventricles to complete their filling and not contract too quickly. This delay also allows the atria to empty completely and provide the atrial kick discussed in Chapter 2. If this delay by the AV node did not occur, the atria and ventricles would contract at the same time thus decreasing stroke volume (SV) and compromising cardiac output. The short isoelectric line on the EKG after the P wave is the indication of the delay that takes place in this node (Fig. 3–6).

> **CLINICAL ALERT**
>
> If the AV node were not present when fast atrial rates are present, such as with **atrial fibrillation**, these dangerously high rates of impulses would feed into the ventricles. This then is a protective section of the whole impulse conducting system.

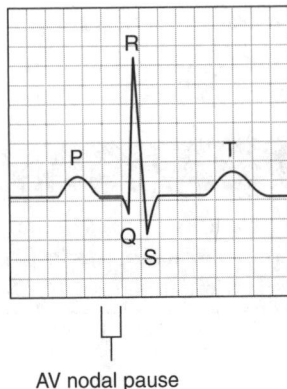

AV nodal pause

FIGURE 3–6 • **Conduction pause at the AV node.** During the pause through the AV node, no activity is seen on the EKG tracing and this is denoted by an isoelectric line.

Bundle of His

The impulse then travels from the AV node, through the AV junction, to the bundle of His. The AV junction is the AV node and the solid or nonbranching portion of the bundle of His that is made up of specialized conduction tissue. The function of the bundle of His is to conduct impulses to the ventricles as they come through the AV node.

CLINICAL ALERT

The bundle of His receives a dual blood supply from the left anterior and posterior descending coronary arteries that makes it less vulnerable to **ischemia**.

Bundle Branches

The bundle of His divides into right and left bundle branches with the right bundle branch continuing on the right side of the interventricular septum, carrying the impulse through the right ventricle. The left bundle branch stretches down the left side of the interventricular septum and is responsible for the impulse to be carried through the left ventricle. The left bundle branch splits even further into three separate branches or subdivisions known as fasciculi (anterior, posterior, and septal). This allows the left bundle branch to deliver impulses more quickly to the thicker, muscular left ventricle than the right bundle branch which feeds the thinner, less muscular walls of the right ventricle. This enables both ventricles to contract at the same time.

BOX 3–2 Heart Pacemaker Sites	
Pacemaker	**Beats per minute**
SA node	60-100
AV junction	40-60
Purkinje fibers	20-40

Purkinje Fibers

The right and left bundle branches divide into smaller branches which end in a network of filaments known as Purkinje fibers. These fibers spread into the endocardium and the papillary muscles to assist in the transference of the impulse. This causes the ventricles to depolarize and contract in a rotating or twisting type of motion that helps to squeeze blood out of the ventricles, forcing it into the arteries to feed the body. When the SA node is damaged and can't send impulses, as in the case of particular myocardial infarctions, the Purkinje fibers will initiate an impulse on their own. These fibers also have pacemaker cells which can fire at a rate of 20 to 40 beats per minute (Box 3–2). Children under the age of three have an inherent rate of 40 to 50 beats per minute in the Purkinje fibers. These activities of the bundle of His, the separate bundle branches, and the Purkinje fibers (known collectively as the **His-Purkinje system**) creates the QRS pattern on the EKG tracing (Fig. 3–7).

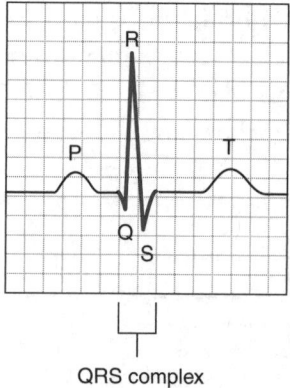

QRS complex

FIGURE 3–7 • **Movement of impulse through His-Purkinje system.** The movement of the initial impulse through the Bundle of His, the Bundle Branches, and the Purkinje Fibers is seen on the EKG as the QRS complex.

ABNORMAL HEART IMPULSES

Abnormal impulses can occur in the cardiac conduction system resulting in aberrant heart rhythms. An EKG or a cardiac monitor strip can electronically demonstrate these dysrhythmias. Causes of abnormal impulses include enhanced **automaticity**, triggered activity, reentry, backward conduction, escape rhythms, and conduction disturbances. These disruptions in normal heart rhythm can be caused by trauma, drug toxicity, electrolyte disturbances, myocardial ischemia, and myocardial infarction.

- **Enhanced Automaticity:** In normal automaticity, pacemaker cells generate impulses automatically without the need for stimulation. The SA node is the preferred pacemaker and its automaticity and faster firing rate inherently supersedes the others. The normal PQRST pattern is derived from this generated impulse (Fig. 3–8). Additional areas in the heart that have the capability to produce impulses are located in other areas of the atria, the AV nodal junction, and the ventricles. In **enhanced automaticity**, cardiac cells that do not typically act as pacemakers depolarize spontaneously, or one of these alternate pacemaker sites increases its firing rate through acceleration of its inherent automaticity to beyond normal and therefore, takes over control of the heart rate. A decrease in the automaticity and firing of the SA node can also allow these substitute pacemakers to seize control. Some disease processes that allow this enhanced automaticity to occur include ischemia (lack of oxygen) of the myocardium, injuries to the heart muscle, increased sympathetic tone, digitalis overdose, low potassium (hypokalemia), high potassium (hyperkalemia), and low calcium (hypocalcemia). This altered automaticity can cause atrial flutter; atrial fibrillation; ventricular fibrillation (Fig. 3–9); ventricular tachycardia (Fig. 3–10); supraventricular tachycardia (Fig. 3–11); junctional tachycardia; accelerated idioventricular rhythm; accelerated junctional rhythm; or premature atrial, junctional or ventricular complexes (Fig. 3–12).

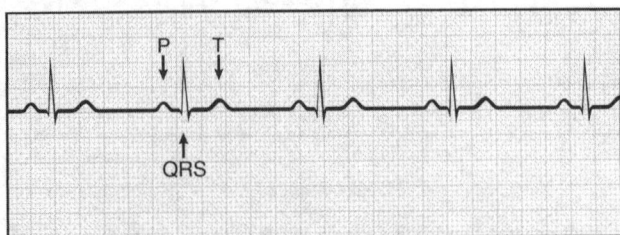

FIGURE 3–8 · Normal PQRST. A normal PQRST pattern from an impulse generated from the SA node. [*Modified From Saladin KS. (2011). Human Anatomy, 3e. McGraw-Hill.*]

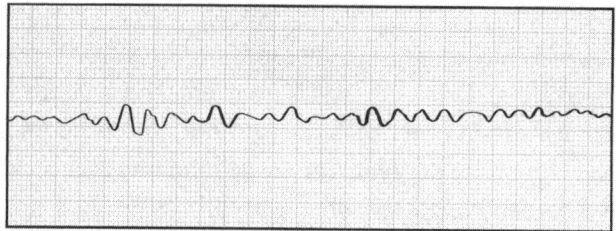

FIGURE 3−9 • **Ventricular fibrillation.** Ventricular fibrillation is indicated on the ECG tracing by a wriggling type of twisted line. No PQRST is occurring when this happens as the ventricular myocardium is contracting in an uncoordinated fashion.

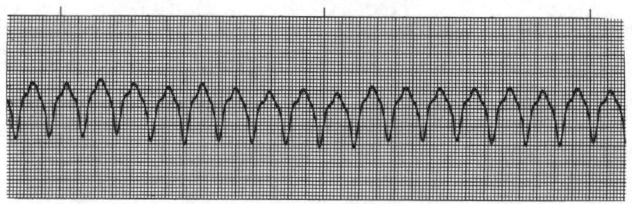

FIGURE 3−10 • **Ventricular tachycardia.** In Ventricular Tachycardia, no PQRST pattern is noted. The ventricles can discharge at rates between 140-250 beats per minute.

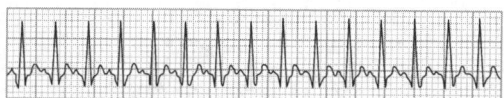

FIGURE 3−11 • **Supraventricular tachycardia.** In Supraventricular Tachycardia the PQRST pattern is visible. The atria are firing very quickly causing an increased rate in the ventricles as well. This can be caused by different disruptions including automaticity and reentry issues.

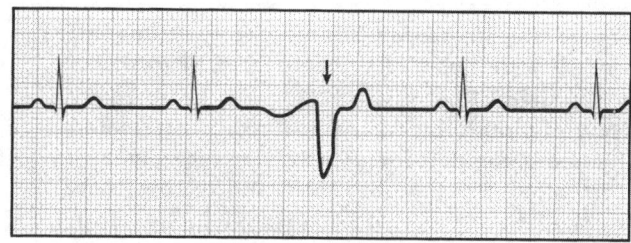

FIGURE 3−12 • **Premature ventricular contraction.** A Premature Ventricular Contraction can have different configurations depending on where it originates in the ventricles. The P wave is absent and the QRST formation is wide and distorted.

- **Triggered Activity:** In triggered activity, abnormal electrical impulses (also called *afterdepolarizations*) are conducted during the normal resting period of repolarization. This occurs when pacemaker cells from an alternative site (from a location other than the SA node) receive a single stimulus, but then can respond by depolarizing more than once. This can occur as both an early afterdepolarization when the cell has not had time to fully repolarize or as a delayed afterdepolarization when it occurs after the cell has had time to completely repolarize. These impulses are known as **ectopic** and can arise from either the atria or ventricles. These beats can occur as a single beat or in pairs (coupling). "Runs" can also be experienced when three or more beats occur in succession and longer "runs" can take place as a sustained rhythm. These individual beats are known as premature atrial, junctional, or ventricular beats (Fig. 3–13). This is another potential cause of ventricular tachycardia. Causes of triggered activity include: hypokalemia, hypercalcemia, slow pacing rates, drug toxicity (especially digoxin), hypomagnesemia, myocardial ischemia, myocardial injury, hypoxia, and increased catecholamine release.

CLINICAL ALERT

Some medications can cause a prolongation of the repolarization process that can produce triggered activity. When this occurs, the potential for a particular rhythm, known as torsades de pointes (twisting of the points) can take place. This is a type of ventricular tachycardia that has a twisting type of baseline. Some of these medications involve antiarrhythmics such as: quinidine (Quinaglute), sotalol (Betapace), and amiodarone (Pacerone), antibiotics such as: erythromycin (E.E.S.), azithromycin (Zithromax), and clarithromycin (Biaxin), and antipsychotics such as: haloperidol (Haldol) and ziprasidone (Geodon).

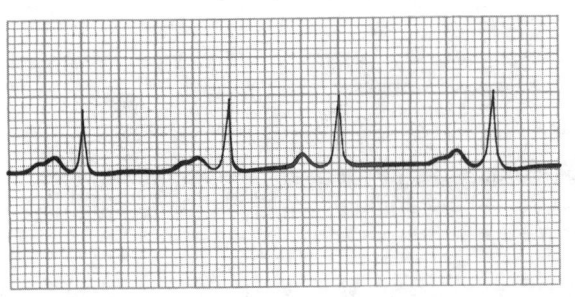

(a)

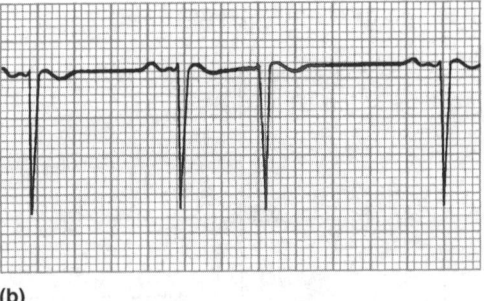

(b)

FIGURE 3–13 • **Premature atrial and premature junctional beats.** (a) Premature atrial contractions (beats) may have a P wave that is slightly different from the other P waves. This beat occurs too quickly in the cycle. (b) Premature junctional contractions (beats) have no visible P wave and the beat is again premature for the sequence of PQRST complexes.

- **Reentry:** In reentry, the impulse spreads through the same tissue again at a faster-than-normal rate that it has previously stimulated. Normally, an impulse spreads through the conduction system and is followed by subsequent impulses. In a reentry variant, this impulse follows its intended route, but then, reenters and begins the depolarization process again in the same area. The original impulse is delayed long enough to allow cells to repolarize, thus creating a situation in which they are available for another impulse. As long as contractile cells of the cardiac muscle continue to accept this impulse, it will follow a circular pathway. One of three factors can be present to activate this process: 1. a potential or accessory pathway; 2. some type of block within the circuit; 3. a delay in the conduction of the impulse. This can cause premature atrial, junctional, and ventricular beats as seen in the figures previously and can precipitate short bursts of fast heart rates such as paroxysmal supraventricular tachycardia and ventricular tachycardia. Causes of reentry are hyperkalemia, myocardial ischemia/injury, an accessory conduction pathway between the atria and ventricles, and some antiarrhythmic medications.

CLINICAL ALERT

When an extra conduction pathway exists, a special form of tachycardia can arise called Wolff-Parkinson-White Syndrome (WPW). In these individuals, the length of the PR interval is very short. Usually the AV node is the only pathway, but, with this abnormality other impulses are directed to the ventricles and then reentered into the circuit again. This extra pathway is found in the bundle of Kent (Fig. 3–14) .

- **Retrograde:** In backward (retrograde) conduction, impulses below the AV node are transmitted in a backward motion so that they then enter the atria in a reverse fashion. This may cause the atria and ventricles to beat asynchronously and an increase in length of time for conduction can occur. This can cause junctional tachycardias. Several changes may take place on the EKG including P wave location changes and a short interval between the P wave and the QRS complex (Fig. 3–15).

- **Escape Rhythms:** Escape rhythms are produced when the SA node slows or fails to initiate the depolarization process and a lower site assumes the task of creating impulses to activate heart function. The AV junction and ventricles act as escape pacemakers to ensure cardiac output is maintained. Escape rhythms include junctional rhythm and idioventricular rhythm (Fig. 3–16). Escape beats can also occur to protect the cardiac output.

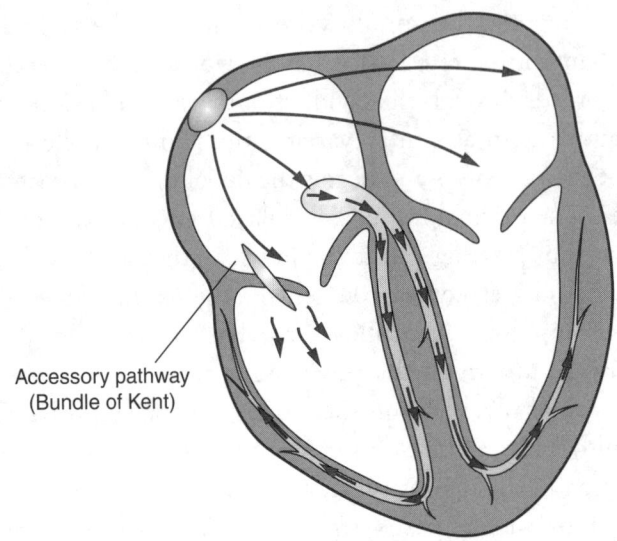

FIGURE 3–14 • **The bundle of Kent.** In Wolff-Parkinson-White Syndrome (WPW), impulses are passed through the Bundle of Kent instead of the normal pathway from the SA node to the AV node.

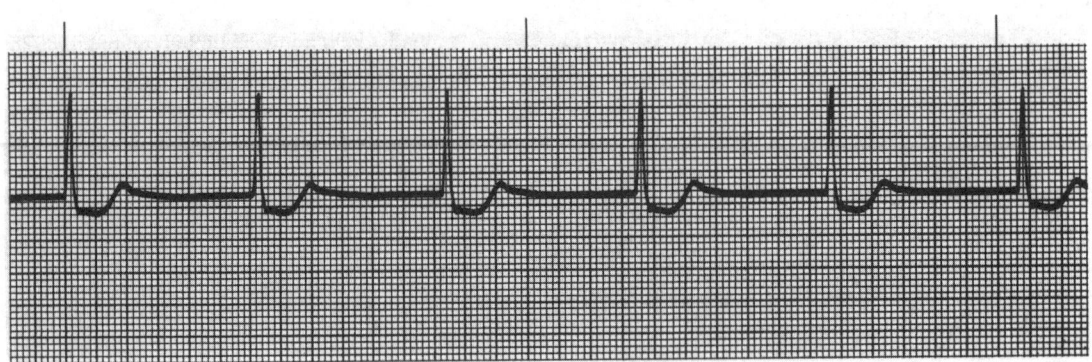

FIGURE 3–15 • **Junctional rhythm.** In a junctional rhythm, no P wave is present. It may be hidden within the QRS complex.

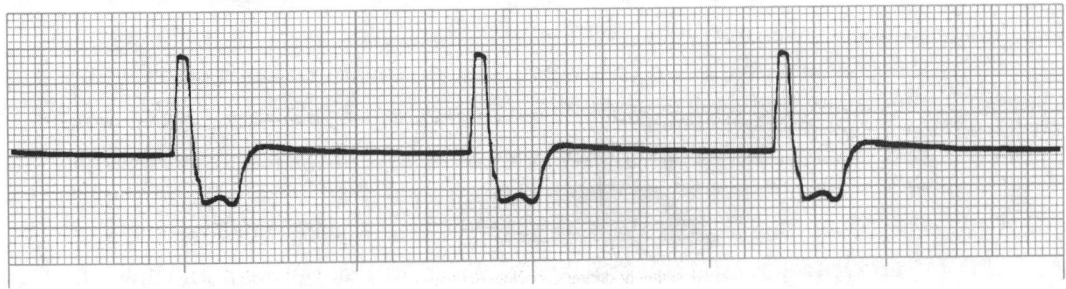

FIGURE 3–16 • **Idioventricular rhythm.** This Idioventricular rhythm has a rate of 35 beats per minute.

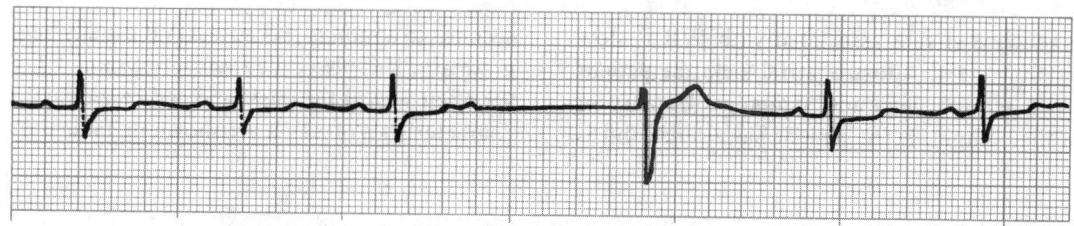

FIGURE 3–17 • Ventricular escape beat. When beats are missed or the heart rate becomes extremely slow, escape beats will attempt to produce heart beats that will preserve cardiac output. Notice the prolonged area with the widened escape beat.

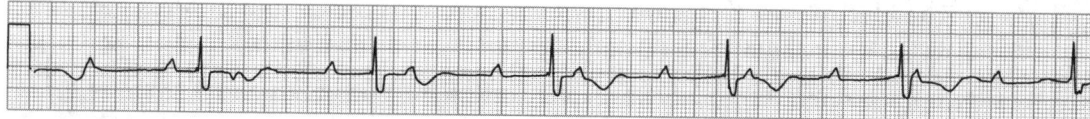

FIGURE 3–18 • Complete heart block. In Complete Heart Block, both P waves and QRS complexes are present but they do not function together. Notice there is not always a P wave immediately preceding each QRS complex.

These would include both junctional and ventricular escape beats that would come into play with very slow rates in an attempt to preserve cardiac output (Fig. 3–17).

- **Conduction Disturbances:** Different etiologies such as trauma, electrolyte disturbances, myocardial ischemia, myocardial injury, and myocardial infarction as well as certain drug toxicities can cause disturbances through the conduction system. This can cause both rapid and slow conduction. One example of this problem in conduction is atrio-ventricular blocks (Fig. 3–18).

Conclusion

The cardiac conduction system is comprised of an electrical system of pathways among the sinus node, atrial tissue, and the AV junction. The EKG is used by health care professionals to monitor phases of the cardiac conduction cycle and to identify rhythm and conduction disturbances. To see this conduction system in action, the electrocardiogram or the rhythm strip is utilized. Note these key points about the cardiac conduction system:

- The heart's cardiac cells have one of two functions: mechanical (contractile) or electrical (pacemaker). The two types of cardiac cells are the myocardial cells and the pacemaker cells.

- An inotropic response relates to the contractility of the heart muscle.
- A chronotropic response relates to the heart rate.
- Action potential describes the electrolyte exchanges that occur across the cardiac cell membranes during depolarization. The resting potential occurs when a fully depolarized cell returns to its resting state and restores its electrical charges to normal in a process called repolarization.
- There are five stages in the depolarization process: rapid depolarization, initial repolarization, plateau, final rapid depolarization, and diastolic depolarization.
- The electrolytes of major importance in the depolarization process are sodium, potassium, and calcium.
- Refractoriness is the ability of cardiac cells to remain unresponsive to stimuli or to reject an impulse. The three refractory stages are: absolute refractory period, relative refractory period, and supernormal period.
- Cardiac cells are especially vulnerable during the relative refractory period.
- The cardiac conduction system ensures the chambers of the heart contract in a coordinated fashion.
- The electrical conduction system normally passes from the SA node to the AV node into the bundle of HIS and the bundle branches ending in the Purkinje fibers.
- Causes of abnormal heart impulses include enhanced automaticity, triggered activity, reentry, backward conduction, escape rhythms, and conduction disturbances.

PRACTICE QUESTIONS

1. **Which cardiac cells can spontaneously conduct electrical impulses without nerve involvement?**
   A. Pacemaker cells
   B. Myocardial cells
   C. Refractory cells
   D. Mechanical cells

2. **The primary pacemaker in a normal heart is the**
   A. AV node
   B. SA node
   C. AV junction
   D. Purkinje fibers

3. A positive inotropic medication would help a patient to increase

   A. heart rate.

   B. contractility.

   C. electrical conduction.

   D. mechanical conduction.

4. The characteristic of conductivity in a heart cell would mean that the cell would be able to

   A. create an electrical impulse.

   B. respond to an electrical impulse.

   C. transmit an electrical impulse.

   D. contract after an electrical impulse.

5. During the plateau phase of the cardiac cycle, which of the following electrolytes is slowly entering the cell?

   A. Potassium

   B. Sodium

   C. Calcium

   D. Chloride

6. Which of the following is the resting phase of the cardiac cycle?

   A. Phase1

   B. Phase 2

   C. Phase 3

   D. Phase 4

7. Which of the following would be a true statement regarding pulseless Electrical Activity?

   A. No electrical activity is noted on the electrocardiogram.

   B. No demonstrable heart beat is present in the patient.

   C. The heart is functioning in a normal manner.

   D. The cardiac conduction cycle is coming from an ectopic source.

8. In which of the following phases would the heart NOT be able to respond to a stimulus?

   A. Supernormal period

   B. Relative refractory period

   C. Absolute refractory period

   D. Pre-relative refractory period

9. Commotio cordis must be treated immediately for which of the following dysrhythmias?

   A. Ventricular fibrillation
   B. Premature ventricular contraction
   C. Asystole
   D. Third-degree heart block

10. The normal generated cardiac impulse is created in the

   A. AV node.
   B. Bundle of His.
   C. Purkinje fibers.
   D. SA node.

11. The QRS complex on the EKG is created by the activity of which of the following?

   A. SA node
   B. AV node
   C. Bachman's bundle
   D. His-Purkinje system

12. Which of the following causes a situation in which cardiac cells respond to a single stimulus by depolarizing more than once?

   A. Enhanced automaticity
   B. Triggered activity
   C. Reentry
   D. Retrograde conduction

13. Which of the following cardiac conduction disturbances is responsible for a condition known as Wolf-Parkinson-White Syndrome (WPW)?

   A. Enhanced automaticity
   B. Triggered activity
   C. Reentry
   D. Retrograde conduction

14. An escape rhythm occurs in an attempt to provide

   A. a decrease in ejection fraction.
   B. a greater impulse generation.
   C. an increase in cardiac output.
   D. a decreased stroke volume.

ANSWER KEY

1. **A.** Pacemaker cells, also called conducting cells or automatic cells, spontaneously generate and conduct electrical impulses without stimulation by a nerve.

2. **B.** The SA node serves as the primary pacemaker in a normal heart.

3. **B.** Medications such as digitalis, dopamine, and epinephrine can improve the heart's ability to contract. This would be considered to be an inotropic response.

4. **C.** Conductivity is the cardiac cell's ability to receive an electrical impulse and transmit it to another cardiac cell.

5. **C.** Calcium slowly enters the cell during the plateau phase.

6. **D.** Phase 4 or diastolic depolarization is the resting phase of the cardiac cycle.

7. **B.** When a patient is in pulseless electrical activity (PEA), electrical activity is seen on the EKG; however, the patient does not have pulses or blood pressure.

8. **C.** Absolute refractory period is when the cardiac cells cannot respond to stimuli.

9. **A.** Commotio cordis causes instantaneous ventricular fibrillation and must be treated immediately with defibrillation.

10. **D.** The SA node or sino-atrial node is referred to as the pacemaker because it reaches potential more quickly than the rest of the cardiac tissue and generates impulses 60 to 100 times per minute.

11. **D.** The activities of the bundle of His, the separate bundle branches, and the Purkinje fibers (known collectively as the His-Purkinje system) creates the QRS pattern on the EKG tracing.

12. **B.** Triggered activity occurs when pacemaker cells from an alternative site (from a location other than the SA node) receive a single stimulus, but then can respond by depolarizing more than once.

13. **C.** When an extra conduction pathway exists, (one of the three factors present for reentry conduction problems), a special form of tachycardia can arise called Wolff-Parkinson-White Syndrome (WPW).

14. **C.** Escape rhythms are produced when the SA node slows or fails to initiate the depolarization process and a lower site assumes the task of creating impulses to activate heart function, thus attempting to preserve cardiac output.

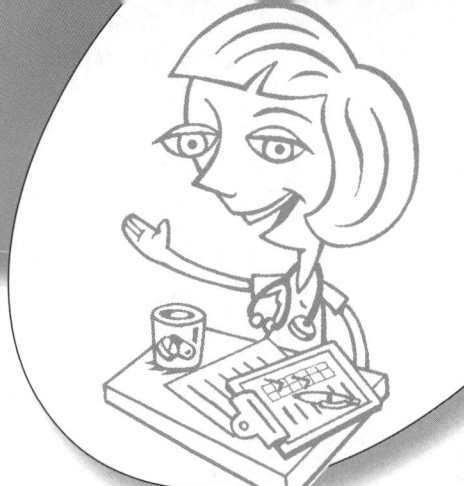

chapter 4

Cardiac Monitoring and 12-Lead EKG Basics

LEARNING OBJECTIVES

At the end of this chapter, the student will be able to:

① Relate the process involved in heart monitoring preparation including the use of electrodes, leads, electrocardiogram (EKG) machine, and cardiac paper.

② Describe the types of cardiac monitoring available to health care professionals.

③ Understand leads and planes associated with cardiac monitoring and 12-lead EKG.

④ Describe Einthoven's Triangle.

⑤ List the components of the 6-limb leads and the 6-chest leads and the views of the heart involved.

⑥ Understand the use of nonstandard leads and EKGs.

⑦ Understand the difference between bipolar and unipolar leads.

Overview

The electrocardiogram (EKG) measures the heart's electrical activity by showing the exact progression of electrical events during depolarization and repolarization. The EKG allows health care professionals to monitor the work of the heart as demonstrated by the unique waveforms it produces. These waveforms demonstrate the phases of contraction and aids in the identification of rhythm disturbances. Health care professionals can also use this to assess for disease and injury related to heart function, to evaluate pacemaker performance, to determine the effects of medications and electrolytes, and as a baseline of normal patient assessment for future reference. To do this, **electrodes** are placed at specific locations on the patient's skin to sense the electrical current and transmit them to an EKG monitor.

> **CLINICAL ALERT**
>
> The EKG is not able to demonstrate the contractile strength of the heart. Other modes of testing, such as an echocardiogram, are available to help with this piece of assessment. Both blood pressure and pulse can provide important evidence of performance of the cardiac system.

Types of Electrocardiograms

There are two types of EKGs: the rhythm strip and the 12-lead. Table 4–1 describes these EKGs.

TABLE 4–1 Types of EKGs	
Rhythm Strip	• Monitors cardiac rhythm status. • Uses one or more leads simultaneously. • Heart activity and heart rate are displayed on monitor. • Uses bipolar leads I, II, III, V_1, V_6, MCL$_1$, and MCL$_6$.
12 Lead	• Provides complete picture of electrical activity. • Provides 12 different views of the heart. • Electrodes are placed on patient's chest and limbs. • Information about the heart's frontal (vertical) plane is provided by six limb leads: I, II, III, aVR, aVL, and aVF. • Information about the heart's horizontal plane is provided by six precordial leads: V_1, V_2, V_3, V_4, V_5, and V_6.

Monitoring Systems

The two EKG monitoring system types are hardwire and telemetry.

Hardwire

Hardwire monitoring is most commonly used in emergency departments, intensive care units, postanesthesia care units, or surgical suites. This type allows for continuous observation. These can also be electronically transmitted to a main console so that more than one patient can be observed at a time. In this type of monitoring, the electrodes are connected directly to the cardiac monitor that is permanently secured to the wall near the patient's bed or they could be mounted on a device similar to an IV pole so that they can be moved between patients and/or rooms. Each monitor is different and may have a variety of attachments or monitoring capabilities depending on the company. Parameters such as blood pressure, pulse oximetry, capnography, and other hemodynamic measurements can be a part of the functionality of the hardwire bedside monitor as well as being able to capture rhythm abnormalities and monitor for injury patterns that may be evolving for the patient. EKG tracings or rhythm strips can be transmitted to the main console so that print copies may be maintained of the patient's cardiac activity. The disadvantages of hardwire monitoring are: patient discomfort due to restricted movement by the monitor cable and electrodes, the disconnection of leads or the presence of extraneous waveforms that may present on the screen as life-threatening dysrhythmias as the patient moves about in the bed, patient discomfort due to electrode placement and removal, especially for men with hair on their chests, the presence of diaphoresis (sweating) on the patient in which electrode attachment becomes difficult, and a feeling of being "tied down" by the patient.

Telemetry

Telemetry is used for more mobile patients in medical-surgical and step-down units. This system monitors only heart rate and rhythm and can be used for detecting dysrhythmias. Telemetry uses electrodes placed on the patient's chest with the electrodes then connected to a small battery-powered transmitter box. The patient can carry this transmitter box in a pocket or a pouch with a strap that can be worn across the shoulder or around the neck. The transmitter sends electrical signals to a monitor screen at a different location where the tracings can be printed and analyzed. One screen can monitor multiple patients. Electrodes are still utilized with this style of monitoring and the same problems can occur as above such as disconnection or the creation of extra waveforms with movement, however, it allows the patient a greater range of mobility and is especially useful in the detection of problems when the patient engages in activities of daily living.

The Process

Electrodes

Electrodes can be made from paper, plastic, or metal (or any combination of the three) and contain conductive material that allows recording of the heart's electrical currents. The types of electrodes that are placed on the skin are the metal disk, metal suction cup, and the disposable disk. The disposable disk is the most common type to be used for continuous monitoring purposes. The metal disks and suction cups are more frequently used for 12-lead EKG purposes (Fig. 4–1).

Lead Wire Systems

Lead wire systems utilize either three or five electrodes. These are also known as three-lead and five-lead systems. In the three-electrode system, there is one positive electrode, one negative electrode, and a ground electrode that prevents accidental shock to the patient. This type of monitoring allows visualization of lead I, lead II, or lead III through either the lead selector button on the monitor or by changing the location of the positive, negative, and ground leads. The most common is lead II. The right arm, left arm, and left leg are the electrode positions in the three-electrode system (Fig. 4–2). Telemetry monitoring usually employs this three-electrode system.

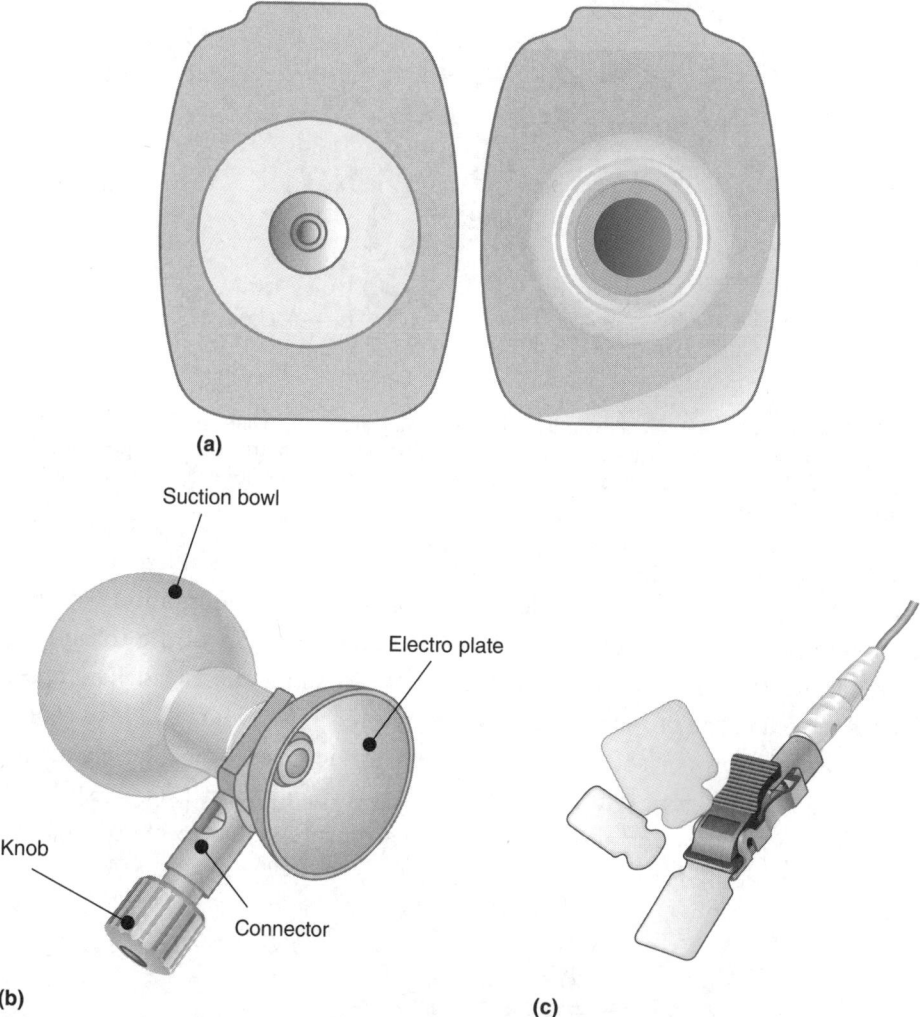

(a)

Suction bowl

Electro plate

Knob

Connector

(b)   **(c)**

FIGURE 4-1 • Types of electrodes. Different types of electrodes used in EKG monitoring and 12-lead EKG. (a) A common type of bedside monitoring electrode showing the electrical conducting gel. (b) A bulb type of electrode (not used as commonly). (c) A metal disk type of electrode used for 12-lead EKGs. The wire is attached by a clip type of end to the electrode.

CLINICAL ALERT

When placing electrodes for monitoring purposes, the lower limb leads are usually placed on the abdomen, however, they can be placed on the limbs themselves if necessary to obtain a good waveform. Consider the comfort of the patient when determining this. Long wires to the legs can cause problems with positioning in the bed. If a patient has extreme hair on his chest, the right and left arm leads can be placed on the shoulder area or upper arm.

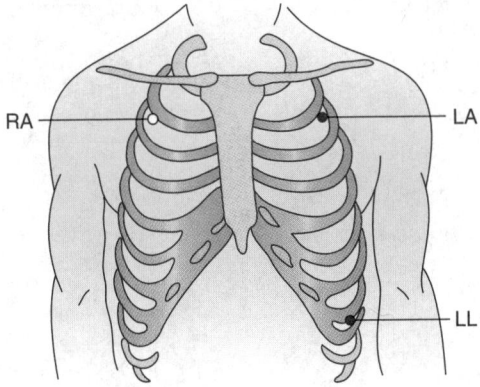

FIGURE 4–2 • **Placement of electrodes for three-lead system.** The white electrode attaches to the right arm area (RA), the black electrode to the left arm area (LA), and the red electrode to the left upper or mid abdominal area to represent the left leg (LL). Electrodes are normally universally color coded.

The five-electrode system is a popular choice due to the ability to monitor any of the 12 leads through the lead selector button on the monitor. For this lead system option, the leads are placed in similar fashion as the three-lead system with the addition of a right leg (RL) lead and a chest lead. The chest lead is moved to the proper position on the chest for each choice of lead monitoring and the proper selection is made on the lead selector. The electrode positions are right arm, left arm, right leg, left leg, and chest (Fig. 4–3). Lead selectors on the monitor allow the health care professional to choose which lead they would like to monitor.

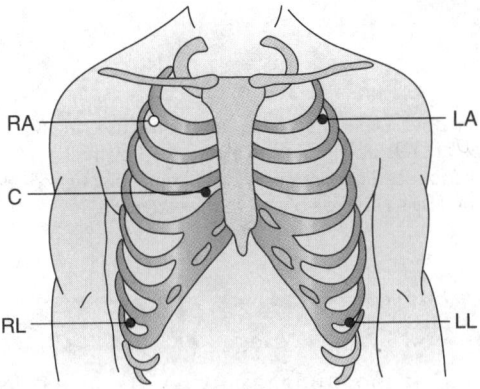

FIGURE 4–3 • **Placement of electrodes for five-lead system.** The white electrode attaches to the right arm area (RA), the black electrode to the left arm area (LA), the red electrode to the left upper or mid abdominal area to represent the left leg (LL), the green electrode to the right upper or mid abdominal area to represent the right leg (RL), and the brown chest lead is placed in the proper position for particular chest leads to be monitored. This chest electrode is placed in the correct position to monitor lead V_1. Electrodes are normally universally color coded.

CLINICAL ALERT

Electrodes are normally universally color coded. Be sure to check in each institution for this color coding, however, the most common is to have red, green, white, black, and brown electrodes. An easy way to remember proper placement is with a mnemonic: "White to the right, red to the bed." This helps to remember that the white electrode is placed on the right side. The black electrode (the opposite of white) is then placed on the opposite side. With the three-electrode system, the red is then placed "to the bed" or on the left abdomen which is closer to the bed. The five-electrode system is the same except the brown electrode usually goes on the mid chest area and the green electrode goes on the left side of the abdomen, therefore, the colors usually associated with Christmas, red and green, are together on the lower abdomen.

Another form of the five-electrode system is known as the EASI system, also known as a reduced lead continuous 12-lead EKG. In this system, electrodes are placed in a particular fashion on the chest and all 12-leads can be monitored simultaneously. The monitor conducts special mathematical calculations to provide a three dimensional view and a total of 12 views as in a 12-lead EKG. The EASI system correlates well with the 12-lead EKG, but, should not be used in place of the conventional 12-lead EKG. Electrode placement is depicted in Fig. 4–4.

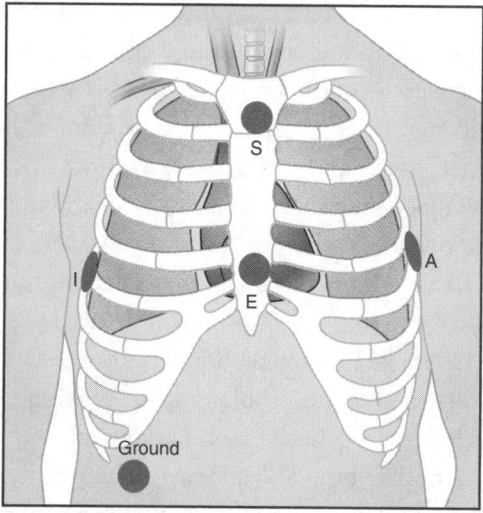

FIGURE 4–4 • **Placement of EASI electrodes.** In the EASI method of monitoring, five electrodes are utilized and placed in the following manner: "E" at the lower sternal area at the level of the fifth intercostal space / "A" at the left chest area at the level of the fifth intercostal space mid axillary line / "S" at the top part of the sternum / "I" at the right chest area at the level of the fifth intercostal space mid axillary line / A ground wire on the torso (placement anywhere on torso). (*ECG Intrepretation Made Incredibly Easy, 5e, Wolters Kluwer/Lippincott William Wilkins.*)

Application of Electrodes

Prior to placing electrodes on a patient for either an EKG or cardiac monitor, be sure to provide privacy and explain the purpose of the monitoring or electrocardiogram. Some patients may have misinformation about the procedure and may express fear or concern, such as being "shocked" or that the machine can control their heart rhythm. Allay those fears with simple explanations that the procedure is used to watch the heart activity and that there is no pain involved. If the patient is being attached to a cardiac monitor, discuss that the monitor is very sensitive and that alarms occasionally occur from the machine itself. Clarify that if the patient moves about in the bed or if a lead wire becomes disconnected from the electrode, the monitor will alarm in the same manner as if a dysrhythmia were detected. Also, other parameters can cause the monitor to alarm such as abnormal blood pressures or faulty respiratory readings. Make sure that the patient is aware that even though the health care professional is not in the room, the patient is on a main monitor screen and that they are being viewed at all times. Always answer questions about the monitor for both the patient and significant others prior to leaving the room and secure the call light in an easy to reach location.

Check all equipment to ensure that the EKG machine or monitor and all cables and lead wires are intact (no breakage or fraying) and functioning. Make sure that the appropriate paper is loaded into the machine and is filled. Next, gather the electrode supplies and ensure the electrode gel in the electrodes is moist and has not dried. This conductive gel is necessary to help to bridge across the dead or dried cells that lie on the surface of the skin. If the gel is dry, electrical contact will be decreased and **artifacts**—waveforms not produced by the heart's electrical activity—can appear. Attach the lead wires to each electrode. It is usually best to apply the lead wires to the electrodes before placing on the patient to reduce patient discomfort. Snap on electrodes must be pushed on to the end of the lead wire and if the electrode is on the patient, this can cause pain as pressure is applied to make this connection. This can also force the conductive gel out of the electrode and cause problems with making good contact. If the system uses clip-on lead wires, they can be attached after the electrodes are attached to the skin. Another type of lead wire is the pinch variation. These are usually used with the EKG machine to attach to the metal disk type of electrodes. These can be used for monitoring but are more often used for EKG tracings. Choose the appropriate lead placement and expose the patient's chest. Make sure the patient's limbs are resting on a supportive structure to reduce muscle tension and tremors which can interfere with proper readings.

> ## CLINICAL ALERT
>
> When exposing the chest, again be aware of privacy and obtain permission from the patient for family members in the room to be present. Do not assume that individuals in the room are spouses or appropriate family members for this type of exposure.

Prepare the patient's skin by rubbing with a gauze pad, a dry washcloth, or the small abrasive area supplied by the manufacturer on the back of the electrode if necessary. Rub each site until it reddens slightly. Soap and water can be used to cleanse prior to application of the electrode. Alcohol is not recommended for this process as it can dry the skin area. Tincture of benzoin and antiperspirant are also not recommended. However, benzoin might be necessary if the patient is very **diaphoretic**. This can help the pad stay on the skin. If this is used, be sure to apply a thin layer only to the area that is making contact with the sticky portion of the electrode and not the center where the conductive gel is present. Benzoin can reduce the conduction of the electrical impulses. Allow the tincture of benzoin to dry before applying the electrode.

If excess hair is present, clip this with clippers or scissors. Some commercially available single use clippers are available for this. Shaving is controversial. Check with the institution to determine if shaving is acceptable in that location.

Remove the backing from the electrode and apply to the site by pressing one side of the electrode against the patient's skin, pulling gently, and then pressing the opposite side of the electrode against the skin. To stabilize the electrode, take two fingers and press the outside of the electrode to ensure it sticks to the patient's chest. Do not apply electrodes over broken skin, joints, scar tissue, burns, rashes, pacemakers, medication patches, other implanted devices, jewelry, bony prominences, skin folds or creases, or thick muscles. Double check lead wires for secure attachment to the electrodes (Fig. 4–5).

Cardiac Monitors and the EKG Machine

Prior to adhering the electrodes and leads to the patient ensure that the EKG machine or cardiac monitor and all involved parts are in sound working order. The electrodes and lead wires for the cardiac monitor are usually all placed on the chest, although the shoulders and upper arms can be used as well. The lower abdomen is used for the lower extremity electrodes. After placing the electrodes and leads and attaching the necessary cables, turn on the cardiac monitor. The EKG waveform should appear.

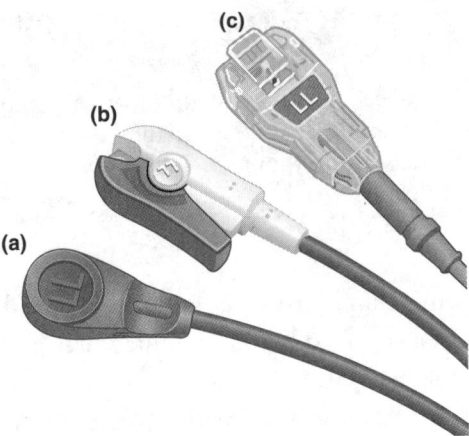

FIGURE 4–5 • **Types of lead wires.** (a) Snap On (b) Clip On (c) Pinch type.

Once the patient is attached to the monitor, select the appropriate lead and make sure that the rhythm is readable. Either touching the screen, pressing buttons, or turning knobs will make needed adjustments. To select different leads on the cardiac monitor in order to obtain varied views of the patient's cardiac rhythm, enable the lead selector button. Reset the **amplitude** if necessary on the machine so that the QRS complexes are captured for correct reading of heart rate. Adjust the size of the waveform by manipulating the gain control and position button.

Reset alarm rates if necessary. Do not turn off alarms. This is a necessary part of monitoring the patient. Set the monitor's heart rate alarms to 10 to 20 beats per minute higher and lower than the patient's heart rate. Be sure to consult your facility's policy for setting these alarms. Consider your patient's condition and age in case the alarms need to be set to different parameters. The pediatric patient's heart rate will be normally higher and therefore the alarms may need to be adjusted for this patient. To make sure the monitor is working properly, take the patient's apical pulse and compare the heart rate you obtain to that which is displayed on the monitor.

CLINICAL ALERT

If a patient is having extra heartbeats such as with premature ventricular contractions, these beats may be counted on the machine, but are not perfusing the patient. By counting the patient's radial pulse, the health care professional can determine which beats are actually carrying oxygenated blood throughout the body.

If necessary make a printed copy for the chart. The record button on the monitor will print the paper record of the patient's cardiac rhythm. The paper strip is either printed from the monitor or from a central console. Be sure to label the rhythm strip with the patient's name, identification number, date of birth, physician's name, date, time, medications administered, presence of chest pain, patient's activity during recording, and interpretation of the rhythm. Again, check on institution policy regarding information necessary on printouts. Some machines may require you to program some of the basic information into the system (such as patient name, date of birth, and date) beforehand so that the information will be automatically printed on the rhythm strip.

CLINICAL ALERT

If situations arise that require interventions for your patient that are related to the readings on the monitor, such as dysrhythmias or heart rates, be sure that the times on the recording are concurrent with the times that are documented in the patient record related to medications given or other treatment regimens that were instituted in response to those problems.

When the multichannel 12-lead EKG machine is used, proper patient identification will need to be entered before the EKG is recorded. (Some cardiac monitors are able to create a 12-lead EKG with the assistance of a special cord that allows the 10 leads to be attached to the patient.) Place the proper electrodes on each limb and across the chest. These are then attached to the lead wires which are marked for the health care professional's convenience. Make sure that the rhythm on the screen on this instrument is clear and legible before pressing the print button. Have the patient lie still and refrain from talking. Encourage them to relax with their head resting comfortably on a pillow. Increased respiratory rates and effort will affect the outcome of the reading. Heavy and erratic baselines, as well as loss of a lead on the screen, need to be resolved before printing. If the patient is in an area such as the emergency department and is being observed for the potential of a heart attack, it is usually best to leave the leads in place on the patient's chest. If a second EKG is requested at a later time, the lead placements will be exactly the same and proper identification of changes between the two can be detected. Make sure that all appropriate identifying information is on the EKG tracing. Ensure that the provider caring for the patient views the EKG. A 12-lead EKG will have all 12 leads on it and most will also provide a lead II rhythm strip at the bottom of the page. Each lead is labeled and it is easy to see the change to a new lead on the page since each lead has particular identifying characteristics.

Problems with Waveforms and Machines

Some problems that can occur with either the cardiac monitor or the EKG machine are listed below.

- **Malfunctioning equipment:** Equipment that is excessively worn or that has broken lead wires and cables can cause incorrect grounding. This can cause an inadvertent electrical shock to the patient.

- **Lack of waveform:** The lack of a waveform can be caused by improper electrode placement, a disconnected electrode, dry electrode gel, or failure of a wire or cable. Rectify these situations by repositioning the electrodes, reapplying disconnected electrodes, and replacing dry electrodes or damaged wires or cables.

- **Waveform abnormalities:** Waveform abnormalities can occur when the electrodes are not connected to the correct electrode wire, therefore changing the normal positive and negative **deflections** that create the complexes. If the monitor picture or the EKG tracing does not look appropriate, check for the correct placement of the wires and electrodes.

- **Baseline issues:** Several different baseline issues can occur. A *wandering baseline* causes a baseline that appears jagged or irregular and isn't stationary (Fig. 4–6). Patient movement that might occur due to chilling associated with fever or ambient room temperature, nerves, uncontrolled muscle tremors, seizures, disease processes such as Parkinson's disease or extra chest wall movement during labored respirations, electrode placement over bone instead of soft tissue, or poor contact between the electrode and the skin can cause a wandering baseline. Rectify these issues by helping the patient relax and remain still, applying warm blankets, treating high fevers, repeating the EKG after treatment for distressed breathing has been accomplished, and by repositioning the electrode. A *fuzzy baseline* is caused by electrical interference from other equipment in the room, such as razors, hair dryers, or radios. This may be seen as a wide, thickened baseline that also has thin, rapid spikings. This is also known as 60-cycle interference (Fig. 4–7). Electrode malfunction and improper grounding of the patient's bed may also be causes. Resolve a fuzzy baseline by ensuring all electrical equipment is attached to a common ground

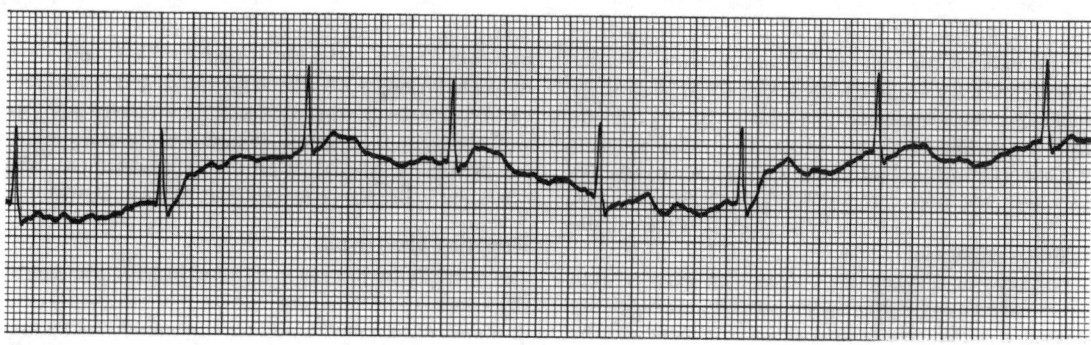

FIGURE 4–6 • **Wandering baseline.** A wandering baseline can be caused by placing the electrodes in any areas of heavy movement when the patient is in distress or if the patient is restless or moving a great deal and the electrodes are on bony areas.

and the patient's bed ground is attached to the room's common ground. Replacing the electrodes and ensuring that three-pronged plugs are not loose may also help. Remove other equipment in the room that may be interfering.

- **Artifact:** Artifact can be manifested in a rough, uneven, wavy type of baseline or in what might appear as extra beats or exaggerated complexes that are not cardiac in origin (Fig. 4–8). Excessive patient movement, as seen in seizures, anxiety, and chills, can cause artifact. Other causes of artifact are static electricity; interference from other electrical equipment; malfunctioning, dirty, or corroded lead wires or cables; hair on the chest; and improper electrode placement. In the case of the patient who experiences seizures, notify the practitioner and provide for patient safety by removing surrounding equipment and ensuring the patient doesn't fall off the examination table or out of the bed. If the patient is chilled or anxious, provide

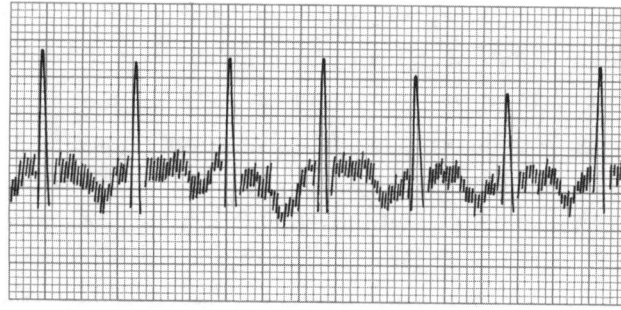

FIGURE 4–7 • **60-cycle interference.** 60-cycle interference can be caused by ungrounded electrical equipment in the room.

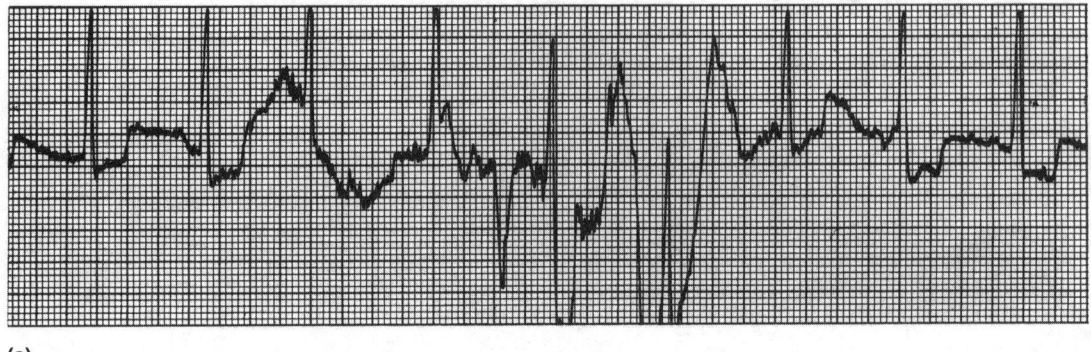

(a)

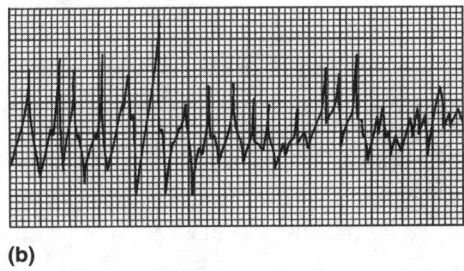

(b)

FIGURE 4–8 • **Artifact.** (a) and (b) demonstrate EKG rhythm strips that show artifact. This can appear in many ways on a rhythm strip and can be caused by many different things.

blankets for warmth and therapeutic communication for relaxation or treat fevers that are present. Replace malfunctioning, dirty, or corroded lead wires and cables. Reposition or replace the electrodes as required. Ensure all electrical equipment is attached to a common ground and check the three-pronged plug for proper functioning. To combat static electricity, humidify the room to 40%. Artifact can also occur with telemetry when the signals are not being received well. Changing the battery may help with this problem. The patient may also have wandered past the established perimeters for the base station.

• **False alarms:** Both high and low false alarms can register for many reasons. This may be due to artifact that is captured on the screen as high voltage, such as with seizures, patient movement, or having the gain or amplitude too high. Lower the gain control when this occurs. Hyperkalemia can be a cause of a false high rate alarm due to the associated high peaked T waves which are then read along with the QRS complex as another heartbeat.

False low rate alarms can occur due to non-contact between the electrode and the skin, dried electrode gel, disconnections between the lead wire and the electrode or the monitor. Low amplitude complexes can also be the cause and in this case, the gain needs to be increased.

• **Weak signal:** Faulty or nonfunctioning wires or cables and improperly applied electrodes can cause a weak signal. Reapply or reposition the electrodes and replace defective equipment. The patient may need to be placed on a different lead. The amplitude or gain on the monitor can also be changed when QRS complexes are very small. When this involves telemetry, checking on the patient location or switching batteries may be helpful.

CLINICAL ALERT

When the monitor registers a rhythm that appears to be a dysrhythmia, be sure to conduct a thorough assessment of the patient to ensure that the abnormal rhythm is actually occurring. Simple patient movements such as sneezing, yawning, laughing, changing positions, or brushing their teeth can be depicted as a life-threatening cardiac event, such as **ventricular tachycardia**. If an electrode has become unattached, the rhythm on the monitor may resemble a straight line or **asystole** (no heartbeat). Always treat the patient, not the machine!

Paper

The EKG machine or cardiac monitor records the voltage (potential difference) that is present between electrodes that are placed on the patient. This voltage is a visible representation of the electrical movement through the myocardial or contractile cells. Depolarization and repolarization is noted as the stylus or needle of the machine creates positive and negative deflections. The final product is a representation of both time, duration of the wave, and voltage, amplitude or height of the wave. Another criterion that is noted is the configuration of the wave, which looks at the contours and final shape of the waveform.

EKG paper is a special type of graph paper made up of small boxes that are 1 mm high and 1 mm wide. Each horizontal 1-mm box represents 0.04 seconds. The large boxes, denoted by the heavier lines on the grid paper, are made up of five of these small boxes and thus represent 0.20 seconds (5 × 0.04 = 0.20).

Five large boxes that are comprised of five small boxes each (25 small boxes total) represent 1 second. Fifteen large boxes equal an interval of 3 seconds while 30 large boxes represent 6 seconds. The 6-second strip consisting of 30 large boxes can be used to calculate the patient's heart rate. This horizontal movement of the machine's needle is a measurement of time and is labeled as seconds.

The voltage or amplitude of the waveform is measured by the vertical axis of the EKG paper. The voltage is measured in millivolts (mV) and amplitude is measured in millimeters (mm). Each small box represents 1 mm or 0.1 mV and each large box represents 5 mm or 0.5 mV. When measuring amplitude, simply count the number of small boxes from the baseline wave (isoelectric line) to the highest point visible of the wave. This can also be used to determine amplitude of intervals or segments. To confirm the accuracy of this measurement, the machine must be calibrated to validate that a 1-millivolt (mV) electrical signal will produce a wave that equals 10 millimeters (mm) in height. This measurement is expressed in millimeters (Fig. 4–9).

CLINICAL ALERT

The paper moves through the machine at a rate of 25 mm per second. This speed can be altered to increase or decrease. If the patient has a rapid heart rate, increasing the paper speed will make it easier to see potential P waves and can assist in the diagnosis of the rhythm. When looking at these faster or slower rates of paper speed, remember that the complexes will be distorted.

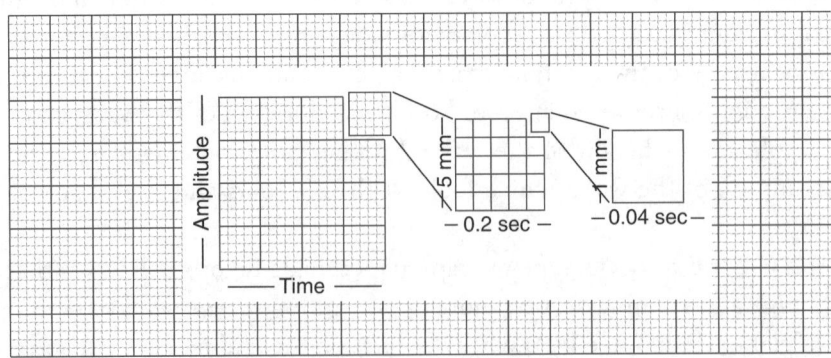

FIGURE 4–9 • EKG paper. The horizontal axis is a measurement of time. The vertical axis is a measurement of amplitude. [*Modified from ECGs Made Easy (2011) by Barbara Aehlert.*]

Leads

The word "lead" is used to mean both a physical object, that is, the lead wire and electrode that is attached to the patient and also to indicate a specific recording of electrical currents between one positive pole and one negative pole, or two electrodes. The direction of the current at a specific time in a portion of the heart is recorded as waveforms on the EKG. This direction of the current is known as a **vector**. A straight line on the EKG means the current is nonexistent or very weak. This occurs when there is not a true negative or positive field within the cell because the charges are balanced. During depolarization, waveforms deflect downward when the current travels to the negative pole and upward when the current travels towards the positive pole. During repolarization, these waveforms create the opposite effect. Current that flows perpendicular (at a 90^0 angle) to the lead is expressed by a **biphasic** (both directions) waveform. The representation on the EKG is the sum of the electrical currents that are passing through the heart at any given time. This picture of electrical activity of the myocytes will correspond to the largest mass of activity, meaning that some activity is masked if a stronger or larger mass is undertaking similar activity at the same time (Fig. 4–10).

Different leads allow the heart's electrical activity to be viewed in planes, or cross-sectional orientations. These include the vertical (frontal or coronal)

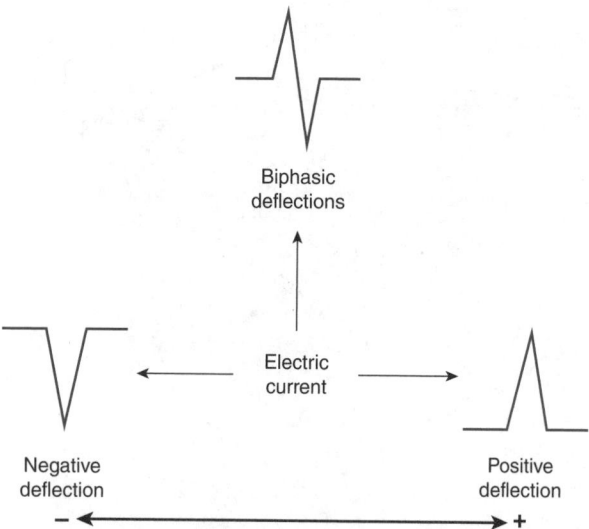

Biphasic
deflections

Electric
current

Negative
deflection

Positive
deflection

– +

FIGURE 4–10 • **Correlation of waveforms and flow of current.** Current flowing in the direction of the positive electrode will create a positive deflection. Current flowing in the direction of the negative electrode will create a negative deflection. Current flowing perpendicular to the line of current will create a biphasic deflection.

and horizontal (transverse) planes. This provides for a complete look at the heart. Twelve leads allow the health care professional to view this three-dimensional view of the electrical activity and this is accomplished with 10 electrodes strategically placed on the body. The EKG machine or the cardiac monitor changes the polarity between the leads to achieve these 12 views instead of the health care professional having to change the positive and negative leads to different places on the body.

Frontal Plane

The six vertical or frontal plane leads are also known as the limb leads and consist of three bipolar and three unipolar leads. The three bipolar leads form a triangle around the heart to show a frontal plane view. This triangle is historically known as Einthoven's triangle. Einthoven's triangle is formed by the axes of the first three limb leads with the heart at the epicenter. The **axis** of the lead is the imaginary connection between the positive and negative electrodes of a lead (Fig. 4–11).

A **bipolar lead** has both a positive and a negative electrode that records the electrical potential difference between the two electrodes. The bipolar leads (also called the standard limb leads) are leads I, II, and III (Table 4–2).

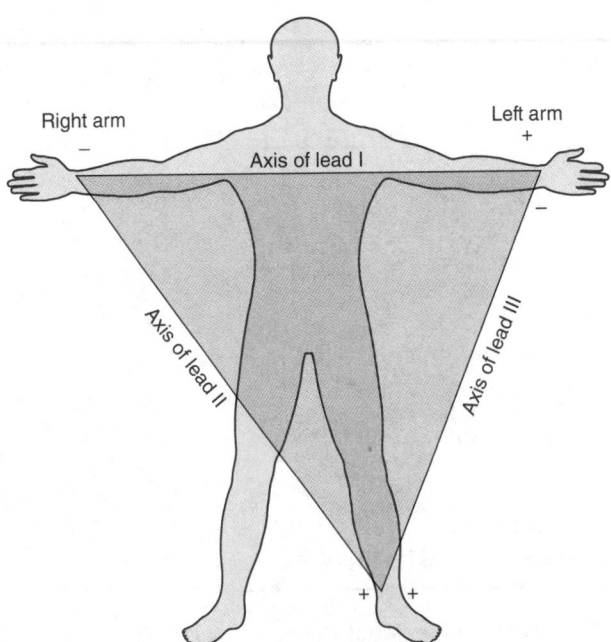

FIGURE 4–11 • Einthoven's triangle. Einthoven's triangle is used as a guide for the 6 vertical or limb leads. [*Elsevier's ECGs Made Easy (2011) by Barbara Aehlert.*]

TABLE 4–2 Standard Limb Leads

Lead I

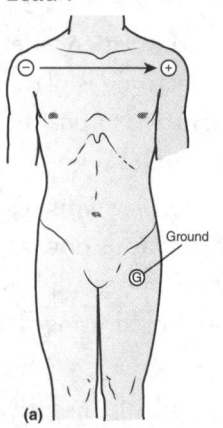

(a)

- Left arm is positive electrode.
- Right arm is negative electrode.
- Third electrode is a ground.
- Axis spans from shoulder to shoulder.
- Views the lateral surface of left ventricle.
- Valuable in looking at atrial rhythms.

Lead II

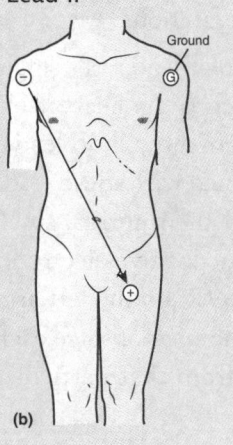

(b)

- Left leg is positive electrode.
- Right arm is negative electrode.
- Axis runs from negative right-arm electrode to positive left-leg electrode.
- Views the inferior surface of left ventricle.
- Commonly used for cardiac monitoring because electrode positioning mirrors the normal current flow in the heart.
- Valuable in atrial dysrhythmias and sinus node problems.

Lead III

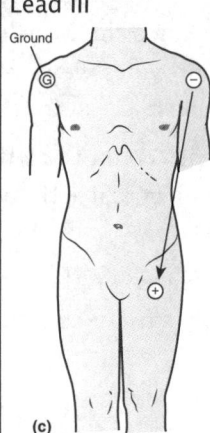

(c)

- Left leg is positive electrode.
- Left arm is negative electrode.
- Axis runs from the negative left-arm electrode to positive left-leg electrode.
- Views inferior surface of left ventricle.

Bipolar leads include a ground electrode to prevent extraneous electrical interference. When cardiac monitoring is utilized, this ground wire is placed on the chest.

- **Lead I:** The positive electrode for this lead is placed on the patient's left arm or on the left side of the chest while the negative electrode is placed on the right arm. This is because current flows from negative to positive. This allows the EKG to show current moving from right to left.

- **Lead II:** The positive electrode is placed on the patient's left leg while the negative electrode is placed on the right arm. The current travels down to the left in this lead and produces a positive deflection that causes tall P, R, and T waves. Sinus node and atrial arrhythmias are monitored using this lead.

- **Lead III:** The positive electrode is placed on the left leg while the negative electrode is placed on the left arm. This lead produces a positive deflection and is used with lead II to view inferior myocardial infarctions.

The last three frontal or vertical leads are unipolar. A **unipolar lead** has a single positive electrode and a relative negative "electrode" which is the heart itself. The unipolar leads (also called unipolar limb leads or augmented limb leads) are aVR, aVL, and aVF. The small letter "a" used in reference with these leads means that they are "augmented" or enhanced because of their normal small amplitude. The "R", "L", and "F" refers to the location of the positive electrode, thus, the positive electrode is placed on the right arm in aVR, on the left arm in aVL, and on the left foot (or leg) in aVF. The "V" stands for vector since each one is looking at the direction of the electrical current from that particular view.

- aVR is augmented vector right. The positive electrode is placed on the right arm and normally produces a negative deflection since the heart's electrical activity moves away from the lead. This lead provides views of the atria and great vessels but no view of the heart's walls.

- aVL is augmented vector left. The positive electrode is placed on the left arm and produces a positive deflection. This lead shows electrical activity coming from the lateral wall of the left ventricle.

- aVF is augmented vector foot. The positive electrode is placed on the left leg and produces a positive deflection. This lead shows activity coming from the heart's inferior wall (Fig. 4–12).

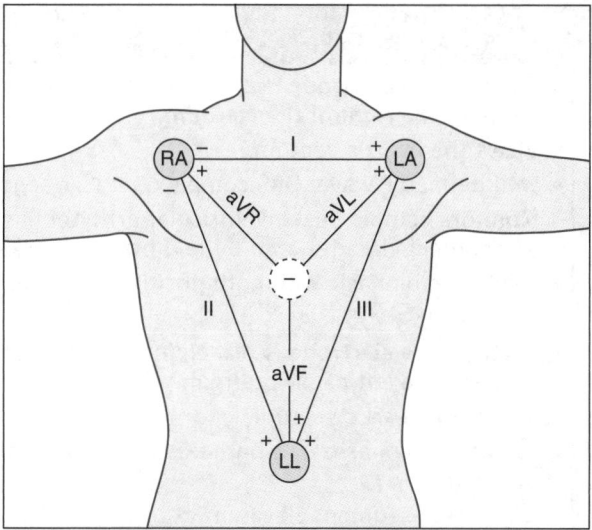

FIGURE 4-12 • **Frontal plane leads.** The frontal plane leads include Lead I, Lead II, Lead III, aVR, aVL, and aVF. [*Elsevier's ECGs Made Easy (2011) by Barbara Aehlert.*]

Horizontal Plane

The chest leads provide information about the heart's horizontal plane and are placed in chronological order across the patient's chest. The view of the heart produced by these leads is as if the body were sliced in half horizontally, providing a left and front side view of the heart. These leads are also unipolar with the center of the heart, as calculated by the EKG machine, serving as the opposing pole for these leads. These are listed in order as: V_1, V_2, V_3, V_4, V_5, and V_6. In the normal EKG, there is a progression of wave formation. This is depicted in Table 4–3 and Fig. 4–13.

> **CLINICAL ALERT**
>
> If leads need to be placed on the torso, position them as close to the appropriate limb as possible to decrease artifact. It is important that the limb leads be placed on the extremity (location does not matter) over tissue and not bony prominences.

Nonstandard Leads

Several leads that are not part of the standard 12-lead EKG can provide valuable information regarding specific situations. These are the right chest leads (right-sided EKG), posterior chest leads (posterior EKG), and modified chest leads.

TABLE 4-3 Precordial Leads

Lead V₁	• The positive electrode is placed in the fourth intercostal space to the right of the sternum. • Views the heart's septum. • Well defined P wave, QRS complex, and ST segment. • Monitors ectopic beats, ventricular arrhythmias, ST-segment changes, and bundle-branch blocks. • Lead V₁ is biphasic with both positive and negative deflections.
Lead V₂	• The positive electrode is placed in the fourth intercostal space to the left of the sternum. • Views the heart's septum. • Lead V₂ is biphasic with both positive and negative deflections. • Detects ST-segment elevation.
Lead V₃	• The positive electrode is placed between V₂ and V₄. • Views the anterior surface of the heart. • Lead V₂ is biphasic with both positive and negative deflections. • Detects ST-segment elevation.
Lead V₄	• The positive electrode is placed in the fifth intercostal space at the midclavicular line. • Views the anterior surface of the heart. • Lead V₄ is biphasic with both positive and negative deflections. • Shows changes in the ST-segment or T wave. • Monitors changes associated with acute myocardial infarction.
Lead V₅	• The positive electrode is placed in the fifth intercostal space at the anterior axillary line. • Views the lateral surface of the heart. • Produces positive deflection on EKG. • Shows changes in the ST-segment or T wave.
Lead V₆	• The positive electrode is placed in the fifth intercostal space at the midaxillary line. • Views the lateral surface of the heart. • Produces positive deflection on EKG.

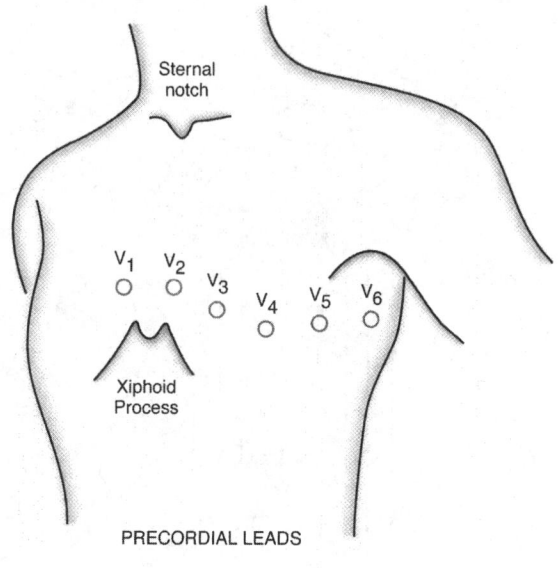

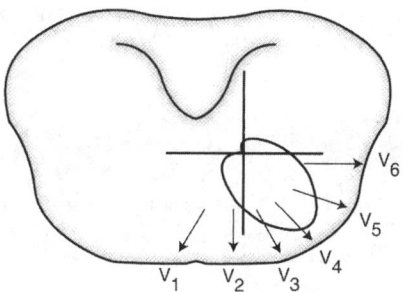

FIGURE 4–13 • **Precordial lead placement.** The precordial leads are placed in chronological order across the patient's chest. [*Modified from Ferry, DR. ECG in 10 Days (2007). McGraw-Hill.*]

- **Right chest leads:** Right chest leads are utilized to assist in the determination of a suspected right ventricular myocardial infarction. A regular 12-lead EKG looks only at the left ventricle. The leads are placed identical to the standard chest leads but all leads are instead placed on the right side of the chest. The right chest leads are V_1R, V_2R, V_3R, V_4R, V_5R, and V_6R. In this situation, the normal V_1 and V_2 switch places. Often only V_4R to V_6R is done to view the right ventricle. This will demonstrate the changes consistent with a myocardial infarction on the right side (Fig. 4–14). Be sure to label this EKG as being right sided. Pediatric patients will have some specific changes on the right-sided EKG that are not consistent with their adult counterparts such as a prominent R wave in V_1R and V_2R that may be present up to age 8.

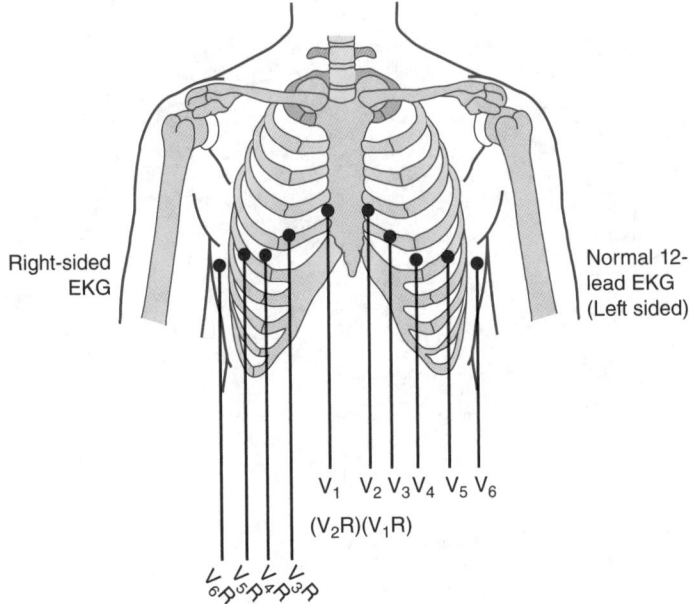

Right-sided EKG

Normal 12-lead EKG (Left sided)

V_1 V_2 V_3 V_4 V_5 V_6

(V_2R)(V_1R)

FIGURE 4-14 • **Right-sided EKG.** A right-sided EKG is an exact mirror image of the normal left-sided EKG. (*Modified from Aehlert, B. ECG's Made Easy, 2011.*)

CLINICAL ALERT

If time does not permit the placement of all six of the right chest leads, V_4R is the lead of choice.

- **Posterior chest leads:** Posterior chest leads are additional leads that are used to specifically view the posterior surface of the heart. These leads are placed on the same horizontal plane as V_4 to V_6, on the left side of the posterior surface (the patient's back). Lead V_7 is placed at the posterior axillary line; lead V_8 is placed at the posterior scapular area (mid-clavicular); and lead V_9 is placed at the border of the spine on the left side. Rarely, a right-sided posterior EKG may be requested by a practitioner. The posterior EKG will help to identify characteristic changes for a posterior wall myocardial infarction. These leads must be identified manually on the EKG printout (Fig. 4-15).

- **Modified chest leads:** Modified chest leads (MCL) are special leads that might be used to assist in detection of bundle branch blocks, premature beats, and supraventricular rhythms. It is often difficult to differentiate between supraventricular tachycardia and ventricular tachycardia.

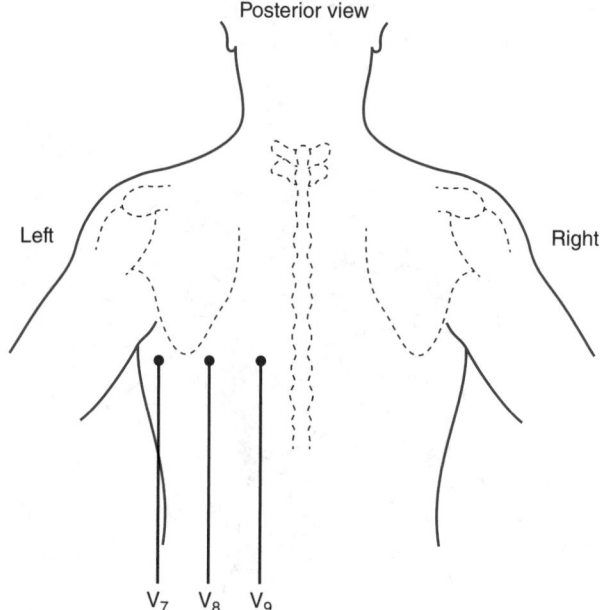

Posterior view

Left

Right

V_7 V_8 V_9

FIGURE 4-15 • **Posterior EKG electrode placement.** Leads V_7, V_8, and V_9 are placed in the same plane as V_6 at the posterior axillary line, the scapular area, and to the left of the spine respectively. (*Modified from Aehlert, B, ECG's Made Easy 4e, 2011.*)

These leads can help in this instance. These modified chest leads are bipolar as opposed to the usual unipolar chest leads. Each lead contains both a positive and negative electrode (Fig. 4–16).

- **MCL₁:** This lead is a variation of chest lead V_1 on the 12-lead EKG where the negative electrode is placed below the left clavicle close to the left shoulder. The positive electrode is placed in the fourth intercostal space to the right of the sternum while the ground is placed on the right upper chest area immediately below the clavicle. Although it is similar to lead V_1, it is a different view of the heart due to the placement of the positive and negative electrodes. In V_1 the heart is the "negative electrode". In MCL₁ the negative electrode is placed below the left clavicle. This lead views the ventricular septum and the QRS complex that is recorded appears negative. Abnormal or ectopic beats will appear as positive deflections. Ventricular and supraventricular tachycardia, bundle-branch defects, and P-wave changes are detected by MCL₁. This lead is also used to confirm pacemaker wire placement.

- **MCL₆:** This lead is a variation of chest lead V_6 where the negative electrode is placed toward the left shoulder and below the left clavicle. The positive electrode is placed in the fifth intercostal space at the left

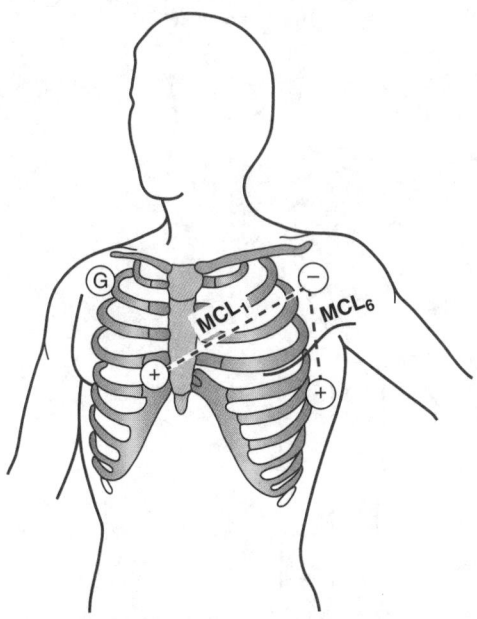

FIGURE 4−16 • Electrode placement for modified chest leads MCL$_1$ and MCL$_6$. Proper placement for positive, negative, and ground electrodes for MCL$_1$ and MCL$_6$. (*Modified from Aehlert, B., ECG's Made Easy 4e., 2011.*)

midaxillary line (similar to lead V$_6$) while the ground is placed below the right shoulder. This lead may be used as an alternative to MCL$_1$ and views the low lateral wall of the left ventricle while monitoring ventricular conduction changes.

Conclusion

Having a clear understanding of the process of applying electrodes and managing the cardiac monitor and EKG machine are important aspects of patient care. There are many different types of machines on the market and each health care professional must become familiar and comfortable with the products utilized in their institutions. The basics of leads including Einthoven's Triangle and the limb and chest leads are essential in understanding how these machines enhance the care of patients through proper diagnosis and observations. Note these key points about cardiac monitoring and the 12-lead EKG;

- The EKG measures the heart's electrical activity by showing the precise sequence of electrical events during depolarization and repolarization.

- EKGs do not measure contractile strength.

- Monitoring systems include both hardwire and telemetry units.

- Electrodes are made of paper, plastic, or metal (or any combination of the three) and contain conductive material that allows the recording of the heart's electrical currents.

- The right arm, left arm, and left leg are the electrode positions in the three-electrode system. The electrode positions in the five-electrode system are right arm, left arm, right leg, left leg, and chest. The EASI system is a specialized system with particular electrode placements.

- Electrodes are traditionally color coded but the health care professional must check at each institution to verify the color coding.

- Always talk to the patient prior to application of leads and lead wires. Allay any fears he or she may have.

- Artifacts can be caused by many different things and must be alleviated before a true reading of the rhythm or the 12 lead can be accomplished.

- Some common causes of problems with the readings from cardiac monitor or EKG machine include: malfunctioning equipment, improper electrode placement, disconnected lead wires, dry electrode gel, frayed or damaged wires, incorrect positioning of either the electrode or the lead wire, movement of the patient, other equipment in the room, bad contact with the skin, false alarms, and weak signals.

- Always check the machine against the patient condition, that is, treat the patient, not the machine.

- Make sure all charting is concurrent regarding times and interventions when dealing with rhythm problems.

- EKG paper measures both time and voltage.

- EKG paper is comprised of small boxes that are 1 mm high and 1 mm wide. Each 1 mm box represents 0.04 seconds.

- Large boxes on the EKG paper measure 0.20 seconds in length.

- Volume or amplitude of the waveform may need to be readjusted for proper readings.

- The term "lead" refers both to the actual physical lead that is placed on the patient and also is indicative of a specific recording of electrical currents between a positive and a negative pole.

- The six frontal plane leads consist of three bipolar leads and three unipolar leads.

- A bipolar lead has a distinct positive and negative lead.

- A unipolar lead has a single positive electrode and a relative negative point.
- The three unipolar limb leads are called augmented leads.
- The chest leads measure the horizontal plane and are unipolar.
- Nonstandard leads include a right-sided EKG, posterior EKG, and the use of modified chest leads, MCL_1 and MCL_6.

PRACTICE QUESTIONS

1. The EKG can be used to assist in diagnosis of all the following **EXCEPT**:
   A. contractile strength of the heart.
   B. rhythm analysis.
   C. myocardial infarction location.
   D. pacemaker performance.

2. Which of the following would be a disadvantage of the use of hardwire monitoring for the patient?
   A. Inability to leave the unit while ambulating
   B. Need for changing of batteries
   C. Wrapping of the strap around the neck
   D. A feeling of being "tied down"

3. Telemetry monitoring usually utilizes which of the following types of electrode wire systems?
   A. Three lead
   B. Five lead
   C. EASI System
   D. Twelve lead

4. Artifact is defined as:
   A. extra beats in the heart.
   B. premature beats.
   C. extraneous waveforms.
   D. a straight line.

5. Which of the following would be the best to use on the skin prior to the application of electrodes?
   A. Tincture of benzoin
   B. Alcohol
   C. Antiperspirant
   D. Dry washcloth

6. Which of the following would be a correct statement regarding the use of a cardiac monitor?

   A. If the complexes are very small, increase the gain.
   B. Turn off warning signals if they keep falsely alarming.
   C. Shave all chest hair prior to applying the electrodes.
   D. Place electrodes over bony prominences.

7. Which of the following would be the best way to troubleshoot for the lack of a waveform?

   A. Replace the ground wire
   B. Treat the patient's chills
   C. Check for disconnected lead wires
   D. Remove extra electrical equipment

8. If extra waveforms are present on the cardiac monitor screen that are obviously not related to the patient's heartbeat, the health care professional may try to rectify this by:

   A. removing extra electrical equipment.
   B. checking for disconnected lead wires.
   C. replacing the ground wire.
   D. treating the patient's chills.

9. Five small boxes on the EKG paper are equal to:

   A. 0.04 seconds
   B. 0.20 seconds
   C. 0.30 seconds
   D. 0.36 seconds

10. Correct calibration of the EKG machine would recognize that a 1 millivolt electrical signal would equal:

    A. 1 mm
    B. 5 mm
    C. 10 mm
    D. 20 mm

11. Biphasic means that the electrical current is causing a waveform that has:

    A. a positive deflection only.
    B. both positive and negative deflections.
    C. a negative deflection only.
    D. no deflections creating a straight line.

12. Which of the following leads is considered to be a bipolar lead?

   A. Lead I
   B. aVR
   C. V_1
   D. V6

13. Einthoven's Triangle is formed by the axes of which of the following?

   A. Augmented leads
   B. Unipolar leads
   C. Standard limb leads
   D. Chest leads

14. Which of the following leads would look at the lateral surface of the heart?

   A. V_1
   B. V_2
   C. V_4
   D. V_6

15. Which of the following leads would be used to determine the presence of a posterior myocardial infarction?

   A. Lead V_4
   B. Lead II
   C. Lead V_8
   D. Lead MCL_1

16. Which of the following would be correct placement for Lead V_4R?

   A. Fifth intercostal space, right mid-clavicular line
   B. Fourth intercostal space, right mid-axillary line
   C. Sixth intercostal space, right mid-axillary line
   D. Fourth intercostal space, right mid-clavicular line

ANSWER KEY

1. **A.** The EKG does not assist with recognition of problems with the contractile strength of the heart. An echocardiogram will help with this aspect of the heart function. EKGs can help determine cardiac rhythms, locations of myocardial infarctions, and the performance of pacemakers as well as assessment for disease and injury, effects of medications and electrolytes and as a baseline for future reference.

2. **D.** Hardwire monitoring can give the patient a feeling of being "tied down" due to the lead wires as they come from the wall unit. It is often difficult to keep these

leads on while in the bed due to turning and movement. Telemetry units can stop working if the patient leaves the unit and wanders beyond the limitations of the perimeter boundaries. They can also need new batteries and the strap that holds the battery unit can wrap around the neck.

3. **A.** Telemetry monitoring utilizes the three-lead system most often. This requires one positive electrode, one negative electrode, and one ground wire.

4. **C.** Artifact can appear in many different ways on the rhythm strip or EKG recording. This is extraneous waveforms that have nothing to do with the patient's underlying rhythm. Premature and extra beats in the heart are actual rhythm disturbances. A straight line could be a rhythm disturbance or a problem with the electrodes.

5. **D.** A dry washcloth or the small abrasive area on the back of the electrode should be used to prepare the skin. Rub the area until it is slightly red. Alcohol can dry out the skin. Tincture of benzoin can be used but it is not a skin prep, rather it is a way to help with adherence to the skin on a patient who is diaphoretic. Antiperspirant is not recommended.

6. **A.** When using a cardiac monitor, check for the size of the complexes. If they are very small, turn the gain control button so that the gain or amplitude is increased so that all of the complexes are counted in the final pulse rate. Alarms should never be shut off. Electrodes should be placed on tissue and not bony prominences. Shaving is controversial and clipping the hair is recommended over shaving. It is not necessary to cut all of the chest hair.

7. **C.** If a waveform is not present, check for disconnected or frayed and worn lead wires. Chills might cause artifact, but not a straight line. Extra electrical equipment in the room might cause 60 cycle interference and replacing the ground wire would not help.

8. **D.** Patient movement such as what might occur with a patient who is chilling from a fever might cause artifact that would appear as extra waveforms on the monitor or EKG. Artifact can also be caused by seizures, muscle tremors, labored respirations, poor contact of the electrode to the skin or the placement of the electrode over a bony prominence instead of tissue. The loss of a waveform, a straight line, could be caused by a disconnected electrode or dry electrode gel, as well as faulty lead wires. Extra electrical equipment in the room could cause problems with the baseline.

9. **B.** One small box on the EKG paper is equal to 0.04 seconds. Each large box contains 5 of these small boxes, therefore, one large box would equal 0.20 seconds.

10. **C.** Calibration is required to make sure that the voltage or amplitude is correct. One mV should equal 10 mm or 10 small boxes (2 large boxes) on the EKG paper.

11. **B.** Biphasic means that both positive and negative deflections would occur on the EKG reading. This occurs when the wave of current flows perpendicular to the lead axis. Movement of the flow of current towards the positive electrode causes a positive deflection and movement towards the negative electrode causes a negative deflection. Straight lines are caused by nonexistent or weak currents.

12. **A.** Bipolar leads have distinct positive and negative electrodes. The standard limb leads, which look at the frontal plane, leads I, II, and III are bipolar leads. The others are unipolar leads which have only a positive electrode and a relative negative "electrode", which is the heart itself.

13. **C.** The standard limb leads, leads I, II, and III, comprise Einthoven's Triangle. The augmented leads are encased within Einthoven's Triangle.

14. **D.** V_6 is the lead that would help to determine damage to the lateral aspect of the heart. V_1 and V_2 would look at the septum and V_4 looks at the anterior surface of the heart.

15. **C.** In order to see the EKG changes that occur with a myocardial infarction involving the posterior aspect of the heart, the posterior leads would need to be utilized. This includes V_7, V_8, and V_9. V_4 looks at the anterior aspect. Lead II provides information about the inferior portion and MCL_1 assists in identifying bundle branch blocks, premature beats and supraventricular rhythms.

16. **A.** The right-sided EKG would be used to determine damage to the right ventricle. V_4R is the best lead to use, although V_1R through V_6R can be performed. The right-sided EKG is a mirror image of the normal left-sided EKG. Therefore, the electrode placement for V_4R would be the fifth intercostal space, right mid-clavicular line.

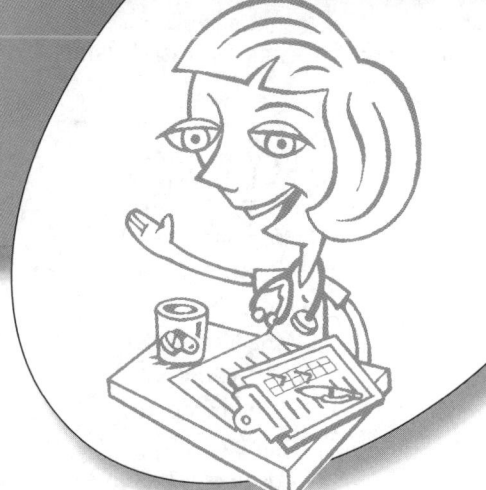

chapter 5

Waves, Complexes, Straight Lines, and Intervals/ Labeling and Interpreting

LEARNING OBJECTIVES

At the end of this chapter, the student will be able to:

❶ Label each of the waves, complexes, straight lines, and intervals found on an electrocardiogram (EKG) or cardiac monitor tracing.

❷ Understand the normals for each of the waves, complexes, straight lines, and intervals in a cardiac cycle.

❸ List the components necessary for interpreting cardiac rhythms.

❹ Interpret a normal sinus rhythm.

KEY WORDS

Aberrant	Patent ductus arteriosus
Addison's disease	Pathological
Antiarrhythmic	Pathophysiologic
Atrial fibrillation	Pheochromocytoma
Bradycardia	Prinzmetal's angina
Cardiomyopathy	Psychotropic
Complex	R prime
Cushing's syndrome	S prime
Duchenne muscular dystrophy	Sarcoidosis
Ectopic	Segments
Interval	Sick sinus syndrome
Lyme disease	STEMI
Notch	Subarachnoid hemorrhage

Overview

In examining a rhythm strip or EKG tracing, the health care professional must understand the waves, complexes, and straight lines that represent the different aspects of the cardiac cycle on the paper. Every waveform has a distinct name and normals that are particular for each. In the previous chapter, the different leads, or views of the heart, were discussed. Since each of these leads looks at a distinct viewpoint of the heart, the waveforms created on each lead will appear differently. Sometimes these variances in positive or negative deflection and shape are significantly different and sometimes they are minor. For purposes of discussion in this chapter, lead II will be used as a reference point. The letters PQRST are used to denote each of the waves on the EKG tracing. Isoelectric lines are present in between and these lines are known as segments. When two or three waves come together, they form a **complex**. Once a clear understanding of the waves, complexes, and straight lines is achieved, information regarding the components of interpretation of the rhythms will be presented.

It is important to remember that every patient is an individual as well. Sometimes there are anatomical differences that are reflected in various inconsistencies in waveforms. These deviations then may not be indicative of disease processes, but rather simply distinctive variations of normal waveforms.

Waves and Complexes

The P Wave

The P wave is the first element of the EKG waveform. This represents depolarization of the atria. (Repolarization is not seen as it has less strength than depolarization of the ventricles and is therefore hidden in the QRS complex.) The beginning upstroke of this wave corresponds to the right atrial activity and the downstroke denotes left atrial activity. In lead II this is characterized by a positive deflection meaning that the wave will be above the isoelectric line. Depending on which lead is viewing the activity of the atria, the P wave can be clearly defined, smaller than others, or have a biphasic configuration. When the electrical activity moves toward the positive pole, a positive deflection will occur. In general, leads I, II, aVL, aVF, and V_2-V_6 usually have an upward appearing P wave. aVR demonstrates a negative deflection and lead V_1 and III commonly have a biphasic (both directions) appearance, although lead III can be variable. The lead depicted in Fig. 5–1 is from lead II.

The P wave should have a smooth, round appearance. The normal width for a P wave is 0.12 seconds or less or 3 small boxes on the EKG paper. (1 mm on the horizontal plane of the EKG paper is equal to 0.04 seconds.) The normal amplitude or height of a P wave is about 0.5 to 2.5 mm depending on the view. In normal sinus rhythm a P wave should be present before each QRS complex. When the P wave is of normal amplitude and length, is upright in lead II, and precedes each QRS, it can be assumed that the original impulse was initiated by the sino-atrial (SA) node. P waves can also originate from different locations of the atria. The term used to describe these altered pacemaker sites is **ectopic**. This ectopic impulse can come from different parts of the atria or from the atrio-ventricular (AV) junction. Ectopic waveforms may appear as smaller than normal, as a wavy line, or may have a sawtooth pattern. P waves that originate from the AV junction will have negative deflections (be seen below the

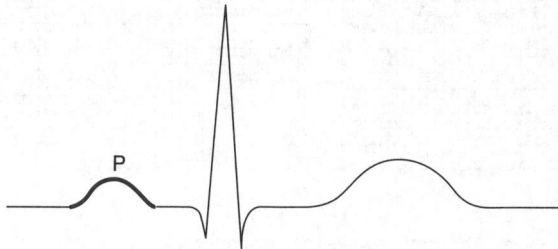

FIGURE 5–1 • The P wave. The P wave is the first deflection noted on the EKG waveform. (*From Huff J, ECG Workout Exercises in Arrhythmia Interpretation, 6e. 2012.*)

isoelectric line) or may appear either after or be hidden within the QRS. When these ectopic P waves occur, certain dysrhythmias, to be discussed later in this book, are created (Fig. 5–2).

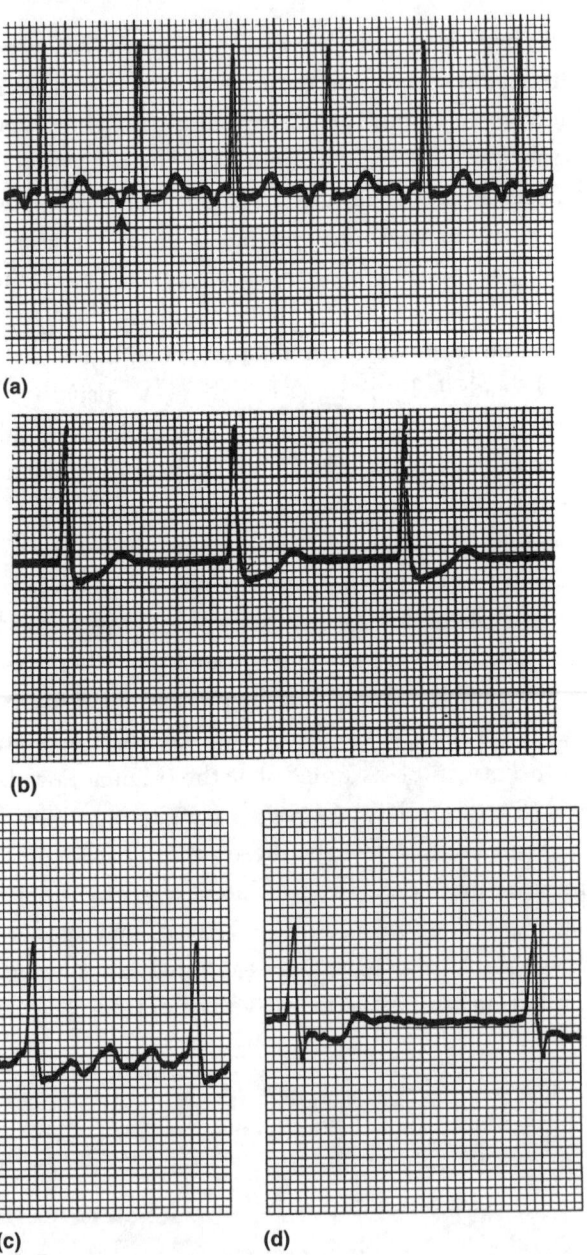

(a)

(b)

(c)   (d)

FIGURE 5–2 • Abnormal P waves. Abnormal P waves can occur for many reasons. (a) Inverted P waves can occur when the impulse is generated from the AV junction. (b) No P waves may be seen when they are most likely embedded within the QRS complex as seen with a junctional rhythm. (c) A sawtooth pattern for the P wave takes place when the atria are beating too fast as in atrial flutter. (d) P waves can appear as only a wavy line in the dysrhythmia atrial fibrillation.

The QRS Complex

When the ventricles depolarize, the QRS complex is generated. It is much larger than the P wave because the ventricles have a much larger muscle mass. Three separate wave deflections comprise this complex known as the QRS. The Q wave and the S wave are smaller negative deflections. The R wave is a larger positive deflection (sometimes called inflection when it is positive) that is present between the Q and S wave. Lead II is again a good view of the QRS complex because the R wave is represented as a strong positive deflection. Other leads in which the R wave is positive are: leads I, III, aVL, aVF, V_4, V_5, and V_6. Negative R waves are seen in leads aVR, V_1, V_2, and V_3 (Fig. 5–3).

There are several different varieties of the QRS complex. The Q wave is always the first negative deflection. The R wave is considered to be the first positive deflection and the S wave is the final negative deflection. Sometimes there is a total QRS complex containing all three deflections and sometimes there is an absence of any one of the components. When looking at this complex, always denoted as the QRS complex, the health care professional may note that it is in reality a QS segment, a QR segment, an RS segment, etc. When

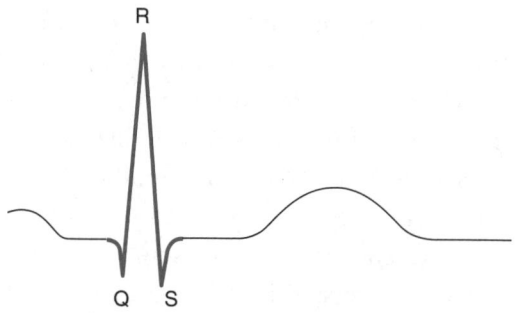

FIGURE 5–3 • The normal QRS complex. The normal QRS has a downward Q, upward R, and downward S wave. Not all QRS complexes have all of these facets. (*From Huff J. ECG Workout Exercises in Arrhythmia Interpretation. 6e. 2012.*)

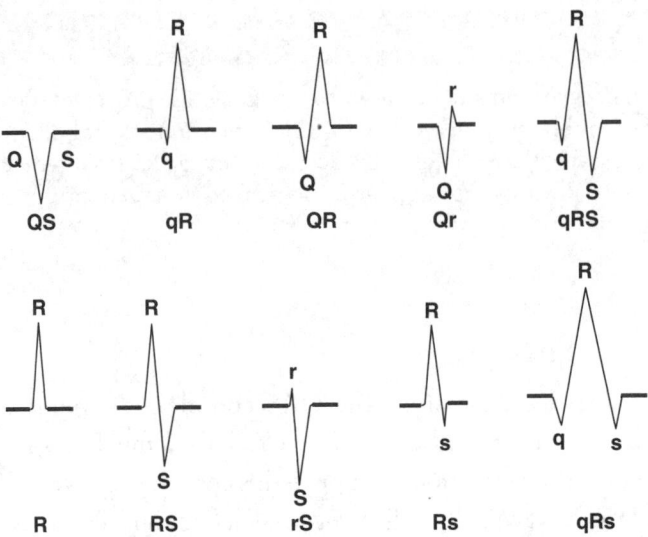

FIGURE 5–4 • **Diverse forms of the QRS complex.** Label each line with either an upper or lower case letter depending on its size. Use lower case if it is under 5 mm in amplitude. Use upper case if it is greater than 5 mm in amplitude. The Q wave is always the first negative deflection. The R wave is always the first positive deflection. The S wave is always the second negative deflection.

one or the other of these waveforms has small amplitude, below 5 mm, then a lower case letter is used to denote it. Those with higher amplitude, greater than 5 mm, are designated with a capital letter. In dealing with this aspect, those segments mentioned above may then become a qs segment, a qR segment, an Rs segment, etc. At times there may only be an R wave present (Fig. 5–4).

Another feature that might be present in the QRS complex is the presence of an extra R or S wave. When this happens, it is called **R prime** or **S prime**. In order to be labeled as R or S prime, the wave must actually touch and cross the baseline (the isoelectric line). If it simply changes directions it is called a "**notch**". R prime is written as R^1 and S prime is written as S^1. Both R and S prime and notching of these waves can be important in diagnosing bundle branch blocks which will be further discussed in Chapter 6 (Fig. 5–5).

Another important aspect of the QRS segment has to do with R wave progression. The R wave should be at its lowest amplitude in V_1 and the largest in V_6. This evolution of the R wave, as it progresses across the chest from right to left, is significant for different diagnostic reasons. One of the most common reasons for poor R-wave progression is the simple misplacement of the chest leads especially leads V_1 and V_2. One of the more common patients for this to occur with is the obese female. There is also a transition point on the EKG

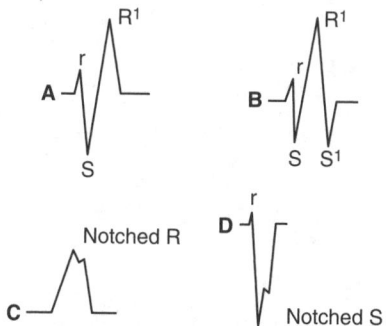

FIGURE 5–5 • **Recognition of R prime (R¹), S prime (S¹), and notched R and S waves.** (A) R prime is written as R¹. (B) S Prime is written as S¹. (C) and (D) Both the R wave and S wave can have notching.

when the R wave begins to become more positive than negative. This usually occurs in either V_3 or V_4. Box 5–1 describes some of the etiologies for poor R-wave progression. Figure 5–6 shows normal progression. Figure 5–7 depicts poor R-wave progression.

The normal duration for the QRS complex is 0.06 to 0.10 seconds. The measurement begins at the Q wave and ends at the end of the S wave. If no Q wave is present, begin the measurement at the beginning of the R wave.

BOX 5–1 Etiologies of Poor R-Wave Progression

- Right bundle branch block
- Left bundle branch block
- Right ventricular hypertrophy
- Left ventricular hypertrophy
- Myocardial infarction
- Pacing rhythm
- Wolff-Parkinson-White Syndrome (WPW)
- Hypertrophic cardiomyopathy
- Muscular dystrophy
- Dextrocardia
- Precordial lead misplacement
- Tension pneumothorax
- Congenital heart disease
- Chronic obstructive pulmonary disease (COPD)(more commonly emphysema)

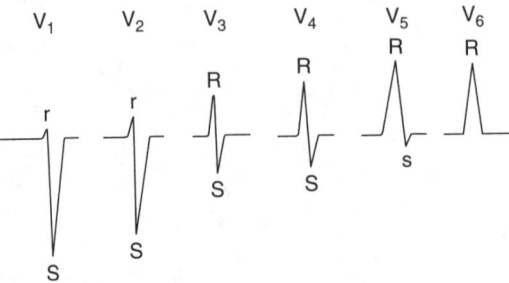

FIGURE 5–6 • **Normal R-wave progression.** The R wave begins as a very small wave in V_1 and progressively enlarges throughout the V leads. The S wave begins as a large deflection in V_1 and progressively disappears in V_6. Note the transition phase in V_3 and V_4.

This measurement is also known as the QRS interval (Fig. 5–8). Widened QRS complexes can suggest delays in ventricular conduction, bundle branch blocks, premature ventricular contractions, and **aberrant** atrial impulses. The absence of a QRS complex could mean ventricular standstill or a conduction block, both requiring emergent intervention. Amplitude or height varies with each lead.

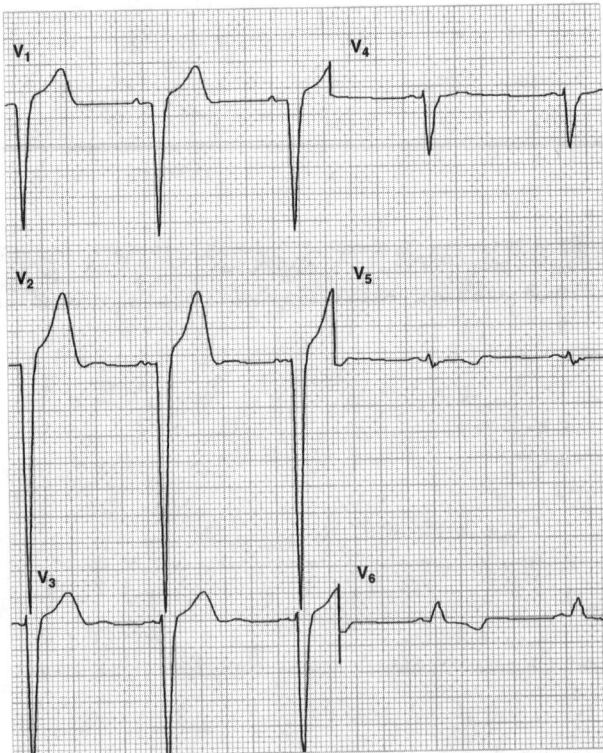

FIGURE 5–7 • **Poor R-wave progression.** This EKG shows poor R wave progression through the V leads.

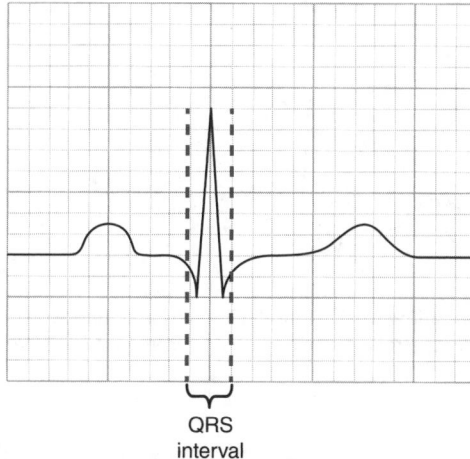

QRS
interval

FIGURE 5–8 • The QRS interval. The QRS interval begins at the initiation of the Q wave and ends at the completion of the S wave. (*Modified from Thaler M The Only EKG Book You'll Ever Need 2010. Wolters Kluwer Lippincott Williams & Wilkins.*)

CLINICAL ALERT

The Q wave carries special significance for a patient experiencing a myocardial infarction. Deep and/or wide Q waves are evidence of infarcted myocardium.

The T Wave

Ventricular repolarization is noted on the EKG as the T wave. The normal T wave is approximately 0.5 mm in height in leads I, II, and III. In the anterior, V_3 and V_4 and lateral views, V_5, and V_6, the amplitude is higher, up to 10 mm. These waves are normally smooth and rounded but are slightly asymmetric as they have an upward slope to the top of the wave and then returns to the baseline or isoelectric line (Fig. 5–9). Remember that the T wave carries the refractory periods and during the relative refractory period stimuli can produce dangerous ventricular dysrhythmias.

Many different processes can cause changes in the T wave. Table 5–1 lists some of these **pathological** diseases. Most of these abnormalities will either have T wave elevation or T wave inversion. Pericarditis, an inflammatory condition of the sac around the heart, actually has both T wave elevation and inversion as patients go through several phases of this disease process. Pericarditis can also cause a notched or pointed T wave configuration.

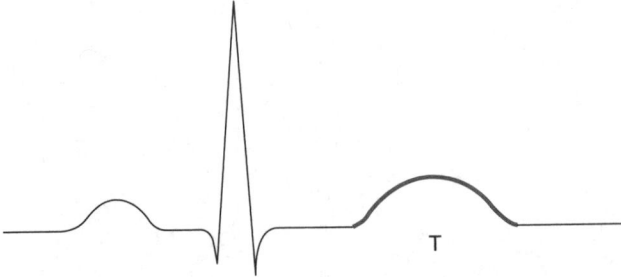

FIGURE 5–9 • **The normal T wave.** The normal T wave has a rounded appearance but is slightly assymetrical with a gradual upstroke at the beginning. (*From Huff J, ECG Workout Exercises in Arrhythmia Interpretation 6e., 2012.*)

TABLE 5–1 Common Etiologies of T Wave Abnormalities	
High or peaked T waves	Hyperkalemia
	Pacemakers
	Myocardial injury
Inverted (depressed) T waves	Myocardial ischemia
	Hypokalemia
	Hypomagnesemia
	Cerebral hemorrhage

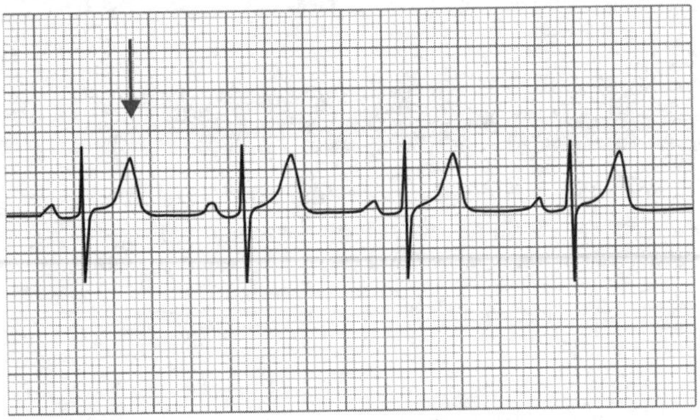

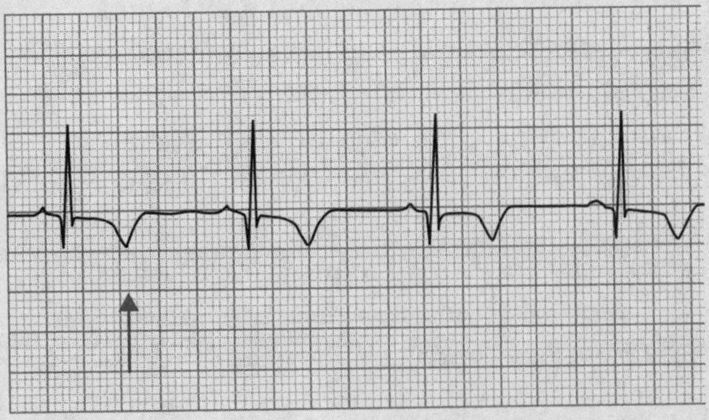

   Normally the T wave will have the same deflection as the prior QRS, that is, if the QRS was positive (above the isoelectric line) the T wave will also run in the positive direction. However, when there is an abnormal ventricular beat or complex, the direction of the T wave will be opposite that of the QRS. This can occur in ventricular dysrhythmias or bundle branch blocks.

> ### CLINICAL ALERT
>
> Patients with significant cerebral bleeding such as that seen with a **subarachnoid hemorrhage** can have "giant" T wave inversion. These are seen as deeply inverted T waves and are also associated with a prolonged QT interval. This pattern can mimic that of an acute myocardial infarction (Fig. 5–10).

The U Wave

The U wave is not always seen and its presence is not necessarily an indicator of disease or wellness. When it is present, it follows the T wave and its background is not totally understood. Theories regarding its origin include

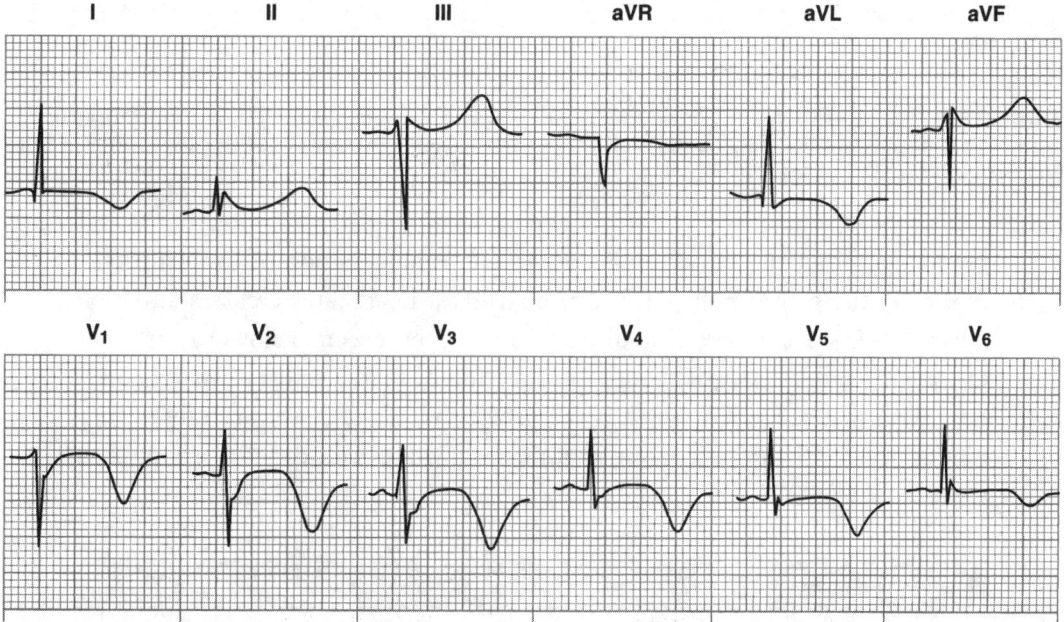

FIGURE 5−10 • T wave changes with cerebral hemorrhage. Giant T wave inversion can be seen with cerebral hemorrhage such as a subarachnoid hemorrhage. QT interval prolongation is also noted. (*From Aehlert, Barbara, ECG's Made Easy 4e. 2011 Mosby JEMS.*)

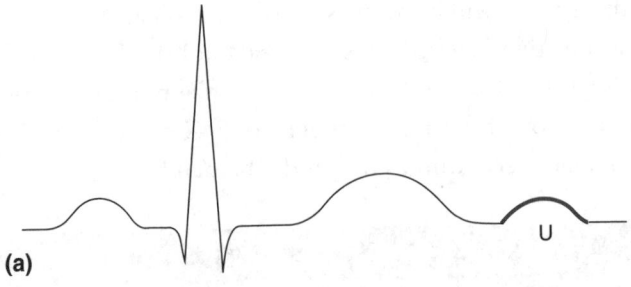

(a)

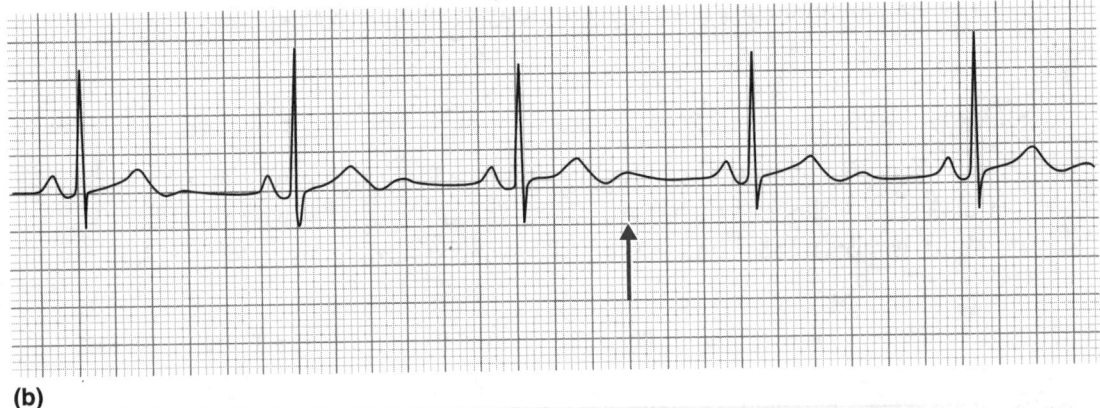

(b)

FIGURE 5−11 • **The U wave.** (a) Location of the U wave. (b) Electrocardiogram with a U wave. Notice that it does look somewhat like a P wave, however, the morphology (shape) is different. (*From Huff J, ECG Workout Exercises in Arrhythmia Interpretation 6e., 2012.*)

repolarization of the Purkinje fibers and late repolarization of the ventricles. Normally these are small (<1.5 mm high). Fast heart rates create a situation where the U wave is very difficult to locate. It is best seen in slower heart rates in leads V_2 and V_3. The deflection or direction of the waveform usually correlates with that of the T wave. It is important to look at these carefully as they may appear to be a P wave. Close examination will reveal a different shape than the P wave (Fig. 5–11).

CLINICAL ALERT

Disorders that can cause tall U waves include: hypokalemia, hypercalcemia, digitalis toxicity, **cardiomyopathy**, left ventricular hypertrophy, certain medications such as procainamide (Pronestyl), quinidine, and amiodarone (Cordarone), hyperthyroidism, central nervous system diseases, and long QT syndrome.

Segments

There are several horizontal straight lines on the EKG tracing. These straight lines are called **segments** and are associated with the wave or complex that precedes it. These segments follow the isoelectric line that is the baseline for the rhythm and represent different periods of time in the cardiac cycle (Fig. 5–12).

- **PR Segment:** The PR segment is the straight line from the end of the P wave to the beginning of the QRS complex. It corresponds to the end of atrial depolarization and the beginning of ventricular depolarization. Atrial repolarization is also taking place during this segment of time. As the impulse conduction is moving through the cells, this denotes its passage through the AV node, the bundle of His, the right and left bundle branches, and the Purkinje fibers. This impulse transmission is too weak to produce discernible voltage and therefore displays as a straight line. A depression of the PR segment can occur with chronic pulmonary issues and ventricular enlargement that can be produced from a chronic excess of pressure being exerted on the ventricular walls. This then creates a thickening of the heart wall known as hypertrophy.

- **ST Segment:** The ST segment begins at the end of the QRS complex and completes at the beginning of the T wave. This "end" of the QRS complex is still named ST whether an S wave is present or not (as stated previously it may end with an R wave). This occurs during the early part of repolarization of each of the ventricles and is usually isoelectric. The J point occurs in this segment and is the point at which the QRS complex itself joins to the ST segment. The J point is important because most people start measuring either depression or elevation of the ST segment at this point. Others may begin the measurement of the segment 0.04 to 0.06 seconds after the J point. Some patients with rapid heart rates or high, peaked T waves that

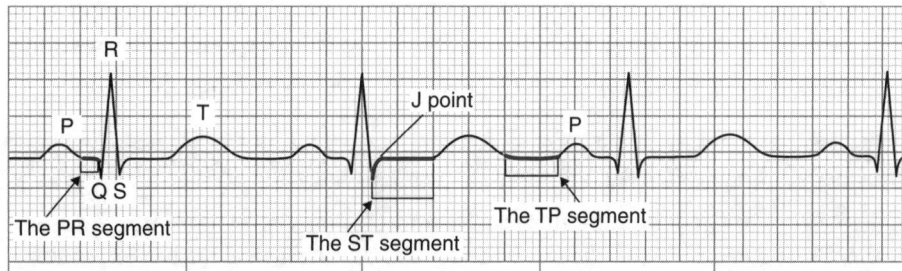

FIGURE 5−12 • **EKG segments.** The PR and the TP segments are used as a guideline to establish the isoelectric line. From this isoelectric line, elevation or depression of the ST segment can be determined.

TABLE 5–2 ST Segment Elevation and Depression

ST segment elevation	
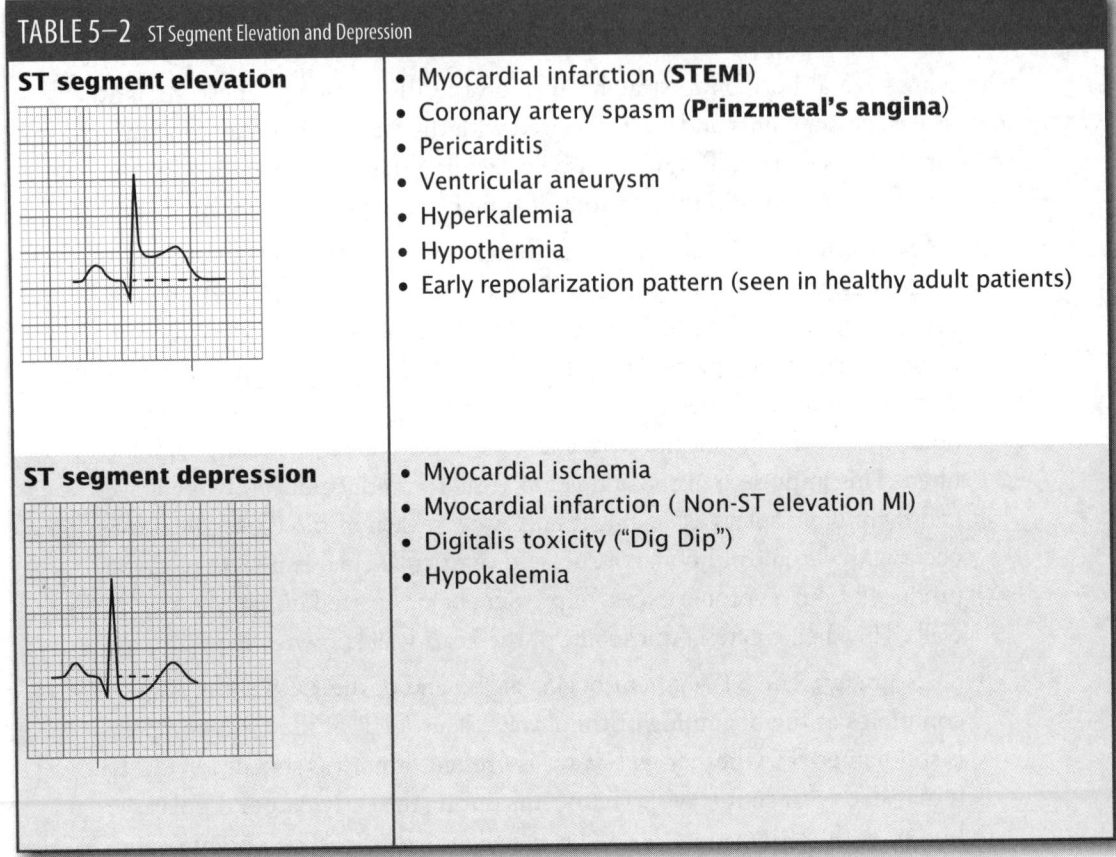	• Myocardial infarction (**STEMI**) • Coronary artery spasm (**Prinzmetal's angina**) • Pericarditis • Ventricular aneurysm • Hyperkalemia • Hypothermia • Early repolarization pattern (seen in healthy adult patients)
ST segment depression	• Myocardial ischemia • Myocardial infarction (Non-ST elevation MI) • Digitalis toxicity ("Dig Dip") • Hypokalemia

may be seen with hyperkalemia do not clearly show the J point. The ST segment is an important factor in determining certain situations. It is of utmost importance in the diagnosis of acute myocardial injury and ischemia. When looking at the ST segment, compare it to the isoelectric line of the PR segment. Table 5–2 shows some of the circumstances that can create either an elevated or depressed ST segment. The ST segment is said to be elevated if it is greater than 1 mm above the isoelectric line. Depression is recognized if it is greater than 0.5 to 1 mm below the isoelectric line.

CLINICAL ALERT

The ST segment is one of the most important pieces of interpretation of the EKG pattern in the diagnosis of an ST elevation myocardial infarction (**STEMI**). It is used in conjunction with laboratory values to determine this diagnosis but, when present in an elevated "coved" type of pattern, is usually considered to be an acute injury pattern in that particular view of the heart. This will be covered in more detail in the chapter on myocardial infarction.

- **TP Segment:** The TP segment begins at the end of the T wave and continues to the beginning of the next cardiac cycle or P wave. This line should be isoelectric and in faster heart rates may be unrecognizable due to the proximity of the T and P waves.

Intervals

An **interval** consists of a combination of a waveform and a segment. Two important intervals exist in the EKG tracing. These are the PR interval and the QT interval.

PR Interval

The PR interval can be abbreviated as PRI. This is measured from the beginning of the P wave to the beginning of the QRS complex and includes the PR segment. The cardiac cycle activity that is represented by the PR interval is that of atrial depolarization to the onset of ventricular depolarization. Normal length for this interval is 0.12 to 0.20 seconds (3-5 small boxes on the EKG graph paper). A fast heart rate can shorten the PR interval.

The PR interval is an important aspect of the EKG. Increases and decreases in the length are associated with cardiac and other **pathophysiologic** abnormalities. Table 5–3 lists several potential reasons for these changes. A shortened PR interval is usually indicative of an impulse generated from an area other than the usual SA node. Conduction defects or delays are characterized by a prolonged PR interval (Fig. 5–13).

CLINICAL ALERT

The pediatric patient is unique in that the PR interval is very short at birth (0.07-0.14 seconds) and reaches a more normal "adult" length by the age of 12 to 16 years (0.09-0.18 seconds). The shorter interval is due to the faster heart rate and the smaller size of the ventricles.

QT Interval

The QT interval starts at the beginning of the QRS complex and ends at the conclusion of the T wave. This is representative of activity within the ventricles inclusive of both ventricular depolarization and repolarization. (The T wave is wider than the QRS indicating that more time is spent in repolarization than depolarization.) Remember that there are times when a Q wave is not

TABLE 5-3 PR Interval Abnormalities

Long PRI	• Use of beta-blocker medications
	• Use of calcium channel blocker medications
	• Atrioventricular blocks
	• Hyperthyroidism
	• Digitalis toxicity
	• Rheumatic heart disease
	• **Lyme disease**
	• Hypothermia
	• **Sarcoidosis**
	• Hypokalemia
	• Septal defects
	• **Patent ductus arteriosus**
	• **Addison's disease**
	• **Sick Sinus Syndrome**
Short PRI	• Wolff-Parkinson-White syndrome
	• **Duchenne muscular dystrophy**
	• Type II glycogen storage disease
	• Junctional dysrhythmias
	• **Pheochromocytoma**
	• **Cushing's syndrome**
	• Adrenalin toxicity
	• Cardiomyopathy

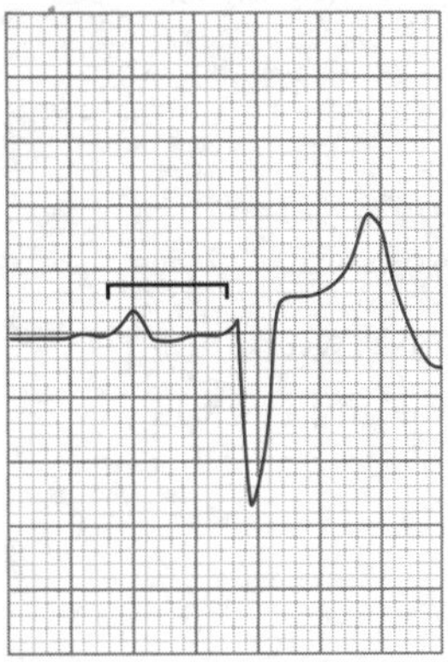

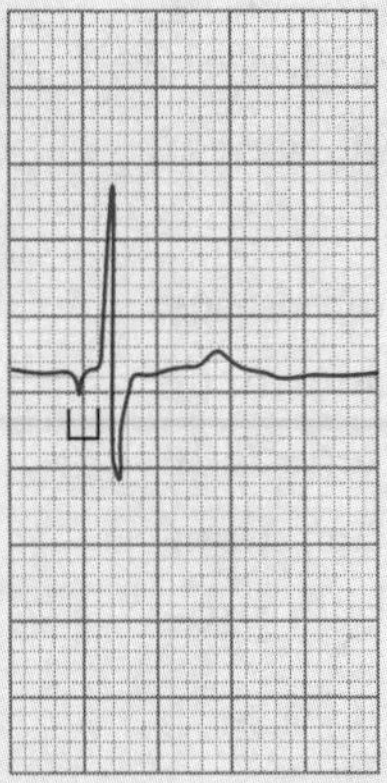

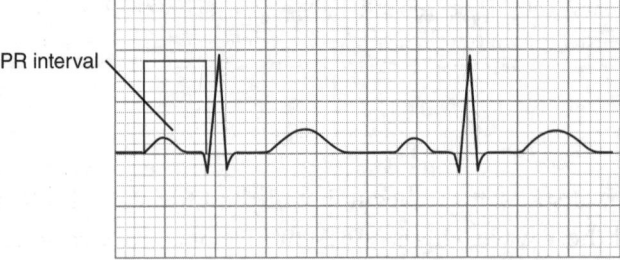

FIGURE 5-13 • **PR interval (PRI).** This PR interval measures 0.24 seconds in length. (0.04 × 6 small squares)

present and this complex begins with an R wave. This measurement is still titled "QT Interval", whether it actually begins with a Q wave or not. This interval is normally less than half of the length of the time from one QRS complex to the next. If it is purely one half the length of the R-R interval, time between one QRS and the next QRS, it is considered to be "borderline". If it is greater than half the of the R-R interval, then it is considered to be prolonged. To measure in this way, the rhythm must be regular, meaning that the same number of boxes between QRS complexes is present consistently. It usually varies between 0.36 to 0.44 seconds. Various factors can impact the QT interval such as age, heart rate, and gender. Slower heart rates will prolong the QT interval. Other causes for a shortened QT interval are digitalis toxicity and hypercalcemia. A prolonged QT interval impacts the relative refractory period which is the vulnerable phase of ventricular repolarization. When it is longer than normal, it can permit an ectopic impulse to seize control of conduction (Fig. 5–14).

CLINICAL ALERT

A prolonged QT interval places patients at risk for a life-threatening dysrhythmia known as torsades de pointes, a type of ventricular tachycardia. Many different situations can cause this increased threat including: hypokalemia, hypocalcemia, hypothermia, **bradycardia**, myocardial ischemia, some **antiarrhythmic** medications, certain antidepressants, specific **psychotropic** medications, particular antibiotics and antimigraine medications, some antinausea agents, genetic factors (hereditary long QT syndrome), and liquid protein diets.

R-R intervals and P-P intervals (measured in the same way as R-R intervals) can be used to establish rate and regularity versus irregularity in rhythms. Regular rhythms will demonstrate the same length between R waves throughout

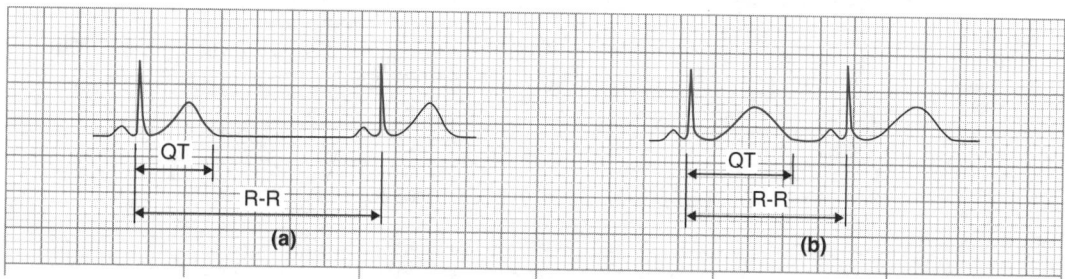

FIGURE 5–14 • QT interval as it compares with R-R interval. (a) Normal QT interval. QT measures 0.44 seconds (0.04 × 11 small boxes), R-R measures 1.4 seconds (0.04 × 35 small boxes). The QT interval is less than half of the R-R interval. (b) Prolonged QT interval. QT measures 0.60 seconds (0.04 × 15 small boxes), R-R measures 0.92 seconds (0.04 × 23 small boxes). The QT interval is greater than half the R-R interval. (*From Aehlert, Barbara, ECG's Made Easy 4e. 2011 Mosby JEMS.*)

the rhythm strip. Atrial regularity can be determined in the same way utilizing the P-P interval.

The Whole Picture

Each piece of the EKG tracing has been discussed. Figure 5–15 is a visual representation of the each of the components of the cardiac cycle as depicted on the EKG strip. This is an important picture to understand as the health care professional begins the process of analyzing and understanding rhythm strips.

Systematic Interpretation

Interpretation of rhythm strips takes time and experience. Each health care professional who works with EKGs will develop his or her own method. It is important to utilize a systematic approach which will then serve as a guideline when reading each patient's particular rhythm. Normal sinus rhythm will be the most common rhythm encountered, but of course there are many abnormal rhythms as well. Understanding normal sinus rhythm will help to identify the aberrant rhythms. With a strong base upon which to build, the individual attempting to interpret rhythms will be successful in accuracy so that correct interventions can be initiated and evaluated. Each of the waves, complexes,

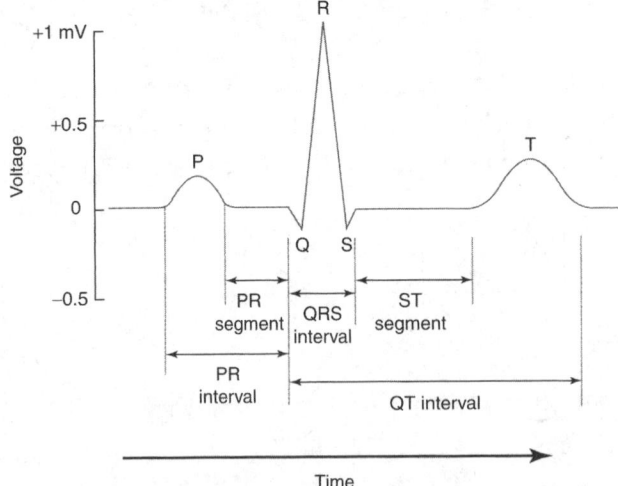

FIGURE 5–15 • The whole picture. All waves, complexes, straight lines, and intervals are labeled in a typical electrocardiogram tracing of one heart beat or cardiac cycle. (*Modified with permission form Mohrman DE, Heller LJ: Cardiovascular Physiology, 6th ed. New York: Lange Medical Books/ McGarw-Hill, 2006.*)

straight lines, and intervals that have been discussed now come together to create a "rhythm". When reading or interpreting rhythms, a 6-second strip is utilized (30 large boxes = 6 seconds). Markings should be present on either the top or bottom of the EKG paper that denotes either 1 or 3 seconds in length to assist with rapid calculations and rhythm analysis.

Verify Regularity

Several methods can be utilized to verify regularity of the rhythm. Basically this is a confirmation of the R-R and P-P intervals as described previously. The same number of small or large squares between each R wave and P wave should be present. This can be accomplished by counting these squares, but other methods can be used to make this easier.

The first technique is to utilize a pair of calipers to measure between two R waves. Calipers have two points that can be pulled apart or pushed closer together determined by the heart rate on a 6-second strip. Choose two R waves and measure that distance with the calipers. Then, without adjusting the calipers, rotate the calipers from the second R wave to the third R wave. The point of the calipers should land on the tip of the third R wave. Walk the calipers across the entire 6-second strip to determine that each R wave is exactly the same distance apart. If the rhythm is regular, they will match all the way across the EKG tracing. If it is irregular, the points will change and it will become apparent that the R waves are not an equal distance apart across the entire strip (Fig. 5–16).

The second technique is to use an index card or a small piece of paper. Hold it against the rhythm and place a mark for each of two R waves. Then use the card or paper in the same fashion as the calipers, checking for distance between each R wave across the entire 6-second strip. Each R wave should fall on a mark on the paper or card with each subsequent R wave then matching up with the

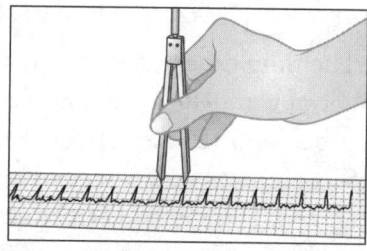

FIGURE 5–16 • **Use of calipers to determine rhythm regularity.** Calipers can help to determine regularity of rhythms. (*From ECG Interpretation Made Incredibly Easy. 5e. 2011 Wolters Kluwer Lippincott Williams & Wilkins.*)

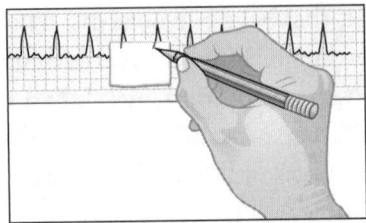

FIGURE 5–17 • Use of index card/paper to determine rhythm regularity. The paper method is another way to determine regularity of rhythms. (*From ECG Interpretation Made Incredibly Easy. 5e. 2011 Wolters Kluwer Lippincott Williams & Wilkins.*)

next mark placed prior from the first two R waves measured. Again, if each R wave matches the marks on the paper across the strip, the rhythm is considered to be regular (Fig. 5–17).

This same procedure can be used to determine atrial regularity by using the P to P intervals as a guide.

CLINICAL ALERT

When assessing for regularity of rhythms, a variance of 0.04 seconds can be considered normal. If the variance is less than 0.16 seconds, the term "essentially regular" may be used. This might happen if ectopic beats are episodically present. If the difference is greater than 0.16 seconds, the rhythm is deemed irregular. Irregular rhythms are then divided into "regularly irregular" and "irregularly irregular". Regularly irregular rhythms might occur if the patient is experiencing ectopic beats at regular intervals. Irregularly irregular rhythms may arise when there is no pattern to the irregularity, such as with **atrial fibrillation**.

Count the Rate

The next step in interpretation of rhythms is to determine the heart rate. This can be accomplished using several different methods. Each of these methods will work with either R waves (ventricular rate) or P waves (atrial rate) (Fig. 5–18).

- **Counting R waves:** The simplest and fastest way to count heart rate is to determine the number of complete QRS complexes (some professionals prefer to use the number of QRS intervals) on a 6-second strip. Multiply the number of QRS complexes in a 6-second strip by 10 to obtain an estimation of the heart rate. This method can be employed for rate calculations for either regular or irregular rhythms. It is most commonly used for irregular rhythms since the other methods can create difficulty in accuracy with irregular rhythms.

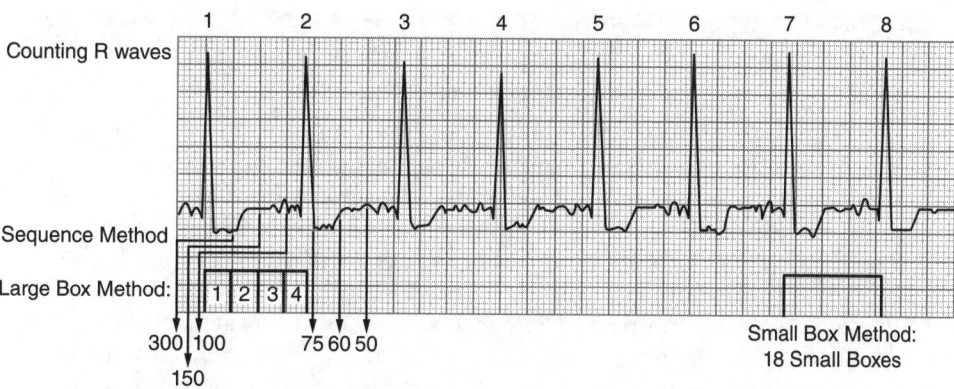

FIGURE 5–18 • **Counting heart rate.** The three main methods of counting heart rate are: Counting R waves — the rate in this 6-second strip is 80 (10 × 8 counted QRS complexes). Large Box Method — the rate will be 75 (300 divided by 4). Small Box Method — the rate will be 84 (1500 divided by 18). Sequence Method — From the first QRS complex on a heavy line (the first QRS in this strip) the next QRS complex comes closest to the heavy line numbered "75". This is the estimated rate.

- **Large box method:** A more accurate way to determine rate is to count the number of large boxes between two R waves that fall closest to a heavy line denoting a large box and then divide that number into 300. So, if there are 5 large boxes in between two R waves, 300 divided by 5 equals a heart rate of 60. If the rhythm is deemed irregular, this method can still be used, but a range is used. Measure the number of large boxes between two of the most distant R waves and the number between two of the closest R waves. That might provide a rate of "60 to 80" beats per minute. Commercial tables are available that have these numbers configured on them for quick reference.

- **Small box method:** In this method, count the number of small boxes between two R waves and divide into 1500. One small box is equal to 0.04 seconds which would then be equal to 1 minute of time per 1500 small squares. If the number of small squares between the R waves is 15, 1500 divided by 15 shows a heart rate of 100 beats per minute. This is a precise measurement and is best used for regular rhythms; however, rate ranges could also be applied to this method.

- **Sequence method:** When utilizing the sequence method, find an R wave (or P wave if atrial rate is desired) that occurs on a heavy black line on the graph paper. Then label the next six heavy black lines with a number from the following sequence starting with the largest number first— 300, 150, 100, 75, 60, 50. The rate is then estimated by finding the point at which the next R wave (or P wave) falls and determining where it lies in relation to the marked dark lines.

Check the P Wave

The next step is to determine that each QRS complex is preceded by a P wave. These P waves should look similar and correlate to the normal parameters for the P wave. Clearly distinguishable upright P waves come from the SA node (depending on the view from the heart). P waves that are absent or inverted in leads that should show positive P waves, means that the conduction probably started in the AV junction.

Establish the PR Interval

Make sure that the PR interval is within normal range. Count the number of small squares that comprise the PR interval and multiply that by 0.04. The PR interval should fall between 0.12 to 0.20 seconds. If the PR interval is not consistent, check for a pattern of inconsistency. Heart blocks are determined by clarifying PR interval changes.

Evaluate the QRS Complex

Measure the duration of the QRS complexes to determine that they are within the normal range of 0.06 to 0.10 seconds. Also check the configuration of these complexes. Make sure they are the same across the 6-second strip.

Assess the QT Interval

Utilize the small squares as a basis to measure the QT interval. It should fall within the normal range of 0.36 to 0.44 seconds. This can be difficult to perform with fast heart rates. Also, remember that, in general, if it is less than half of the R-R interval, it is considered to be normal. A corrected QT interval can be accomplished using a formula based on a heart rate of 60. This is known as the QTc.

Consider the T Wave

Check the T wave for configuration and size. If the QRS and the T wave are in opposite directions, it is most likely an ectopic beat. Another consideration with the T wave includes inversion of the T wave which can signify ischemia to the area of the heart which the lead is viewing. Hyperkalemia (high potassium) can be seen in high peaked T waves.

Notice the ST Segment

The ST segment should be analyzed for either elevation or depression. The normal ST segment should be on the same line as the PR and TP segment. If it is above or below this line, it can carry significance for a potential acute myocardial infarction.

CLINICAL ALERT

Senior members of the patient population may have normal changes to these aspects of EKG tracings. Prolonged PR, widened QRS, and lengthened QT intervals can be normal variances for this age group.

Normal Sinus Rhythm

The most common rhythm to be assessed is Normal Sinus Rhythm, abbreviated NSR. This indicates a heart rhythm that originated in the SA node and traveled correctly through the heart (SA node → atria → AV node → Bundle of His → Bundle Branches → Purkinje Fibers). Every other rhythm is compared to NSR. Remember that sometimes the underlying rhythm is NSR with ectopic beats or short bursts of other rhythms entering the picture.

Normal sinus rhythm will have the following distinctive characteristics: (Fig. 5–19)

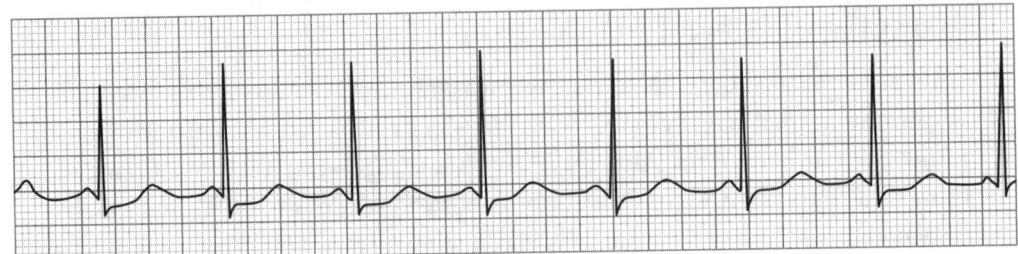

FIGURE 5–19 • Normal sinus rhythm.

- Both atrial and ventricular rates are regular.
- Rate will be between 60 and 100 beats per minute (rates greater than 100 beats per minute are named tachycardias and rates less than 60 beats per minute are called bradycardias).
- A normal P wave precedes each QRS.
- PR interval is within normal limits.
- QRS complexes are normal in configuration and width.
- QT interval is within normal limits.
- T wave is normal in configuration.
- ST segment lies on the isoelectric line.
- No ectopic beats are present.

Conclusion

Understanding the different parameters of the electrocardiograph or cardiac monitor strip is essential in caring for patients. Cardiac abnormalities must be discovered and attended to in order to maintain optimal health for those who are entrusted to health care professionals. In order to recognize abnormalities, normals must be comprehended. A standard systematic method of interpretation will assist the health care provider in assessing rhythm strips easily and quickly, especially when an emergent or urgent situation arises. Key points of this chapter include:

- Each waveform, segment, interval, and complex has its own identifying characteristics and normals.
- The letters PQRST are used to denote each waveform.
- Isoelectric lines are known as segments.

- A grouping of waveforms is a complex.
- The P wave is the first waveform and is representative of the depolarization of the atria.
- A P wave is normal if it is above the isoelectric line (positive deflection) in lead II.
- P waves can have a biphasic configuration.
- Some leads will normally have a negative or biphasic P wave.
- Normal width for a P wave is 0.12 seconds or less.
- One small square on the EKG graph paper is equal to 0.04 seconds in width and height.
- An ectopic P wave is one which originates from another source other than the SA node.
- Some disease processes can cause abnormalities to occur with the P wave.
- Ventricular depolarization is noted on the EKG tracing in the QRS complex.
- Not all QRS complexes have a Q, R, and S wave.
- The R wave is always a positive deflection. The Q and S waves are negative deflections.
- An R or S prime is the presence of an extra R or S wave. This is written as R^1 or S^1.
- A notched R wave is different than an R prime. This happens when the R wave simply changes directions and does not come back to the isoelectric line before the second R wave occurs.
- R wave progression should occur with the lowest amplitude in V_1 and the highest amplitude in V_6.
- Normal duration for a QRS complex is 0.06 to 0.10 seconds.
- A widened QRS may be indicative of delays in ventricular conduction, bundle branch blocks, premature ventricular contractions, or aberrant atrial impulses.
- Deep or wide Q waves can be indicative of a myocardial infarction.
- The normal T wave is positive in lead II.
- The refractory periods occur during the T wave.
- Many disease processes can cause abnormal T waves.
- The T wave should normally have the same deflection as the QRS.

- Patients who are experiencing a subarachnoid hemorrhage may have "giant" T wave inversion.

- A U wave may or may not be present.

- Tall U waves can be caused by a variety of disease processes and medications.

- Segments include the PR segment, the ST segment, and the TP segment.

- The ST segment is very important as a diagnostic tool with myocardial infarction.

- The PR interval (PRI) is important in the diagnosis of conduction defects or delays.

- The normal length for a PR interval is 0.12 to 0.20 seconds.

- Both shortened and prolonged PR intervals are important in certain disease processes.

- The QT interval normal length is between 0.36 to 0.44 seconds.

- The QT interval should be less than the R-R interval to be normal.

- Heart rate can impact the QT interval.

- A prolonged QT interval can influence the relative refractory period and cause a life threatening dysrhythmia known as torsades de pointes, a type of ventricular tachycardia.

- When interpreting an EKG rhythm, it is best to have a systematic way to perform this.

- The steps in interpretation of an EKG rhythm include: verification of regularity, counting the rate, checking the P wave, establishing the PR interval, evaluating the QRS complex, assessing the QT interval, considering the T wave, and noticing the ST segment.

- There are two ways to verify regularity—the use of calipers or the use of a file card or piece of paper.

- There are four ways to count the rate—counting R waves, the large box method, the small box method, and the sequence method.

- Every QRS should have a P wave to be normal.

- The most common rhythm to identify is normal sinus rhythm and is the benchmark to which all other rhythms are evaluated.

PRACTICE QUESTIONS

1. **Which of the following represents depolarization of the atria?**
   A. P wave
   B. Q wave
   C. R wave
   D. T wave

2. **The P wave in lead II will have which of the following characteristics?**
   A. Negative deflection
   B. Isoelectric
   C. Positive deflection
   D. Horizontal

3. **The QRS complex is indicative of:**
   A. repolarization of the atria.
   B. depolarization of the ventricles.
   C. depolarization of the atria.
   D. repolarization of the ventricles.

4. **Which of the following is a true statement regarding the QRS complex?**
   A. The QRS complex will always have a Q wave, an R wave, and an S wave.
   B. The QRS complex normal duration is 0.24 seconds.
   C. The QRS complex will show a negative deflection in lead II.
   D. The QRS complex may actually be only a qs complex.

5. **For an R wave to have an R^1, it must have which of the following characteristics?**
   A. The second R wave must cross the isoelectric line.
   B. The second R wave will have a notch in it.
   C. The first R wave will simply change directions.
   D. The first R wave will be shorter than expected.

6. **Poor R wave progression may be caused by:**
   A. transposition of the limb leads.
   B. hyperkalemia.
   C. cerebral hemorrhage.
   D. precordial lead misplacement.

7. **High peaked T waves will most likely be seen in:**

   A. hyperkalemia.
   B. myocardial ischemia.
   C. verebral hemorrhage.
   D. hypomagnesemia.

8. **Deeply inverted T waves may be present with which of the following processes?**

   A. Subarachnoid hemorrhage
   B. Hyperkalemia
   C. Myocardial injury
   D. Sick sinus syndrome

9. **The point at which the QRS complex meets the ST segment is known as the:**

   A. U point
   B. J point
   C. A point
   D. Z point

10. **The ST segment is crucial in the diagnosis of:**

    A. sick sinus syndrome.
    B. premature ventricular contractions.
    C. myocardial infarction.
    D. lyme disease.

11. **The normal parameter for the PR interval is:**

    A. 0.06-0.10 seconds.
    B. 0.12-0.20 seconds.
    C. 0.28-0.32 seconds.
    D. 0.36-0.44 seconds.

12. **Which of the following patients would normally have a very short PR interval?**

    A. 84-year-old male
    B. 36-year-old female
    C. 18-year-old male
    D. 1-month-old female

13. **A prolonged QT interval places a patient at risk for which of the following life-threatening dysrhythmias?**

    A. Third-degree AV block
    B. Torsades de pointes
    C. Ventricular standstill
    D. Asystole

14. Which of the following pieces of equipment would be useful in determining regularity of a heart rhythm?

A. Magnifying glass

B. Fine point tweezers

C. Calipers

D. Scissors

15. A patient has nine QRS complexes on a 6-second rhythm strip. Which of the following would be the correct estimated heart rate?

A. 60 beats per minute

B. 75 beats per minute

C. 90 beats per minute

D. 100 beats per minute

16. A patient has 22 small boxes in between two QRS complexes. Which of the following would be the correct heart rate?

A. 13 beats per minute

B. 60 beats per minute

C. 68 beats per minute

D. 76 beats per minute

17. In order for the QT interval to be considered normal it should be:

A. greater than half the R-R interval.

B. equal to the R-R interval.

C. less than half the R-R interval.

D. has nothing to do with the R-R interval.

18. Which of the following would be correctly identified in a normal sinus rhythm?

A. P wave follows each QRS complex

B. PR interval is 0.18 seconds

C. ST segment is above the isoelectric line

D. QRS width is 0.24 seconds

ANSWER KEY

1. **A.** Depolarization of the atria is reflected in the P wave. The QRS shows depolarization of the ventricles and the T wave represents repolarization of the ventricles.

2. **C.** Lead II is the best lead to clearly see the PQRST deflections. The P wave in this lead is positive or above the isoelectric line.

3. **B.** Depolarization of the ventricles is shown in the QRS complex. Repolarization of the atria is lost in the QRS complex because depolarization of the ventricles is

stronger than the atrial repolarization. The P wave represents atrial depolarization and the T wave reflects the repolarization of the ventricles.

4. **D.** The QRS complex is unique in that it does not always have each component. Many variations occur. The qs complex means that the R wave is not present and the Q and S waves have negative deflections which are denoted with lower case lettering. The normal QRS duration is 0.6 to 0.10 seconds. The QRS should show a positive deflection in lead II.

5. **A.** An R prime, written as R^1, must cross the isoelectric line in order for it to be considered to be an R prime. If it simply changes directions, and looks like a notch on top of the R wave, it is called "notched".

6. **D.** R wave progression is seen in V_1 through V_6. Therefore, the precordial leads must be placed correctly in order to see good R wave progression.

7. **A.** Hyperkalemia, high potassium, is often associated with high peaked T waves. Myocardial ischemia, cerebral hemorrhage, and hypomagnesemia would be noted to have depressed T waves.

8. **A.** A subarachnoid hemorrhage may have deeply inverted T waves known as "giant" T wave inversion. Hyperkalemia would have high peaked T waves. Myocardial injury would be represented by elevated ST segments. Sick sinus syndrome would have a prolonged PR interval.

9. **B.** The point at which the QRS complex joins to the ST segment is known as the J point.

10. **C.** The ST segment is routinely used to look for both elevation and depression in association with an acute myocardial infarction. The P wave and PR interval would provide information about sick sinus syndrome. The ST segment would not be crucial in the diagnosis of a premature ventricular contraction. Lyme disease can cause a prolonged PR interval.

11. **B.** Normal length of time in seconds for the PR interval is 0.12 to 0.20. This would be represented on the EKG graph paper as 3 to 5 small squares.

12. **D.** The infant normally has a short PR interval. It gradually lengthens until it reaches normal adult dimensions by the age of 12 to 16 years.

13. **B.** Torsades de pointes is a life threatening form of ventricular tachycardia that can occur if the QT interval is prolonged. A prolonged QT interval would not impact an AV block, ventricular standstill, or asystole.

14. **C.** Calipers or a piece of paper or index card can be used to help with determining regularity of heart rhythm.

15. **C.** To estimate heart rate from a 6-second strip, count the number of R waves in 6 seconds and multiply by 10.

16. **C.** To obtain an accurate heart rate, count the number of small boxes in between two R waves and divide that number into 1500. 1500 divided by 22 equals 68. When large boxes are used to count between the R waves, the number to use is 300.

17. **C.** The QT interval should be less than half the length of the R-R interval to be considered normal.

18. **B.** Normal sinus rhythm should have a normal PR interval as demonstrated by the PR interval in this question of 0.18 seconds in length. P waves should precede the QRS complexes. The ST segment should remain on the isoelectric line and normal QRS width would be 0.6 to 0.10 seconds.

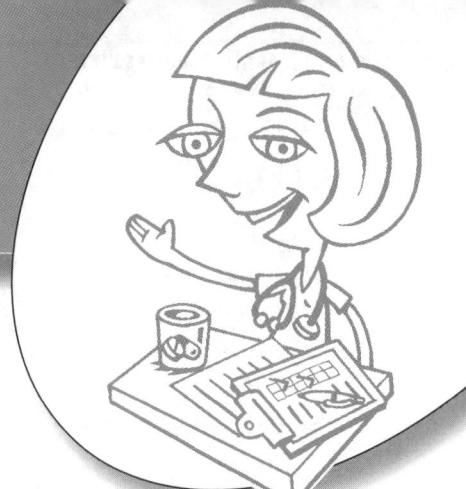

chapter 6

Axis, Hypertrophy, and Bundle Branch Blocks

LEARNING OBJECTIVES

At the end of this chapter, the student will be able to:

1 Define normal axis.

2 Understand the difference between right and left axis deviation.

3 Distinguish between hypertrophy and enlargement.

4 Identify left and right atrial enlargement and left and right ventricular hypertrophy on a 12-lead EKG.

5 Understand bundle branch blocks (BBB) and the clinical implications associated with BBB and hemiblocks.

Overview

Axis is a term that is used to help the health care professional glean a greater amount of information from the 12-lead EKG. Determining whether a patient has a normal axis or not can help to diagnose increases in muscle mass of the left ventricle (**hypertrophy**), dilation (enlargement) of chambers, proper diagnosis of wide QRS tachycardias, hemiblocks, identification of accessory pathways, and myocardial infarctions (MI). The identification of bundle branch blocks (BBB) can also assist the health care provider in the correct analysis of certain conditions for the patient.

Normal Axis

The term axis takes into consideration the vectors that illustrate the direction of depolarization of the ventricles. A vector is, in essence, an arrow that shows the direction of the electrical current. It also depicts the strength of the impulse that is traveling. In the normal heart, the greatest amount of current is headed downward and to the left in the direction of the left ventricle because it is thicker and larger. The sum or average of all the vectors that are occurring simultaneously as the impulse travels through the heart muscle is called the **mean vector**. The vectors originate in the AV node so vectors are always drawn from the site of the AV node as the beginning point of the arrow (Fig. 6–1).

The **mean electrical axis** is then the direction that the mean vector is taking when it is looked at from a perspective of a circle of degrees in the frontal plane (Fig. 6–2). This is known as the hexaxial reference system and is derived from Einthoven's Triangle described in Chapter 4. A circle representing 360° surrounds the heart. It is then divided into four segments. The upper segments are negative degrees and the bottom portion carries positive degrees.

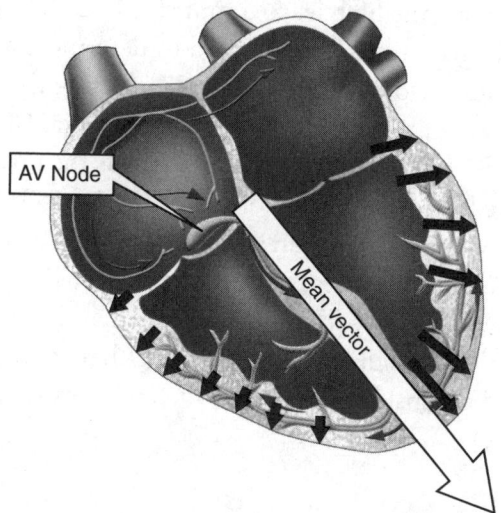

FIGURE 6–1 • **Mean vector.** The Mean Vector is the sum of all simultaneously occurring vectors in the ventricles.

The mean electrical axis is important in that it demonstrates whether or not ventricular depolarization is occurring in a normal fashion. Normally the mean electrical axis should fall within the scope of 0° to +90°. (Some cardiologists may recognize the scope of the mean electrical axis to extend up to −30°.) By determining the axis, abnormalities can be recognized.

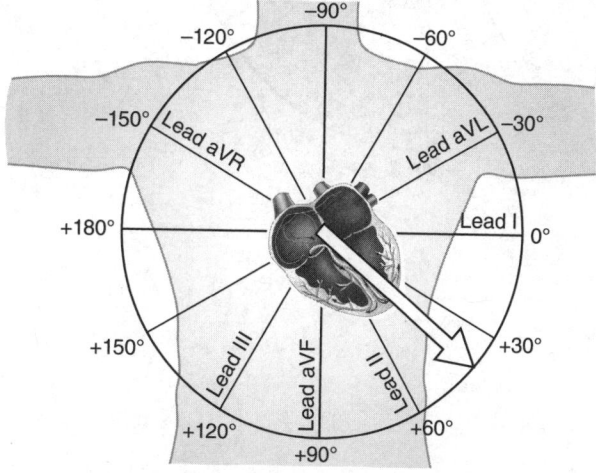

FIGURE 6–2 • **Mean electrical axis.** The mean electrical axis is the mean vector when described in degrees on the frontal plane. The mean electrical axis in this figure is about +40°.

The frontal planes are the limb leads comprising leads I, II, III, aVR, aVF, and aVL. The two leads that are commonly used to determine axis deviations are leads I and aVF. These two leads are perpendicular to each other with lead I lying at 0° on the plane and aVF lying at +90° on the hexaxial reference system. Lead I's positive electrode is on the left arm. aVF has the positive electrode on the left "foot" or the left lower portion of the body (Fig. 6–3). The most powerful period of time within the depolarization process is illustrated by the tip of the R wave, thus the mean electrical axis is noted through the R wave. Positive R wave deflections in these two leads will indicate that the axis is normal. (This is a simplified manner of reading axis deviation. Other aspects of the complete 12-lead EKG can be considered which will render exact measurements of degrees of variance.)

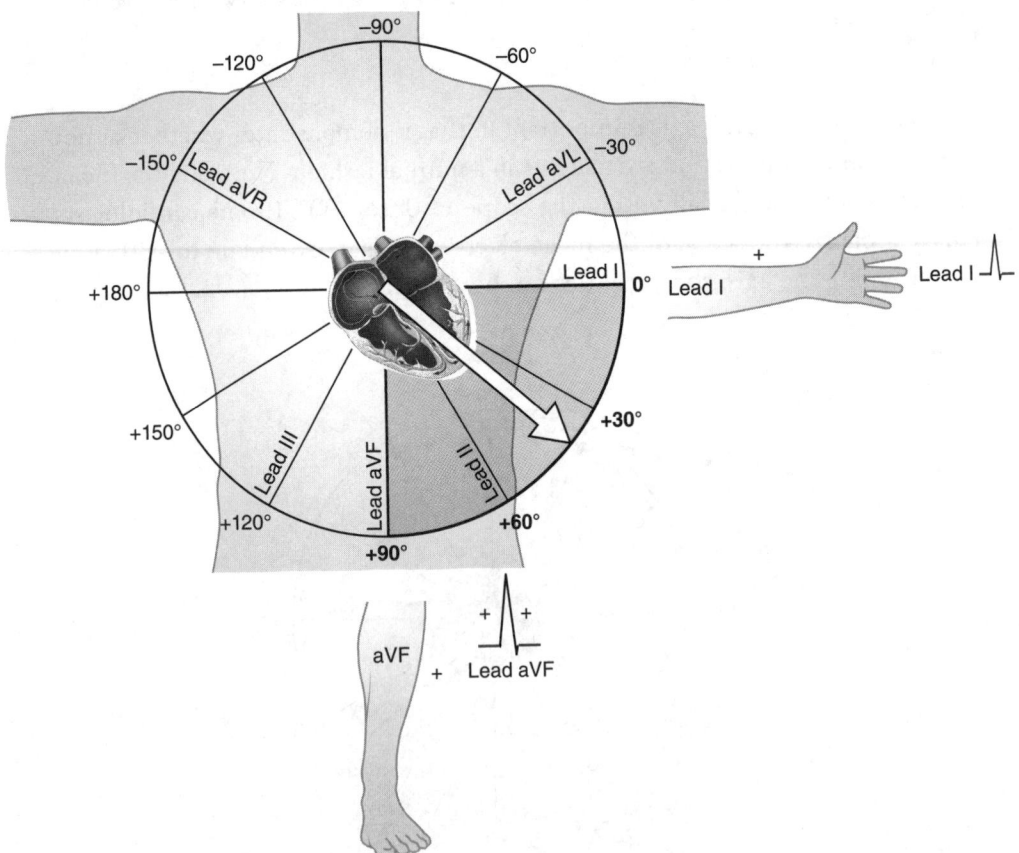

FIGURE 6–3 • Leads I and aVF on the hexaxial reference system. The positive electrode records positive deflections on Leads I and aVF in a normal axis.

> **CLINICAL ALERT**
>
> Axis deviation can be important in helping to diagnose a variety of conditions as well as hypertrophy of the ventricles and an actual **infarction** of the heart. In general, the mean vector will point toward hypertrophy and away from the infarcted portion of the heart wall.

Right Axis Deviation

Right axis deviation (RAD) is signified when lead I displays a negative QRS complex and aVF continues to show a positive QRS complex. This shows that the mean vector is pointing in the direction +90° to +180° (Fig. 6–4).

> **CLINICAL ALERT**
>
> RAD may be normal for some patients who are tall and slender. Their heart can actually be displaced vertically causing this variation. Also RAD would be present (along with decreasing R wave progression in the chest leads V_1-V_6) in patients with **dextrocardia** where the heart is in the right side of the chest. In this situation a right-sided EKG would produce a normal axis and proper R wave progression across the chest leads.

Extreme Right Axis Deviation

Extreme RAD is said to occur when both lead I and aVF have negative QRS deflections. This would be represented on the hexaxial reference system in the range of +180° to −90° (Fig. 6–5). This is exactly opposite of the normal conduction through the heart muscle and is considered to be a rare occurrence. It is also known as "indeterminate."

Left Axis Deviation

Left axis deviation can be noted when lead I shows a positive deflection and lead aVF is now negative. This corresponds to −90° to 0° on the hexaxial reference system (Fig. 6–6). This can be normal in older individuals or those who are obese. The heart in obese patients can become more horizontally placed due to pressure from the diaphragm pushing upward and shifting it in this more level or horizontal position.

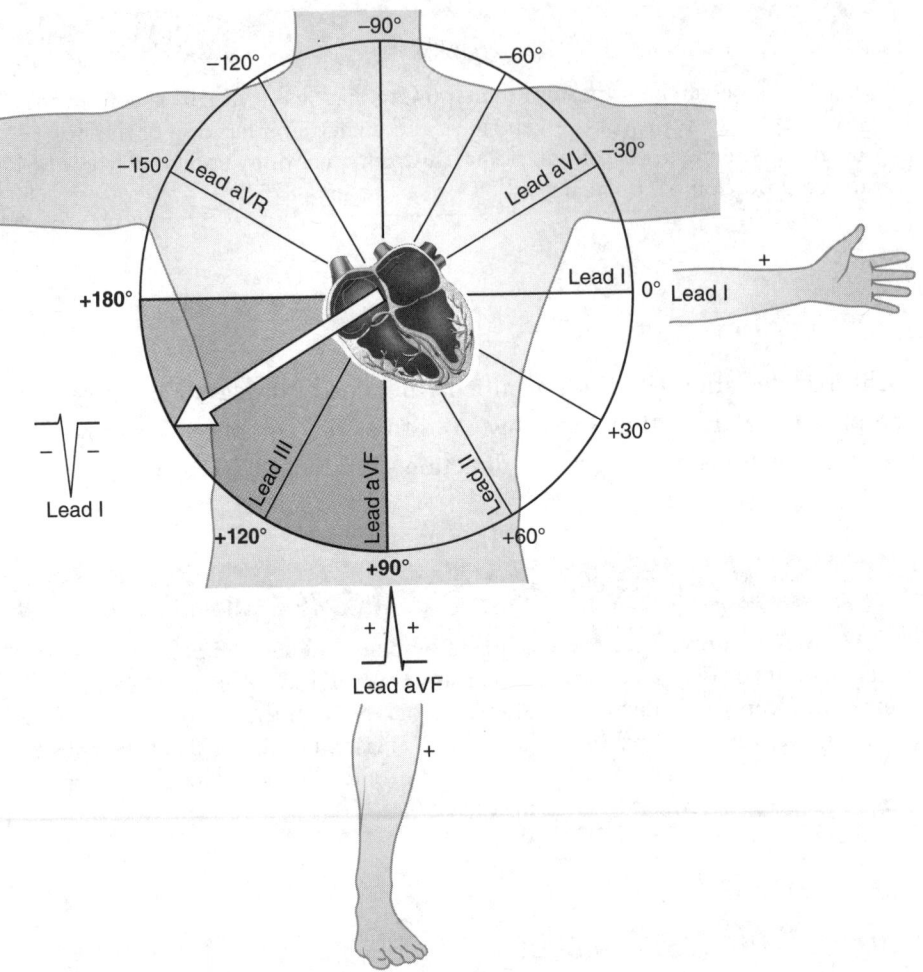

FIGURE 6–4 • Right axis deviation. In right axis deviation, the QRS in lead I will have a negative deflection and lead aVF will remain as a positive deflection.

Table 6–1 shows the changes that occur in the leads and some of the etiologies for each of the axis deviations.

Hypertrophy and Enlargement

Hypertrophy and enlargement of the chambers of the heart are two somewhat synonymous words. However, there is a difference between the two and they very often exist simultaneously.

- *Enlargement* reflects an expansion or dilation of a chamber. This can be caused by situations such as volume overload where the chamber has

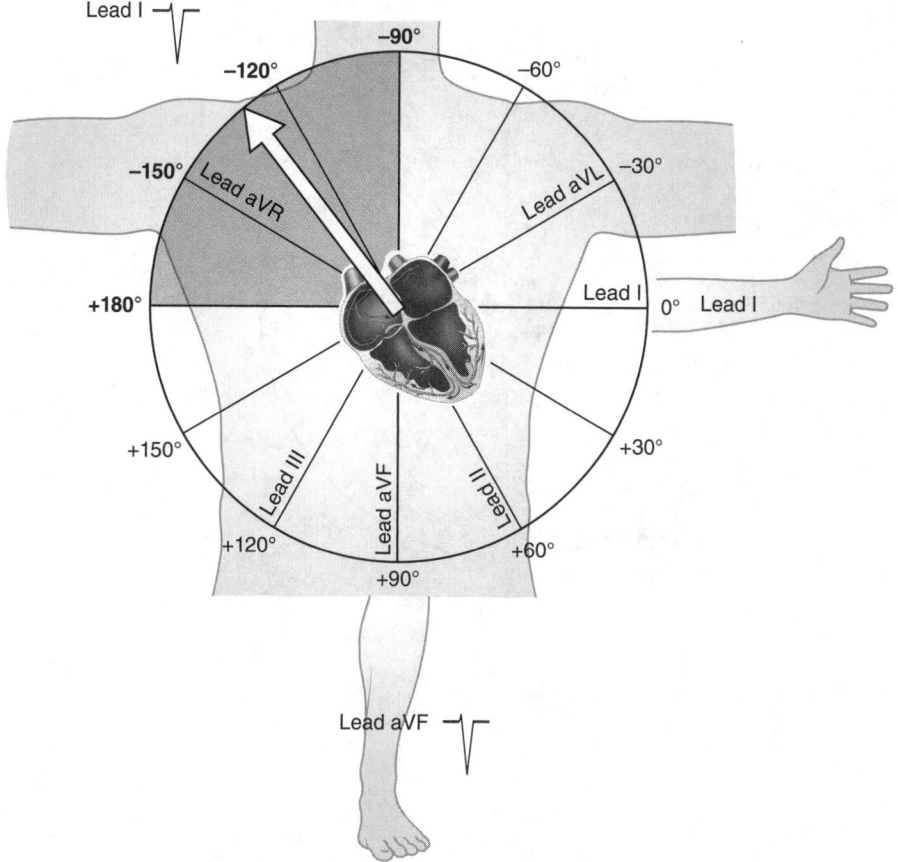

FIGURE 6–5 • **Extreme right axis deviation.** In extreme right axis deviation, both leads I and aVF will have negative QRS deflections.

stretched to accommodate the extra volume of blood. This can also be an acute or chronic situation. Aortic insufficiency could cause left ventricular enlargement as it sits at the point where blood should be expelled into the aorta and therefore, causes an overload of blood volume in the left ventricle. Another potential area of enlargement would be in the left atrium due to mitral valve problems as the diseased valve does not allow good emptying of the left atrium into the left ventricle.

- *Hypertrophy* relates to muscle mass itself. This is caused by an increase in pressure rather than volume. As the heart attempts to work against increased pressures that can be caused by hypertension or aortic stenosis, the muscle gains mass and becomes thicker. This makes the wall of the ventricle stronger and more powerful.

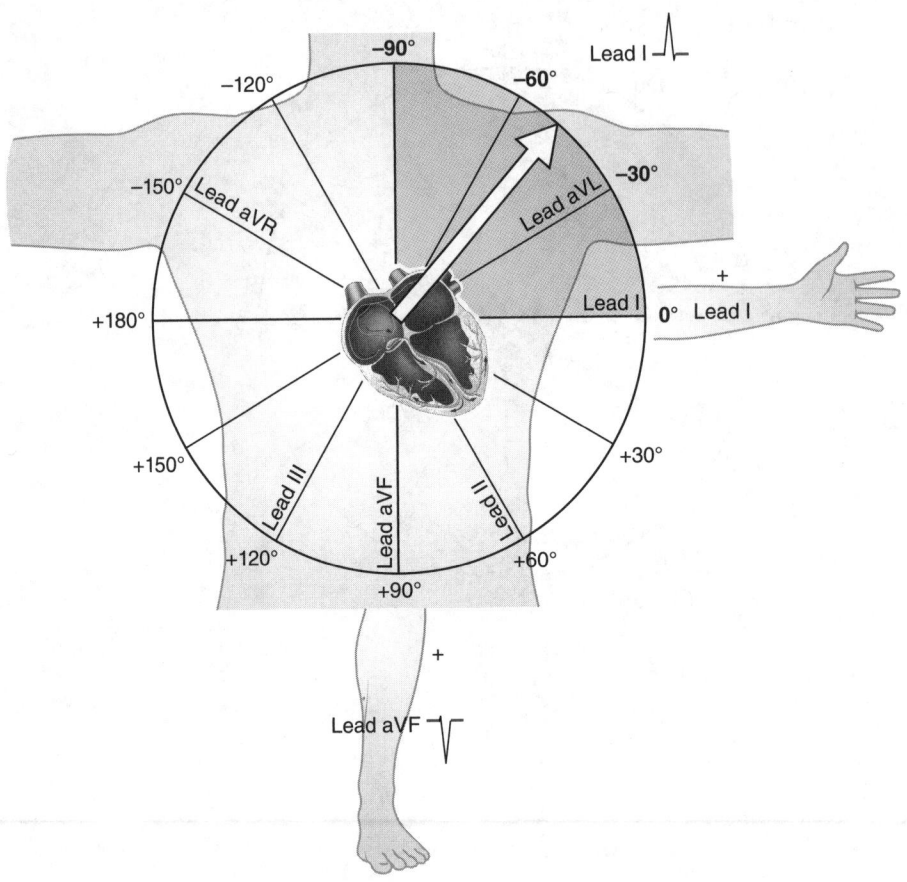

FIGURE 6−6 • Left axis deviation. Left axis deviation will show a positive deflection in lead I and negative deflection in aVF.

The 12-lead EKG can provide clues to these changes in chamber walls. In general, the term enlargement is utilized when the atria are examined and the term hypertrophy is used to designate ventricular changes. The P wave is an expression of atrial activity. Consequently, changes are noted in this waveform for atrial enlargement. The QRS complex correlates to ventricular activity and is therefore used to seek information regarding ventricular hypertrophy.

Atrial Enlargement

Atrial enlargement is seen through increased amplitude of the P wave. In order to visualize this amplitude correctly, it is important that calibration of the machine is checked. 1 mV should be equal to 10 mm (10 small squares) in height. As stated in previous chapters, the P wave should be less than

TABLE 6–1 Axis Deviations			
Axis	Lead I	Lead aVF	Causes
Normal	Positive	Positive	-----------
Right axis deviation	Negative	Positive	• Emphysema • Loss of electrical conduction in left ventricle (acute myocardial infarction) • Wolff-Parkinson-White (WPW) syndrome • **Pulmonary embolism** • Normal variant in thin individuals • Right atrial enlargement • Congenital heart defects • Lateral myocardial infarction • Tricyclic overdose • Right ventricular hypertrophy • Right bundle branch block • Ventricular ectopic rhythms • Dextrocardia
Extreme right axis deviation	Negative	Negative	• Potential incorrect lead placement • Electrolyte disturbances • Cardiomyopathies • Ventricular ectopic rhythms
Left axis deviation	Positive	Negative	• Pregnancy (high diaphragm) • Older adult • **Ascites** • Abdominal distention (tumors/obesity) • Hyperkalemia • Left atrial enlargement • Emphysema • Inferior myocardial infarction • Left bundle branch block • Left ventricular hypertrophy • Ectopic ventricular rhythms • Pacemaker

0.12 seconds in duration and the amplitude should be 2.5 mm or less. The best leads to determine atrial enlargement are leads II, III, aVF, and V_1.

Right atrial enlargement is seen in the upswing of the P wave since this is the portion of the P wave that represents right atrial contraction. This initial portion of the P wave will be tall and peaked. The duration of the P wave does not change because the latter portion of the P wave signifies left atrial activity,

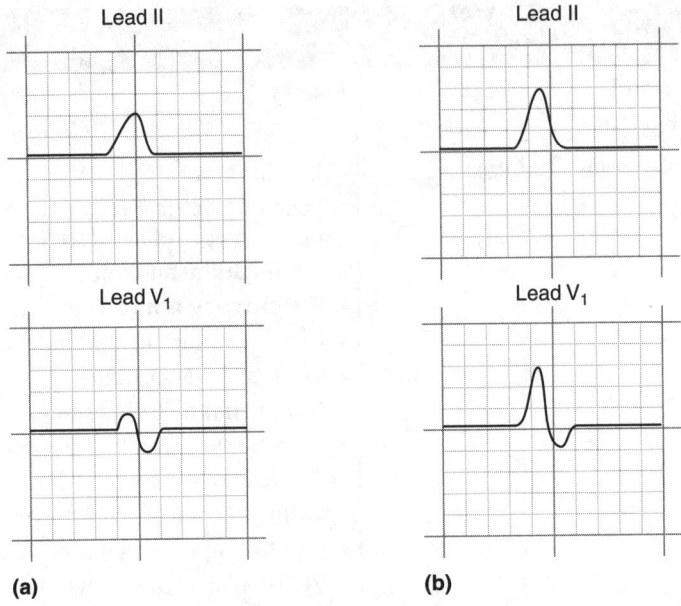

FIGURE 6−7 • **Right atrial enlargement.** (a) Normal P wave configurations in leads II and V$_1$. (b) P wave changes as seen in right atrial enlargement in leads II and V$_1$. Lead II has increased amplitude and is peaked. Lead V$_1$ shows a biphasic P wave with the largest component of this wave being first demonstrating enlargement of the right atrium. (*Modified From Thaler, M, The Only EKG Book You'll Ever Need 6e. 2010.*)

which is unchanged. This type of P wave is also known as **P pulmonale** because of etiologies of the enlargement which originate from pulmonary problems such as chronic obstructive pulmonary disease, pulmonary hypertension, congenital heart diseases, or failure of the right ventricle. The P wave in V$_1$ will be biphasic with the largest portion being the first component of the waveform. This can indicate right atrial hypertrophy or increase in muscle mass as well if it is enlarged and peaked. The other aspect that can be noted in right atrial enlargement is that of axis deviation of the P wave to the right. It may extend beyond +90°. When this happens, the P waves with greatest amplitude will be seen in leads III and aVF (Figs. 6–7 and 6–8).

Left atrial enlargement will be exhibited by prominence in the final portion of the P wave which is indicative of activity of the left atrium. In V$_1$ the second portion of the biphasic P wave will be deep and extend at least 1 mm past the isoelectric line. In this situation, the P wave is widened, as opposed to right atrial enlargement. The enlarged left atrium requires more time to depolarize and is greater than 0.12 seconds in width. Notching of the P wave is seen in leads I, II, aVL, V$_4$, V$_5$, and V$_6$. Causes of left atrial enlargement include mitral stenosis, hypertension, failure of the left ventricle, and mitral regurgitation.

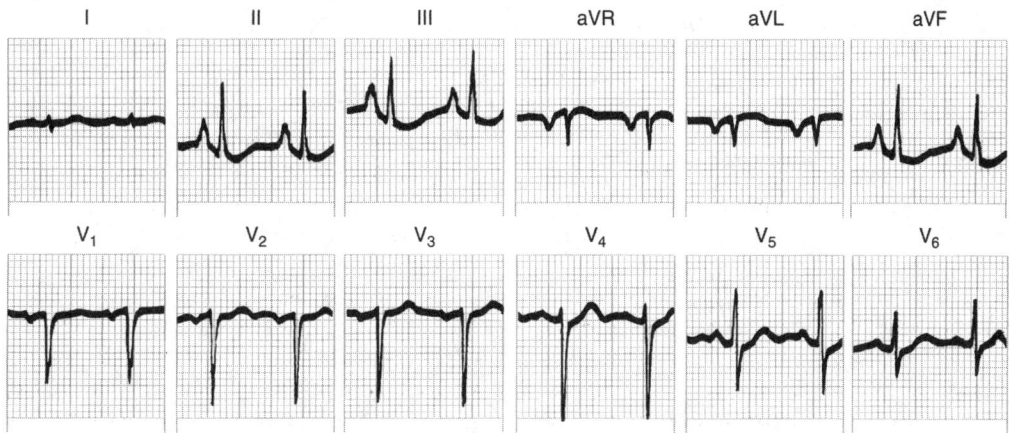

FIGURE 6–8 • Right atrial enlargement on EKG. Note the P pulmonale pattern with the high peaked P waves in leads II, III, and aVF. (*Modified from Aehlert, B ECG's Made Easy 4e., Mosby JEMS, 2011.*)

The notched P wave that can be seen with left atrial enlargement is also known by the term **P mitrale**. There is usually no axis deviation associated with left atrial enlargement (Fig. 6–9).

> **CLINICAL ALERT**
>
> Always correlate the P wave abnormalities with patient history and clinical assessment. Some EKG changes are normal for the patient and may simply be a sign of a nonspecific conduction irregularity.

Ventricular Hypertrophy

The ventricles can become both hypertrophied as demonstrated by an increase in the muscle mass due to an increase in the pressure and enlarged from a continuous volume surplus. The term used with the ventricles is usually hypertrophy. The QRS complex provides information about the work of the ventricles and is therefore impacted when ventricular hypertrophy occurs. The changes in the QRS have to do with amplitude and axis deviation.

> **CLINICAL ALERT**
>
> The QRS can exhibit changes due to factors other than hypertrophy. Lung disease, age, and weight can also create these changes. Very thin and/or young adult patients may have increased QRS amplitude simply because the chest leads are geographically closer to the heart.

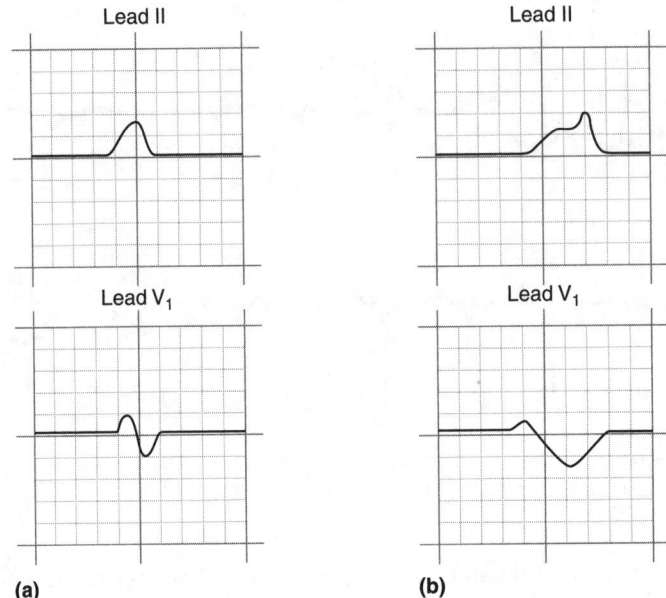

FIGURE 6–9 • Left atrial enlargement. (a) Normal P waves in leads II and V₁ (b) Increased duration of the P wave is seen in lead II. The amplitude of the negative portion of the biphasic P wave in lead V₁ falls below the isoelectric line by at least 1 mm. (*From Thaler, M, The Only EKG Book You'll Ever Need 6e. 2010.*)

Right Ventricular Hypertrophy (RVH) is noted on the 12-lead EKG through right axis deviation. Usually the left ventricle is the stronger of the two and carries the axis. When the right ventricle increases in size, it can then become more prominent and the left ventricle becomes subservient. The normal axis should be between 0° and +90° and will now demonstrate a deviation toward the right, between +90° and +180°. Lead I will become more negative and lead V_1 will have a much larger R wave than usual. The normal R wave progression will also reverse. V_1 lies over the right ventricle and it will now take the lead in R wave height rather than the left ventricle (leads V_5 and V_6). R waves will be larger in leads V_1 and V_2 and smaller in leads V_5 and V_6. The S waves also reverse being smaller in V_1 and larger in V_6. Etiologies of right ventricular hypertrophy are chronic pulmonary disease processes such as chronic obstructive pulmonary disease (COPD), pulmonary hypertension, valvular problems, and congenital heart disorders. When the right ventricle is performing its duty of delivering blood to the pulmonary circulation, anything (such as pulmonary hypertension) that causes it to pump against a strong resistance can become an etiology for hypertrophy in the right ventricle (Fig. 6–10).

Left Ventricular Hypertrophy (LVH) is a more difficult diagnosis to make on EKG tracings because the left ventricle normally predominates. At times the

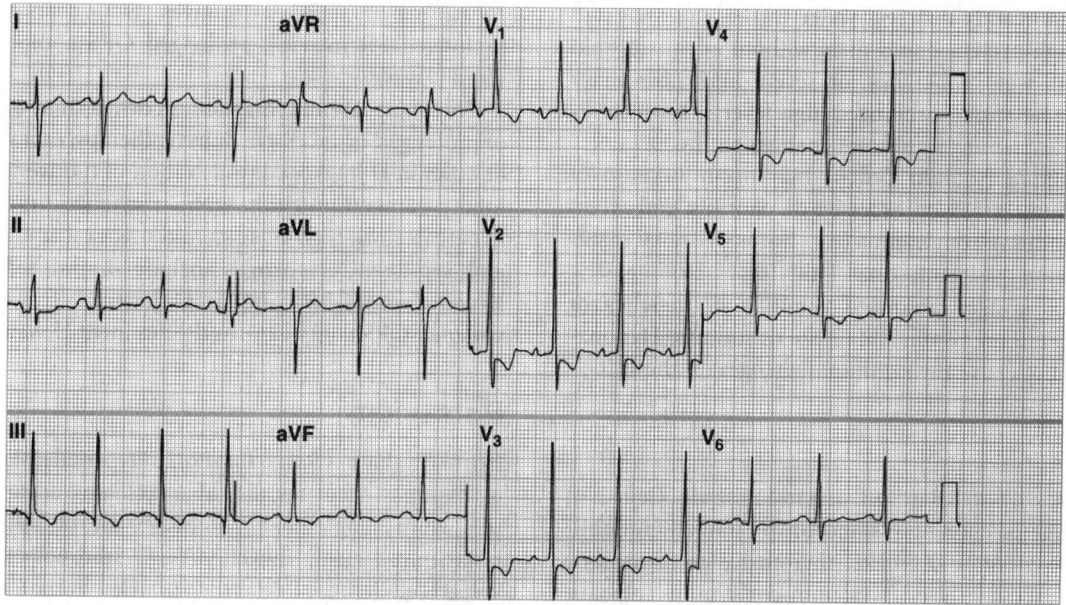

FIGURE 6-10 • **Right ventricular hypertrophy.** Right axis deviation is seen in this EKG tracing. Note the prominent R waves in lead V_1 and the loss of normal R wave progression. Lead I shows a more negative QRS than normal.

axis will deviate beyond −15°. Changes in the chest leads that might be present include

- Large S wave in V_1
- Large R wave in V_6 (greater than 18 mm)
- Large R wave in V_5 (greater than 26 mm)
- Combined amplitude of S wave in V_1 or V_2 and R wave in V_5 or V_6 is equal to greater than 35 mm in height
- R wave height in V_6 is greater than that in V_5

When assessing for left ventricular hypertrophy, the more of the above criteria that are met, the greater the chance that it is actually present (Fig. 6–11). Limb lead changes can also occur, though the chest lead changes are more common. In the limb leads, the R wave will be greater than 13 mm in lead aVL, 21 mm in aVF, and 14 mm in lead I. Also the R wave in lead I and S wave in lead III combined will surpass 25 mm. Etiologies for left ventricular hypertrophy include systemic hypertension, valvular disease processes, cardiomyopathies, and aortic insufficiency and stenosis. When looking at the possible causes, consider the anatomy and physiology of the heart. The left ventricle is responsible for delivering blood to the systemic circulation; therefore, if something is

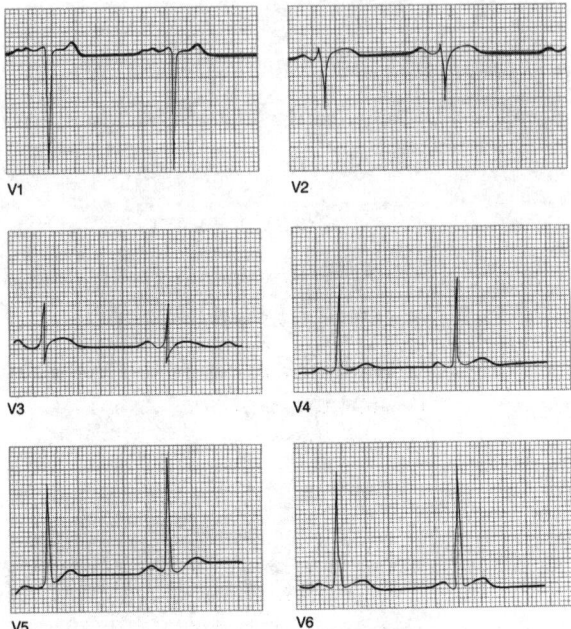

FIGURE 6–11 • Left ventricular hypertrophy. Left ventricular hypertrophy is best seen in the chest (precordial) leads. Note the large S wave in V_1. The R wave in V_6 is greater than 18 mm. The combined amplitude of the S wave in V_1 and R wave in V_6 is greater than 35 mm. The R wave in V_5 is large but is not greater than 26 mm. (*From Thaler, M, The Only EKG Book You'll Ever Need 6e. 2010.*)

causing the left ventricle to exert more pressure in order to deliver, such as systemic hypertension, it can cause hypertrophy.

> ## CLINICAL ALERT
>
> Both ventricles can possess hypertrophy. When this happens, changes for left ventricular hypertrophy would be present in the chest leads as well as RAD in the limb leads.

Another feature that might present on the EKG related to right and left ventricular hypertrophy is strain. This is also known as secondary repolarization abnormality. The T wave will have a gradual dipping or downstroke and a quick upswing on the return to the isoelectric line. The T wave then demonstrates both inversion and asymmetry. This can also be seen with a depressed ST segment that is also "humped." Right ventricular strain would obviously be present in the initial chest (V) leads, V_1 and V_2, while left ventricular strain would be manifested in leads V_5 and V_6 (Fig. 6–12).

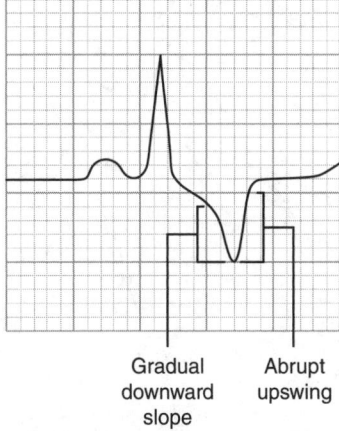

Gradual   Abrupt
downward   upswing
slope

FIGURE 6–12 • **Strain or secondary repolarization abnormality.** Both inversion and asymmetry are seen in ventricular strain or secondary repolarization abnormality. The upward slope has an abrupt upswing. The downward portion is gradual. (*Modified from Thaler, M, The Only EKG Book You'll Ever Need 6e. 2010.*)

Bundle Branch Blocks

When normal conduction is present, the electrical impulse travels from the AV node to the bundle of His into the bundle branches. As the current sweeps through the ventricles, contraction of the ventricles occurs and the QRS complex is created. This happens extremely quickly producing the narrow complex that is less than 0.10 seconds in width. The left ventricle is dominant due to the larger mass of this ventricle as opposed to the right ventricle, thus presenting the normal leftward axis of 0° to +90°. When a **bundle branch block** occurs, these normalities change (Fig. 6–13).

In normal conduction both ventricles are depolarized at the same time. When either of these branches is blocked, the conduction will be normal for the branch that was spared. The branch that is blocked will have a conduction pause as it comes around the blocked area and then proceeds normally again once it is past the block. Depolarization of the unblocked branch is then more rapid than that of the blocked branch. This asynchronous depolarization creates a widened QRS (greater than 0.10 seconds or 2 1/2 small squares) and two QRS complexes in one. This creates the R^1 (R prime) type of complex discussed in Chapter 5. R^1 is produced by the ventricle that has delayed depolarization. The QRS width will be at least 0.12 seconds or 3 small squares. The limb leads are the best leads to interpret this variance in width. If the measurement is 0.10 to 0.12 seconds, it is called an incomplete bundle branch block. Therefore, the $R-R^1$ may be

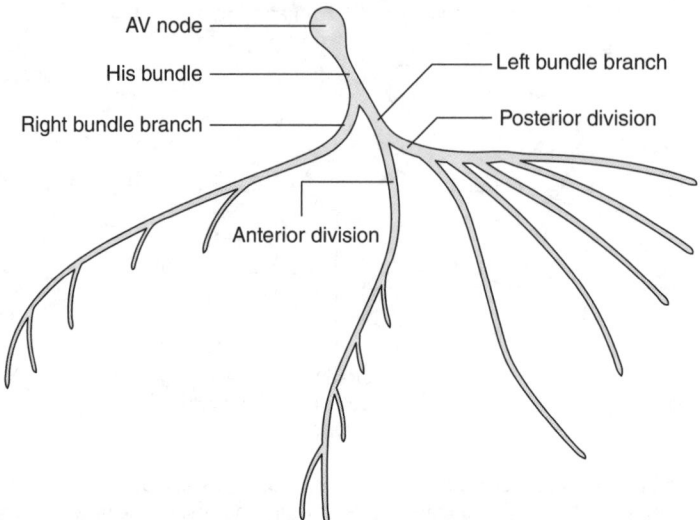

FIGURE 6-13 • Normal bundle branches. The right and left bundle branches divide after the Bundle of His. The left bundle branch has two major subdivisions known as the anterior and posterior divisions or fascicles. (*From Dubin, D. Rapid Interpretation of EKG's 6e. 2000.*)

present but the width is not greater than 0.12 seconds (incomplete BBB). Greater than 0.12 seconds will generate the term complete bundle branch block. The chest leads will provide better information regarding the R-R[1].

> **CLINICAL ALERT**
>
> If a patient has a bundle branch block (BBB) with tachycardia that is derived from an area above the ventricles (supraventricular), the complexes can be very wide and can be misdiagnosed as ventricular tachycardia. Treatment is different for each of these rhythms.

Right Bundle Branch Block

In right bundle branch block, the left ventricle depolarizes normally. Therefore, this first depolarization is the "R" and constitutes the activity of the left ventricle. The R[1] is the right ventricle as it is the delayed conduction. This is best noted in the right chest leads, V_1 and V_2. Usually a small R wave will be produced first, followed by an S wave and then the second R wave. This may be written as rSR[1]. This is also known as an "M" pattern or "rabbit ears" (Fig. 6–14). Right bundle branch block can be a normal variation for some individuals. It can also be caused by conduction defects.

Another aspect of right bundle branch block is that deep S waves are found in the left lateral chest leads, V_5 and V_6, known as reciprocal changes.

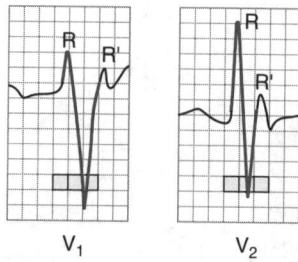

V_1 V_2

FIGURE 6–14 • **RR¹ in right bundle branch block.** RR¹ as seen in V_1 and V_2 representing a right bundle branch block. Note that the width is also at 0.12 seconds. (*Modified from Dubin, D. Rapid Interpretation of EKG's 6e. 2000.*)

These can also be present in leads I and aVL (Fig. 6–15). Repolarization is also affected and will be noted as ST segment depression and inversion of the T wave in the right precordial leads (V_1 and V_2).

Left Bundle Branch Block

In left bundle branch block, the left ventricular impulse is delayed. The first R wave seen is the right ventricle which will produce a smaller R wave first. The R prime (R¹) is not always present in this block. Sometimes it is noted as a wide, notched R wave with an increase in the final upswing. The leads to see this in are V_5 and V_6. In this variation, the widened QRS will again be seen. ST segment depression and T wave inversion can also be seen in the left chest leads (V_5 and V_6). Reciprocal deep S waves will be seen in the anterior leads (V_1 and V_2) (Figs. 6–16 and 6–17). Left axis deviation can also occur.

> **CLINICAL ALERT**
>
> There are times when a BBB is not apparent unless the rate increases and a critical rate is achieved. This reflects that the conduction to the right and left branches moves at a normal pace when the rates are slower, however, when the heart rate increases, the conduction defect becomes apparent. This will cause an intermittent type of BBB with the wide complex and rabbit ear morphology only present when the rate surpasses the "critical rate."

Variations in EKG tracings are noted in Table 6–2 for both right and left bundle branch blocks. When determining the presence of bundle branch block, first look at the width of the QRS complex. If it is greater than 0.10 seconds, a block is present. Establish whether it is a right or left block by noting which leads carry the "rabbit ears" or RR¹. Right bundle branch block will distinguish itself in leads V_1 and V_2. Left bundle branch block will be characterized in leads V_5 and V_6.

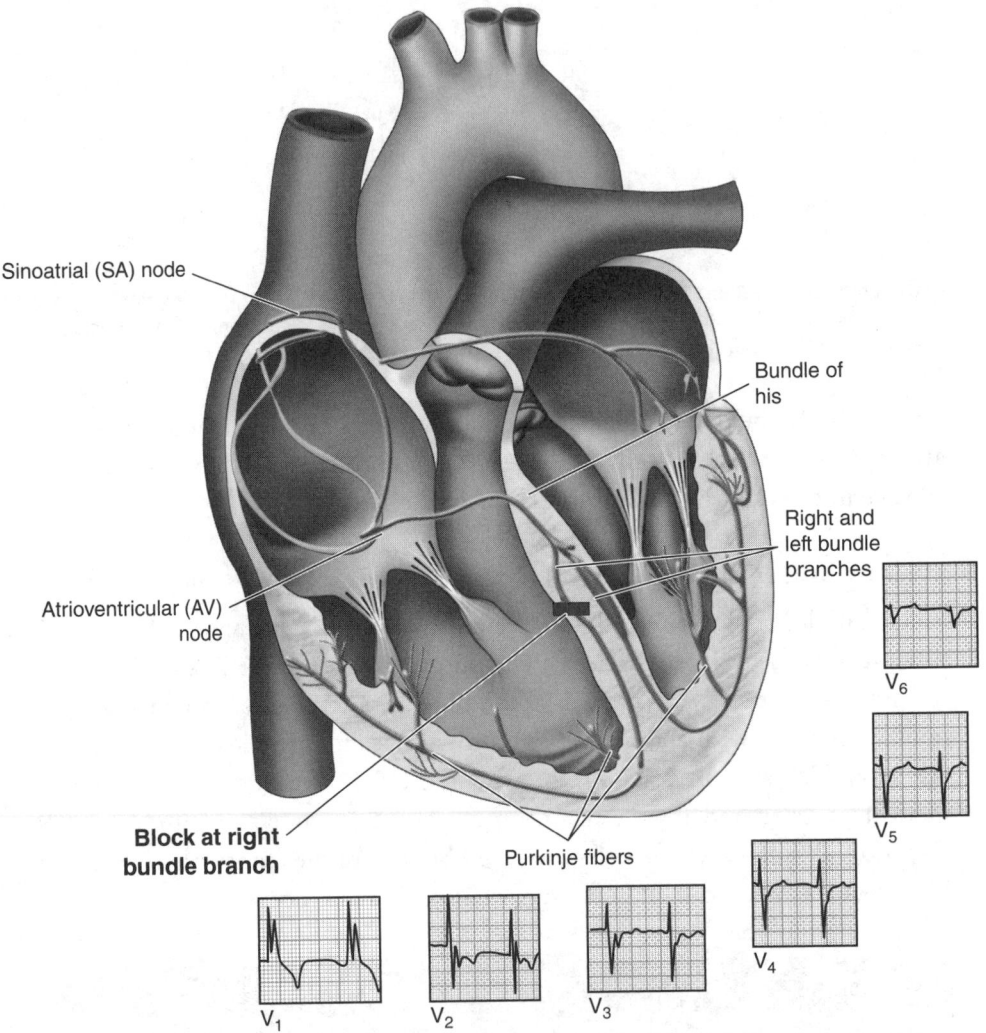

FIGURE 6–15 • **Chest leads depicting right bundle branch block.** Note the RR[1] (rabbbit ears) and increased width of the QRS in leads V_1 and V_2. Deep S waves are present in leads V_5 and V_6. (*Modified from Thaler, M, The Only EKG Book You'll Ever Need 6e. 2010.*)

CLINICAL ALERT

Due to the effects that are present with the R waves, it is difficult to diagnose right ventricular hypertrophy in the presence of right bundle branch block. Left ventricular hypertrophy is also precluded by left bundle branch block. Also, when a patient presents with a left bundle branch block, the diagnosis of acute myocardial infarction becomes very difficult based on EKG changes alone. Other challenges with diagnosing BBB occurs with junctional rhythms, Wolff-Parkinson-White (WPW) syndrome, hyperkalemia, and other disease processes that can widen the QRS complex.

Left bundle branch block

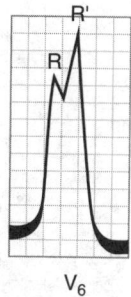

V_6

FIGURE 6–16 • RR^1 in left bundle branch block. RR^1 as seen on V_6 in left bundle branch block. Note that the first R wave is smaller. (*Modified from Dubin, D. Rapid Interpretation of EKG's 6e. 2000.*)

Hemiblocks

A conduction block can also occur in any of the three fascicles or subcomponents of the left bundle branch (Fig. 6–18). When a block occurs in any of these sets of fibers, axis deviation will manifest. The anterior and posterior fascicles are the most common and can be important in the diagnosis of acute myocardial infarction. (The third fascicle of the left bundle is the septal fascicle. The right bundle branch does not have separate fascicles.) This is dependent on which coronary vessel is occluded. It is important to compare a present EKG to a previous EKG in order to correctly diagnose a hemiblock. Since an anterior hemiblock will present with a left axis deviation, other causes of this axis deviation (left ventricular hypertrophy, inferior myocardial infarction, or an overweight individual with a "horizontal" lying heart) must be included in the differential diagnosis. Neither anterior nor posterior hemiblocks will have a widened QRS. No ST or T wave changes will appear. Only axis deviation will arise and other causes of this axis deviation must be ruled out. For the anterior hemiblock, left axis deviation of −30° to −90° will be presented. The posterior hemiblock will have right axis deviation. Other EKG changes that can occur include a wide S in lead I and Q wave in lead III with a posterior hemiblock and a Q wave in lead I and wide S wave in lead III in the anterior hemiblock.

CLINICAL ALERT

When blocks are combined, serious outcomes can take place. A posterior hemiblock in association with a right bundle branch block can lead the patient into atrioventricular blocks. These blocks in the AV node or the Bundle of His cause serious bradycardias and immediate interventions must occur.

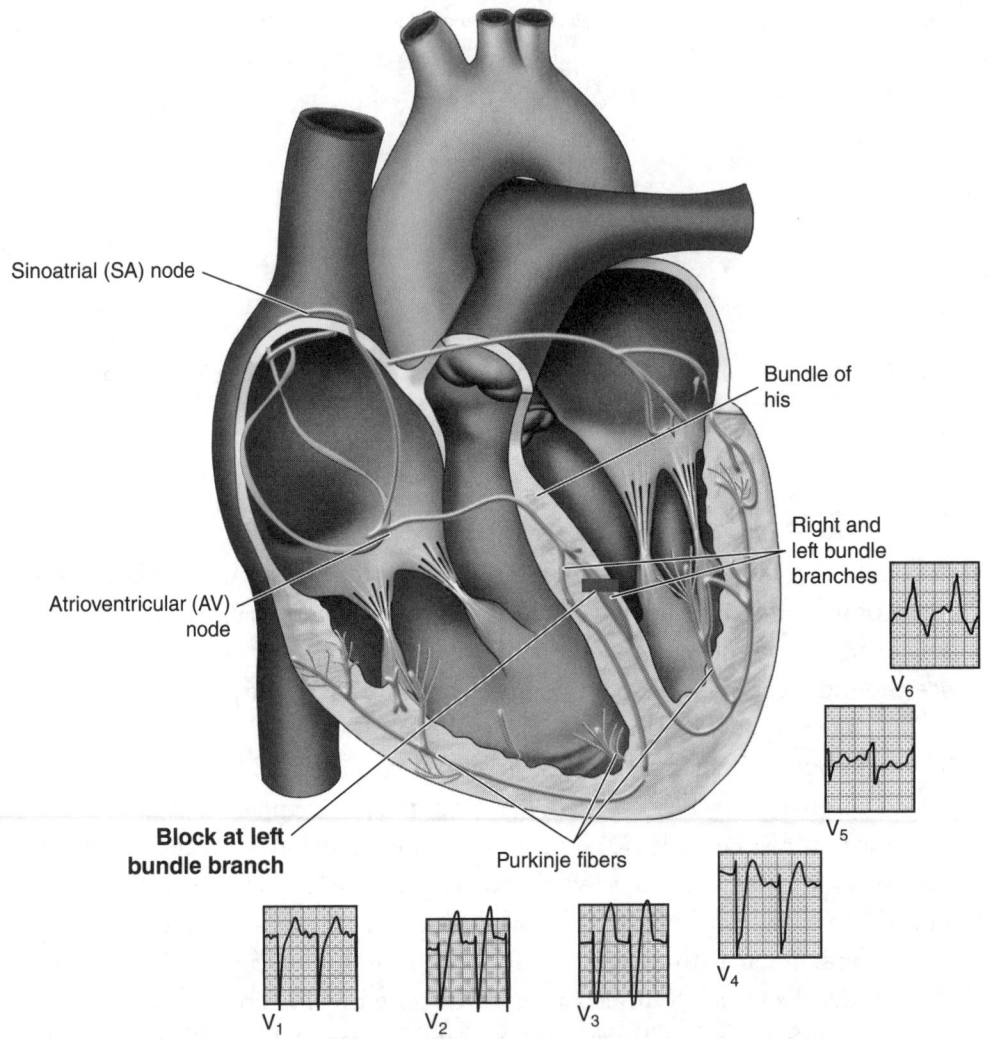

FIGURE 6-17 • **Chest leads depicting left bundle branch block.** Note the width and change in configuration of the QRS in leads V_5 and V_6. Sometimes a clear RR^1 is not noted, but rather a notching effect occurs. Also note the broad and deep S waves in V_1 and V_2. Also seen are the repolarization issues as reflected in the ST segment depression and T wave inversion in leads V_5 and V_6. (*Modified from Thaler, M, The Only EKG Book You'll Ever Need 6e. 2010.*)

The manifestations of a combination of the right bundle branch and the posterior fascicle would include a widened QRS and an RSR^1 in the anterior leads (V_1 and V_2), which would indicate the right bundle branch was involved and a RAD to provide information regarding the left posterior hemiblock. When the right bundle branch is blocked along with a hemiblock, the term "bifascicular" is used. Blocks of the right bundle branch and both anterior and posterior fascicles are termed "trifascicular" (Fig. 6–19).

TABLE 6-2   Bundle Branch Block Features

Bundle Branch block	QRS Width	V_1 and V_2	V_5 and V_6	Repolarization Changes
Right bundle branch block	>0.10 seconds	RR[1] (rabbit ears or "M" pattern)	Deep S waves (Reciprocal)	ST segment depression and T wave inversion in V_1 and V_2, lead I, and aVL
Left bundle branch block	>0.10 seconds	Deep S waves (Reciprocal)	RR[1] (rabbit ears or "M" pattern) May show as only a notched or broad R wave	ST segment depression and T wave inversion in V_5 and V_6

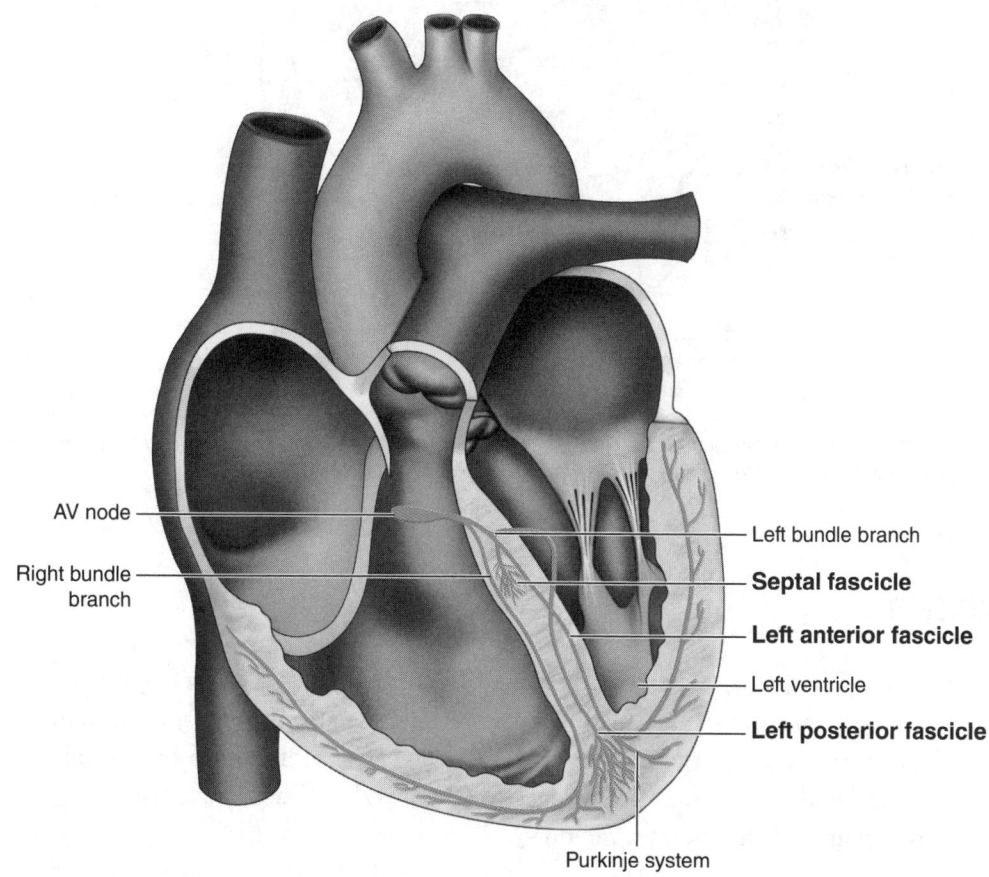

AV node

Right bundle branch

Left bundle branch

Septal fascicle

Left anterior fascicle

Left ventricle

Left posterior fascicle

Purkinje system

FIGURE 6-18 • Fascicles of the left bundle branch. The left bundle branch divides into three sets of Purkinje fibers: the septal fascicle, the anterior fascicle, and the posterior fascicle. (*Modified from Thaler, M, The Only EKG Book You'll Ever Need 6e. 2010.*)

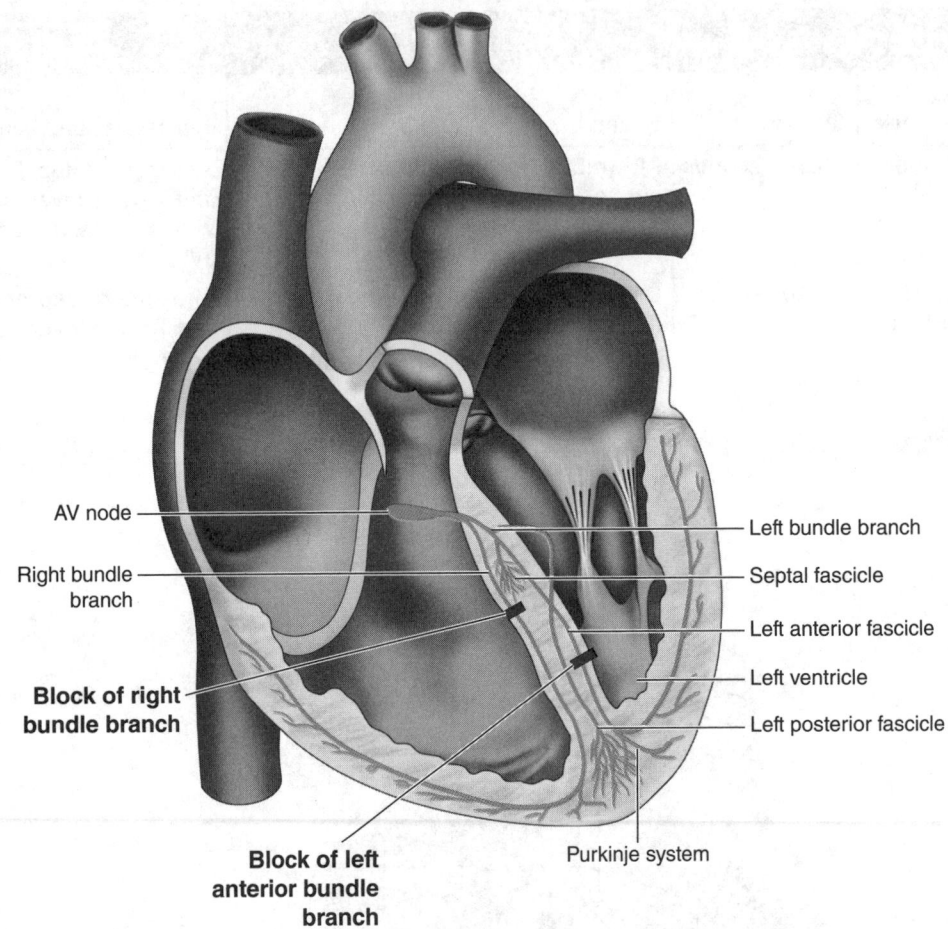

AV node

Right bundle branch

Block of right bundle branch

Block of left anterior bundle branch

Left bundle branch

Septal fascicle

Left anterior fascicle

Left ventricle

Left posterior fascicle

Purkinje system

FIGURE 6–19 • Bifascicular block. A bifascicular block involving the right bundle branch and the anterior fascicle of the left bundle branch. (*Modified from Thaler, M, The Only EKG Book You'll Ever Need 6e. 2010.*)

Conclusion

Understanding axis, hypertrophy, and BBB can be difficult concepts, but are important in identifying potentially lethal situations for the patient. Hypertrophy and enlargement of chambers can cause problems in cardiac output and are therefore significant pieces of the puzzle of cardiac disease.

Key points of this chapter include:

- A vector is an arrow that shows the direction of the electrical current.
- The mean vector is the sum or average of all vectors that are occurring simultaneously.

- The mean electrical axis is the direction in which the mean vector is traveling.

- The normal mean electrical axis would be in a downward and left direction.

- The hexaxial reference system is derived from Einthoven's Triangle and is the circle of degrees in the frontal plane that is used to determine the mean electrical axis.

- The mean electrical axis helps to identify that normal ventricular depolarization is occurring.

- The mean electrical axis should lie within the scope of 0° to +90°.

- The two leads most commonly used to identify the mean electrical axis are leads I and aVF.

- Leads I and aVF are perpendicular to each other.

- Lead I lies at 0°.

- Lead aVF lies at +90°.

- The R wave is used to assess the mean electrical axis. Positive R wave deflections in leads I and aVF means that the axis is normal.

- The mean vector will point toward hypertrophy and away from infarction.

- Right axis deviation (RAD) is signified on the 12-lead EKG by a negative QRS complex in lead I and a positive QRS complex in lead aVF.

- Tall slender individuals may have a normal right axis deviation.

- Dextrocardia would have a right axis deviation.

- A right-sided EKG would produce a normal axis and normal R wave progression across the chest leads in a patient with dextrocardia.

- Extreme RAD is in the range of +180° and −90° and would show negative QRS deflections in both lead I and aVF.

- Left axis deviation will be manifested with a positive deflection in lead I and a negative deflection in lead aVF.

- An obese patient might have a normal left axis deviation.

- Enlargement indicates an expansion or dilation of a chamber.

- Enlargement is caused by volume overload.

- Hypertrophy indicates an increase in muscle mass.

- Hypertrophy is caused by an increase in pressure.

- Enlargement is usually used to discuss the atria. Hypertrophy is used to describe changes in the ventricles. These can also happen simultaneously.
- Enlargement is noted on the EKG in the P wave, an indicator of atrial activity.
- Right atrial enlargement is seen as a tall peaked first upswing of the P wave. Another name for this is P pulmonale.
- Axis deviation of the P wave to the right is also seen in right atrial enlargement.
- Left atrial enlargement will be shown on the 12-lead EKG as a prominence in the final portion of the P wave. This is also known as P mitrale.
- The QRS complex is used to visualize hypertrophy of the ventricles.
- Right ventricular hypertrophy is noted by RAD on the 12-lead EKG.
- Left ventricular hypertrophy is noted by several aspects of the 12-lead EKG including the presence of an S wave in V_1, and the amplitude of the R wave in the lateral leads as well as the combined amplitude of the S wave in the anterior (V_1 or V_2) leads and the R wave in the lateral (V_5 or V_6) leads.
- Strain is noted on the 12-lead EKG in the T wave and the ST segment.
- Strain is also known as secondary repolarization abnormality.
- Right ventricular strain would be seen in leads V_1 and V_2.
- Left ventricular strain would be seen in leads V_5 and V_6.
- A bundle branch block can occur in either the right or left bundle branch.
- A widened QRS would indicate a bundle branch block.
- The presence of an R^1 (R prime) is also indicative of a bundle branch block.
- RR^1 is also known as "rabbit ears."
- Reciprocal changes, seen as deep S waves will also be seen in bundle branch blocks.
- ST segment depression and T wave inversion can also be seen with bundle branch blocks.
- Right bundle branch block is noted in the right chest leads, V_1 and V_2.
- Left bundle branch block is noted in the lateral chest leads, V_5 and V_6.
- A left bundle branch block may have a notching on the R wave.
- Intermittent bundle branch blocks (BBB) can also be seen.
- Left bundle branch block will cause difficulty in diagnosis of acute myocardial infarction.

- The left bundle branch is subdivided into three fascicles.
- When one of these fascicles becomes blocked, the patient has a hemiblock.
- Hemiblocks will not have QRS widening. Only axis changes are indicative of hemiblocks.
- Other causes of axis deviations must be ruled out to diagnose a hemiblock. EKGs must be compared to prior EKGs.
- Left axis deviation can indicate an anterior hemiblock.
- RAD can indicate a posterior hemiblock.
- Bifascicular blocks are a combination of a right bundle branch block and one of the fascicles of the left bundle branch.
- Trifascicular blocks are a combination of a right bundle branch block and both the anterior and posterior fascicles of the left bundle branch.
- A posterior hemiblock in the presence of a right bundle branch block is a dangerous combination and can lead the patient to an atrioventricular block which can cause a profound bradycardia.

PRACTICE QUESTIONS

1. **Which of the following is the proper definition of the mean vector?**
   A. The atrioventricular node where all impulses must pass
   B. The sum of all the arrows showing the direction of the impulse
   C. The direction of the arrows as noted on the hexaxial reference system
   D. The thick, large left ventricular wall during contraction

2. **The normal mean electrical axis would lie between which of the following degrees on the hexaxial reference system?**
   A. 0° to +90°
   B. +90° to +180°
   C. +180° to −90°
   D. −90° to 0°

3. **Which of the following two leads are used to determine axis deviation?**
   A. Leads III and aVL
   B. V_1 and V_6
   C. Leads I and aVF
   D. Leads II and V_4

4. In relation to an acute myocardial infarction, the vector will lead:

   A. away from the infarction.

   B. toward the infarction.

   C. in the same direction as the infarction.

   D. perpendicular to the infarction.

5. Dextrocardia would show which of the following variations on the 12-lead EKG?

   A. Left axis deviation

   B. Increasing R wave progression

   C. Positive QRS complex in lead I

   D. Right axis deviation

6. An obese individual might be prone to showing which of the following axis deviations?

   A. Right axis deviation

   B. Left axis deviation

   C. Extreme right axis deviation

   D. No axis deviation

7. Hypertrophy is caused by:

   A. the volume of blood in a chamber.

   B. an increase in pressure within a chamber.

   C. mitral valve disease processes.

   D. aortic insufficiency.

8. Right atrial enlargement would be seen as:

   A. a prominence of the final portion of the P wave.

   B. a P wave that is greater than 0.12 seconds in width.

   C. the presence of a left axis deviation.

   D. a tall peaked initial portion of the P wave.

9. Which of the following would be an indicator of left ventricular hypertrophy?

   A. Small S wave noted in leads V_1 and V_2

   B. R wave height in V_6 greater than in V_5

   C. Combined S wave (V_1) and R wave (V_6) of 26 mm

   D. R wave in lead V_6 of 32 mm

10. Which of the following would be a true statement regarding right ventricular hypertrophy?

    A. Normal R wave progression will be present in right ventricular hypertrophy.
    B. Left axis deviation will be present in right ventricular hypertrophy.
    C. Pulmonary hypertension can cause right ventricular hypertrophy.
    D. Aortic stenosis can cause right ventricular hypertrophy.

11. Which of the following would be a possible etiology for left ventricular hypertrophy?

    A. Systemic hypertension
    B. Emphysema
    C. Pulmonary hypertension
    D. Chronic obstructive pulmonary disease

12. Which of the following would be present in a complete bundle branch block?

    A. QRS width of greater than 0.12 seconds
    B. P wave of greater than 0.10 seconds
    C. T wave of greater than 0.20 seconds
    D. U wave of greater than 0.04 seconds

13. The 12-lead EKG will show reciprocal changes in the form of deep S waves in a right bundle branch block in which of the following leads?

    A. Leads II and aVF
    B. Leads V_5 and V_6
    C. Leads V_1 and V_2
    D. Leads I and aVL

14. A diagnosis of an acute myocardial infarction is difficult to make when a patient presents with which of the following on the 12-lead EKG?

    A. Left bundle branch block
    B. Right bundle branch block
    C. Left atrial enlargement
    D. Right atrial enlargement

15. Which of the following can lead the patient to develop a dangerous atrioventricular block?

    A. Anterior hemiblock with a left bundle branch block
    B. Posterior hemiblock with a left bundle branch block
    C. Posterior hemiblock with a right bundle branch block
    D. Anterior hemiblock with a right bundle branch block

16. **Which of the following would be termed "trifascicular"?**
    A. Blockage of the right bundle branch and anterior and posterior fascicles
    B. Blockage of the left bundle branch and the anterior fascicle
    C. Blockage of the right bundle branch and the posterior fascicle
    D. Blockage of the left and right bundle branches

ANSWER KEY

1. **B.** The sum of all the vectors or arrows as the impulse travels through the heart is the mean vector. The atrioventricular node is the starting point for all vectors. The direction of the arrows represented on the hexaxial reference system is the mean electrical axis. The left ventricular wall is the strongest and thickest and the mean vector will travel in that direction in normal axis.

2. **A.** The mean electrical axis on the hexaxial reference system will head in the direction of the left ventricle which lies within the scope of 0° to +90°.

3. **C.** The two most common leads used to assist in determining axis deviation are leads I and aVF. They lie perpendicular to each other and lie within the scope of 0° to +90°.

4. **A.** When an acute myocardial infarction is present, the vector will be directed away from the infarcted or dead tissue.

5. **D.** Dextrocardia occurs when the heart is misplaced and is situated in the right side of the chest instead of the left. RAD will be present with this anomaly as well as a decreasing R wave progression in the chest leads.

6. **B.** An obese individual can have left axis deviation simply because the diaphragm is pushed upwards and it places the heart in a more horizontal position. This causes the vectors to be misplaced to a mean electrical axis between −90° and 0° on the hexaxial reference system.

7. **B.** An increase in pressure within a chamber causes hypertrophy. Extra volume in a chamber can lead to enlargement of the chamber itself. Mitral valve disorders and aortic insufficiency contribute to increased volumes within the left atrium and left ventricular chambers respectively.

8. **D.** Right atrial enlargement is characterized by a tall peaked initial upswing of the P wave. This first portion of the P wave is representative of the right atrium. The final portion of the P wave represents the left atrium. Right atrial enlargement will cause a right axis deviation. No change in duration of the P wave occurs in right atrial enlargement. Left atrial enlargement will increase the width of the P wave.

9. **D.** Left ventricular hypertrophy will show an R wave in lead V_6 of greater than 18 mm. Other criteria include a large S wave in V_1, R wave height that is greater in V_5 than in V_6, and a combined S wave amplitude in V_1 or V_2 and R wave amplitude in V_5 or V_6 that is greater than 35 mm in height.

10. **C.** Pulmonary hypertension would cause an increase in the pressure at which the right ventricle would need to exert in order to push blood into the pulmonary circulation. Aortic stenosis would be a cause of left ventricular hypertrophy since the left ventricle would have to push harder to propel blood into the systemic circulation against a diseased aortic valve. RAD would be present in right ventricular hypertrophy and R wave progression would be reversed.

11. **A.** Hypertrophy is caused by an increase in pressure. The left ventricle is responsible for pushing blood out into the systemic circulation; therefore, an increase in systemic hypertension would increase the pressure at which the left ventricle would have to exert against. Emphysema, a form of chronic obstructive pulmonary disease and pulmonary hypertension will affect the right ventricle.

12. **A.** QRS width is one of the defining characteristics for bundle branch block. A width greater than 0.12 will indicate a complete bundle branch block.

13. **B.** Reciprocal changes in a right bundle branch block would be seen in the left or lateral chest leads, V_5 and V_6. This reciprocal change is in the form of deep S waves. Right bundle branch block would show changes in leads V_1 and V_2 of the R' QRS complex.

14. **A.** A left bundle branch block can mask some of the changes that are noted with an acute myocardial infarction.

15. **C.** A right bundle branch block with a posterior hemiblock of the left bundle branch fascicle can lead the patient to develop dangerous and potentially lethal atrioventricular blocks.

16. **A.** A trifascicular block would occur when the right bundle branch and two of the fascicles of the left bundle branch become blocked at the same time. A bifascicular block occurs when the right bundle branch and either the anterior or posterior fascicle become blocked at the same time.

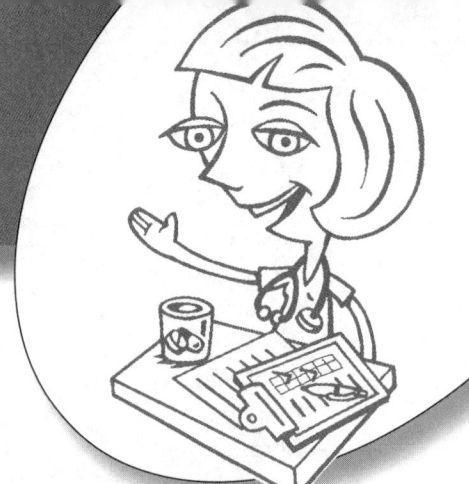

chapter 7

Sinus Node Related Dysrhythmias

LEARNING OBJECTIVES

At the end of this chapter, the student will be able to:

1. List etiologies of dysrhythmias.
2. Understand symptoms that can occur with dysrhythmias.
3. Identify sinus node related dysrhythmias on an electrocardiogram (EKG) tracing or cardiac monitor.
4. Relate pathophysiologic effects of sinus node related dysrhythmias.
5. List general treatment options for sinus node related dysrhythmias.

KEY WORDS

Angina	Huffing
Asymptomatic	Hypotension
Cardiac tamponade	Hypoxia
Cardiogenic shock	Myocarditis
Diaphoresis	Oliguria
Dyspnea	Pneumothorax
Fibrosis	Pulmonary embolus
Flail chest	Tension pneumothorax
Foci	Toluene
Hemothorax	Valsalva maneuver

Overview

Dysrhythmias occur in patients for many different reasons. Although a myocardial infarction (MI) is one of the most common reasons for abnormal heart beats to arise, many other disease processes and injuries can also precipitate rhythms that do not provide for the best cardiac output. Table 7–1 lists some of the etiologies of dysrhythmias.

Health care providers must be ready to interpret these rhythm disturbances and intervene appropriately. Some dysrhythmias are dysfunctional causing interruptions in normal vital signs. Some dysrhythmias are benign and though they may make the patient feel uncomfortable, are not dangerous. Some dysrhythmias are incidental and the patient may not even be aware of it. Some dysrhythmias are beneficial and must be present in order for the patient to survive. Some dysrhythmias are fatal and require life-saving interventions. Symptoms that patients may present with when experiencing a dysrhythmia are listed in Box 7–1.

CLINICAL ALERT

A common sign, especially with faster rhythms, is a feeling or perception of the heartbeat. These palpitations may feel like their heart is beating fast or the patient may describe either a fluttering type of sensation in the chest or the feeling of missed or extra beats. These palpitations can also create anxiety which can contribute to the patient's feeling of impending doom.

TABLE 7–1 Etiologies of Dysrhythmias

Factor	Examples of Etiologies
Hypoxia	• Pulmonary disease processes • Chronic obstructive pulmonary disease • **Pulmonary embolus**
Ischemia	• Myocardial infarction • **Angina**
Irritability	• **Myocarditis** • Inhalation of Toluenes (**Huffing**)
Sympathetic stimulation	• Hyperthyroidism • Heart failure • Anxiety • Exercise
Drugs	• Tricyclic overdose • Beta-adrenergic blocker toxicity • Calcium channel blockers • Psychogenic medications • Antibiotics • Antiarrhythmics • Digitalis toxicity
Electrolytes	• Potassium • Magnesium • Calcium
Bradycardias	• Atrioventricular blocks • Drug overdoses or toxicities • Hypothyroidism • Increased intracranial pressure
Enlargement and hypertrophy	• Pulmonary edema • Valve disorders • **Cardiogenic shock**
Trauma	• Hypovolemia • Blunt cardiac injury • Commotio cordis • **Cardiac tamponade** • **Pneumothorax** • **Tension pneumothorax** • **Hemothorax** • **Flail chest** • Penetrating cardiac injuries • Great vessel injuries

Dysrhythmias (also known in medical terminology as arrhythmias) occur whenever there is an interruption or disruption in the rate, regularity, originating impulse, or conduction of that impulse. These can appear as a single or occasional extra beat, as a prolonged rhythm that the patient maintains for a period of time (or their lifetime) or which may recur intermittently for particular patients throughout their life span, or as a significant acute crisis that can precede sudden death.

This chapter will begin the discussion of dysrhythmias with a glimpse into those rhythms that are sinus in origin.

Sinus Rhythms

Normal sinus rhythm is the most common rhythm and is not a dysrhythmia at all. Identifying information and criteria for this essential heartbeat was provided in Chapter 5. This is the standard by which all other rhythms are judged.

Sinus Bradycardia

Bradycardia means a slow heart rate (HR). When sinus bradycardia (SB) is present, the SA node is still the pacemaker for this rhythm, but it is discharging at a much slower rate than normal. Conduction of the impulse follows the usual pathway. Sinus bradycardia may naturally be present in healthy adults during sleep. It can also be a common presentation in athletes. When examined, the rhythm strip will basically have all the same features as normal sinus rhythm except the rate. The following will be typical EKG characteristics for sinus bradycardia (Fig. 7–1):

- **Regularity:** Regular rhythm
- **Rate:** Less than 60 beats per minute
- **P wave:** Present for each QRS complex
- **PR interval:** 0.12 to 0.20 seconds
- **QRS complex:** Less than 0.10 seconds in width
- **QT interval:** May be longer due to slower rate
- **T wave:** Normal configuration and size
- **ST segment:** Normal configuration and size

Sinus bradycardia (as well as other bradycardias to be discussed in Chapter 9) can frequently occur with an inferior or posterior MI. Another etiology of this slow rate is that of vagal stimulation. When the vagus nerve is stimulated, which can occur with cough, straining, vomiting, or extended standing positions, bradycardia can manifest due to the relationship of the vagus nerve to the parasympathetic nervous system. When the vagus nerve is stimulated, the heart rate will slow or become bradycardic. When patients have some types of fast heart rates, vagal stimulation is often used in an attempt to decrease the pulse. This can be done by having the patient cough, hold their breath and push downward as if having a bowel movement (**Valsalva maneuver**), or placing their face in ice cold water. Stimulation of the carotid artery will also slow the heart rate and produce this dysrhythmia. These treatment options for fast heart rates are performed by the physician or other mid-level provider. Box 7–2 lists some causes of sinus bradycardia.

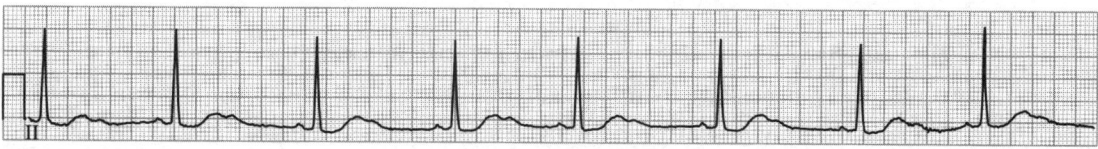

FIGURE 7–1 • Sinus bradycardia. Each QRS is preceded by a P wave and all other parameters are normal except for the rate of 47 beats per minute.

BOX 7—2   Causes of Sinus Bradycardia

- SA node syndromes/disease
- Cardiomyopathy
- Myocarditis
- Neurogenic shock (parasympathetic nervous system takes over)
- Hypoxia
- Myocardial ischemia
- Glaucoma
- Hypothermia
- Inferior and posterior myocardial infarction
- Increased intracranial pressure
- Hypothyroidism
- Heart transplant
- Hyperkalemia
- Sleep apnea
- Normal sleep
- Carotid sinus massage
- Vomiting
- Beta-blockers
- Calcium channel blockers
- Digitalis (Lanoxin)
- Sotalol (Betapace)
- Lithium (Lithobid)
- Amiodarone (Cordarone)
- Propafenone (Rythmol)
- Quinidine

CLINICAL ALERT

Patients who are on beta-blocker medications will often have bradycardic rhythms when the health care provider would expect the heart rate to be fast such as in hypovolemic shock. Beta-blockers keep the heart rate slow in these patients. It is important for the health care provider to be aware of medications patients are taking during assessment.

If the patient is not having any symptoms (**asymptomatic**), no immediate interventions are necessary. Symptomatic bradycardia may need to be treated with the administration of atropine which should increase the heart rate. When patients have a low pulse rate, the only way to improve cardiac output (CO) is to increase the stroke volume (SV) (CO = SV × HR). With many patients, this may not be an option. Atropine improves not only the rate at which the SA node is firing, but also strengthens the conduction of the impulse. A pacemaker may also be required. If the patient has a very low pulse rate, that is, 30 to 40 beats per minute, but is tolerating the low heart rate as evidenced by normal blood pressure, no chest pain, no dizziness or other symptomatology, a pacemaker may still be necessary, but is not emergent. As stated in previous chapters, treat the patient, not the machine. Low heart rates associated with an acute MI may actually be advantageous since it can reduce the oxygen requirements for the heart at that time. Always provide oxygen and make sure that a patent intravenous line is in place when patients display low heart rates.

> ### CLINICAL ALERT
>
> Infants normally have a faster heartbeat. An infant with a heart rate less than 90 to 100 is considered to be bradycardic. Very sick infants or children presenting with bradycardia is an ominous sign. When children attempt to compensate for low cardiac output, they speed the heart rate up as they have a fixed SV. Inability to compensate in this way is a dangerous pattern.

Sinus Tachycardia

Sinus tachycardia (ST) occurs when the SA node sends impulses at a faster than normal rate. Tachycardia is recognized at rates greater than 100 beats per minute. Other tachycardias can also be present, but these have **foci** or impulse generating tissue other than the SA node. Sinus tachycardia can be exhibited in otherwise normal, healthy adults when experiencing anxiety or stress. It can also occur as a response to a disease state such as hemorrhage, pain, a hyperthyroid state, a pulmonary embolus, or other pathologic disorders. When this is present, patients may state that they have a "pounding" feeling in the chest region or may feel like their heart is racing. A radial pulse with very fast heart rates may feel weak and thready to the health care provider. The following list features characteristics of sinus tachycardia as seen on a cardiac monitor or 12-lead EKG (Fig. 7–2):

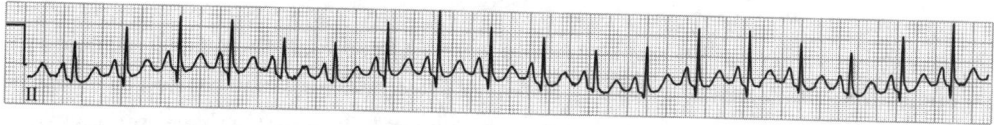

FIGURE 7–2 • Sinus tachycardia. Each QRS is preceded by a P wave and all other parameters are normal except for the rate of 110 beats per minute.

- **Regularity:** Regular rhythm
- **Rate:** Greater than 100 beats per minute (under 180 beats per minute)
- **P wave:** Present for each QRS complex (may be difficult to distinguish P waves from T waves in extremely rapid rates)
- **PR interval:** 0.12 to 0.20 seconds (may be shorter in faster rhythms)
- **QRS complex:** Less than 0.10 seconds in width
- **QT interval:** May be shorter due to faster rate
- **T wave:** Normal configuration and size
- **ST segment:** Normal configuration and size

Sinus tachycardia can occur as a reaction to any demand on the body for increased oxygenation. When the heart beats faster, the ventricles do not have time to fill adequately. This then reduces the amount of blood that is available to be delivered to the lungs and the body during contraction of the ventricles, which in turn equates to a decrease in cardiac output. This decrease in cardiac output may be seen through a decline in the blood pressure and reduced oxygenation of the periphery since perfusion has dropped. Coronary arteries are also filling at a reduced rate due to the decrease in diastolic time. Normally this is the time that the coronary arteries are receiving their burst of blood flow. Patients may complain of chest pain due to the insufficient oxygenation of the heart muscle itself. While many tachycardic rhythms can be easily explained and treated, tachycardias associated with MIs can be an early sign of impending cardiogenic shock or heart failure.

Box 7–3 provides a listing of etiologies of sinus tachycardia.

Determining proper treatment for sinus tachycardia is aimed at identifying the underlying cause and treating this causative factor appropriately. It may require something as simple as providing medications to alleviate anxiety until the basis for the anxious reaction can be corrected. Resting after exercise will reduce the heart rate back to a normal rate. Other therapeutic regimens that may be required could include fluid and electrolyte replacement, stop active internal or external bleeding, pain relief, temperature control, discontinuance of medications or street drugs that increase heart rates such as cocaine, amphetamines, or "bath salts", decrease intake of caffeine or nicotine, or cessation of alcohol intake. If the tachycardia is producing negative cardiac output symptoms such as hypotension or a decreased level of consciousness, medications such as beta-blockers (Metoprolol [Lopressor], Atenolol [Tenormin], Diltiazem [Cardizem], Labetalol [Normodyne]) may be used to bring the heart rate into a normal rate. Symptoms of heart failure such as increased jugular venous distention or crackles during auscultation of lung sounds may preclude the use of these medications.

BOX 7–3 Etiologies of Sinus Tachycardia

- Anxiety
- Fever
- Pain
- Fear
- Lack of oxygen (**hypoxia**)
- Heart failure
- Dehydration
- Exercise
- Stimulation of sympathetic nervous system ("fight or flight" response)
- Hypovolemic shock
- Cardiogenic shock
- Septic shock
- Anaphylaxis
- Over the counter cold remedies or nasal drops
- Hypovolemia
- Infectious processes
- Anterior myocardial infarction
- Pulmonary embolus
- Hyperthyroidism
- Epinephrine
- Atropine
- Dopamine (dopamine hydrochloride)
- Alcohol
- Caffeine
- Nicotine
- Street drugs such as cocaine, amphetamines, ecstasy, cannabis, bath salts

CLINICAL ALERT

Children respond to illness by increasing their heart rate. As stated previously, the two factors that create cardiac output are stroke volume and heart rate. Children, including infants, will increase their heart rate in an attempt to increase their cardiac output when circumstances arise that place them at risk. This occurs because children and infants are unable to change their stroke volume. This fixed stroke volume will cause them to respond to perceived or real threats by increasing the heart rate in an attempt to increase cardiac output. This is an important concept to keep in mind when caring for children. This normal compensatory response to disease states such as dehydration and fever, as well as anxiety and fear of strangers, coupled with the fact that children and infants normally have higher pulse rates, can be considered to be "normal" and therefore, health care professionals should be careful to not become complacent about these high pulse rates in the pediatric population. Increased heart rates in the absence of fever or other disease situations should alert the health care professional to an underlying problem that often requires intense exploration. A toddler with a heart rate of 180 with no fever or distinguishable reason for the tachycardia demands diagnostic attention. A heart rate of 200 beats per minute in an infant and 160 beats per minute in a child under age 5 is considered to be tachycardia.

Sinus Arrhythmia

Sinus arrhythmia is a rhythm which can be normal for particular populations. This is a normal phenomenon in children and some adults up to the age of 30 that is usually associated with respirations. During inspiration the heart rate increases and during the expiratory phase of breathing, the heart rate decreases. Changes in intrathoracic pressure that affects the vagus nerve is the etiology of this type of sinus arrhythmia. The vagus nerve, which is part of the parasympathetic nervous system, reduces its tone during the inspiratory stage of the respiratory cycle due to an increase in the amount of blood flow returning to the heart. This allows for an increase in pulse rate. During expiration, this return decreases and allows the vagal tone to increase causing a decrease in pulse rate. Having the patient hold their breath will cause their rhythm to return to a regular pattern during that time.

Another type of sinus arrhythmia, nonrespiratory sinus arrhythmia, may occur in older adults due to the normal aging process, the presence of an acute inferior MI, the use of medications such as morphine or digoxin (Lanoxin), or an increase in intracranial pressure. A patient receiving digoxin (Lanoxin) who suddenly develops this dysrhythmia should be considered as a potential candidate for digitalis toxicity. Be sure to notify the patient's provider if this dysrhythmia suddenly appears.

In this type of dysrhythmia, all aspects are normal except for the irregularity which takes place. When discussing the rate, it may be recorded as a range, such as "sinus arrhythmia at 52 to 78 beats per minute" (Fig. 7–3).

- **Regularity:** Irregular rhythm
- **Rate:** Normal, between 60 to 100 beats per minute
- **P Wave:** Present for each QRS complex
- **PR interval:** 0.12 to 0.20 seconds/nonvariable
- **QRS complex:** Less than 0.10 seconds in width

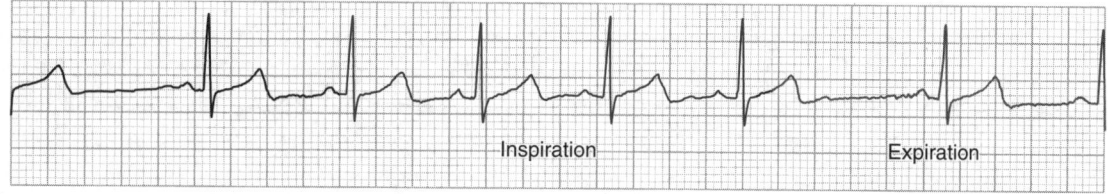

FIGURE 7−3 • **Sinus arrhythmia.** Each QRS is preceded by a P wave and all other parameters are normal except for the variation in regularity associated with inspiration and expiration. The rate in this rhythm strip is 54 to 88 beats per minute.

- **QT interval:** Normal length, may vary slightly
- **T wave:** Normal configuration and size
- **ST segment:** Normal configuration and size

Sinus arrhythmia usually does not require treatment. However, in cases of sudden onset, do consider the causes as listed above.

CLINICAL ALERT

Be sure to correctly identify sinus arrhythmia. This may require a longer than usual observation of the cardiac monitor. A longer rhythm strip may be necessary to determine that it is not a different rhythm such as atrial fibrillation, premature atrial contractions, a block of some type, or sinus pauses. Watch to see that the breathing pattern is in concert with the rates on the rhythm strip or cardiac monitor. Another type of serious sinus dysrhythmia can occur in older adults known as *sick sinus syndrome*. In this case there is wide variation of the P-P intervals.

Sinus Arrest

Sinus arrest occurs when the SA node fails to produce an electrical impulse. Other names for this dysrhythmia are atrial standstill, sinus pause, and sinoatrial arrest. In this disease process, the SA node fails and no PQRST complex or contraction is created. The term sinus arrest is usually used when three or more beats are omitted from the rhythm strip. The EKG tracing or cardiac monitor will have normal appearance except that complete PQRST complexes are missing (Fig. 7–4).

- **Regularity:** Irregular rhythm—however it can be called regular except for the event of the missing PQRST complexes
- **Rate:** Usually normal will vary due to the loss of complexes

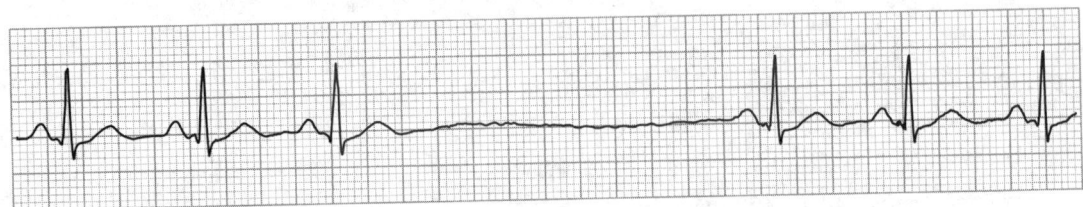

FIGURE 7–4 • Sinus Arrest. Sinus Arrest is noted when there are no PQRST complexes present where they would be expected. The rate for this rhythm is noted as range of 24 to 81 due to the irregularity.

- **P wave:** Present for each QRS complex that is present
- **PR interval:** 0.12 to 0.20 seconds and constant with each beat present
- **QRS complex:** Less than 0.10 seconds in width and constant with each beat present
- **QT interval:** Normal length
- **T wave:** Normal configuration and size when present
- **ST segment:** Normal configuration and size when present

In the absence of the impulse from the normal pacemaker site, other sites such as the AV junction or ventricular tissue may produce an impulse in an attempt to rescue the situation; however, this does not always happen. When these areas of the heart attempt to assist, a junctional or ventricular beat will occur on the EKG tracing or cardiac monitor at some point in the arrest period. These escape beats are essential to the patient's heartbeat at this time (Fig. 7–5).

Patients who are experiencing occasional sinus arrests or pauses may be asymptomatic. These require no immediate treatment except for determining

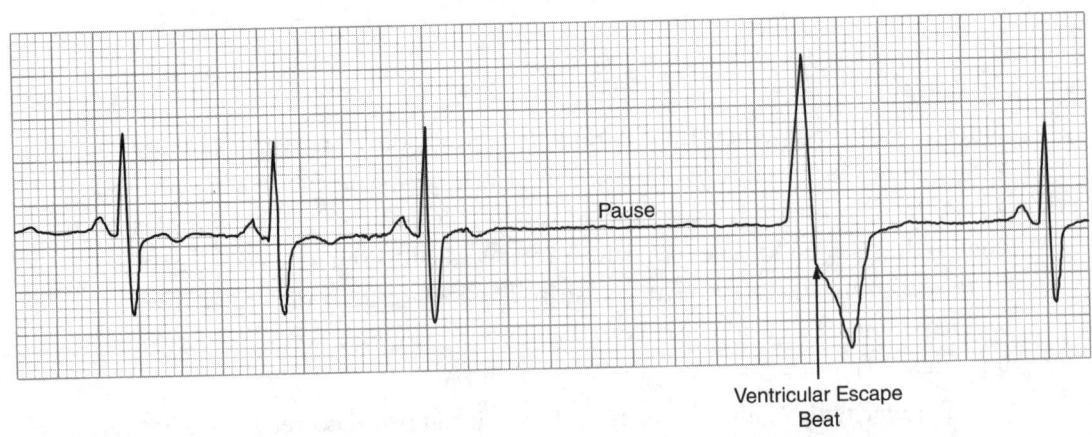

Pause

Ventricular Escape
Beat

FIGURE 7–5 • Sinus arrest with ventricular escape beat. When sinus arrest occurs, an escape beat can be created by either junctional or ventricular tissue. This figure demonstrates a ventricular escape beat during a sinus arrest situation.

the cause and properly treating the process. If these events occur during sleep, they may not have significant value. However, if these episodes become more numerous or are repeated and prolonged, the patient may complain of generalized weakness, dizziness, lightheadedness, or may describe syncopal episodes. Immediate treatment may be necessary for these prolonged or frequent incidents. A prolonged episode of sinus arrest will constitute asystole. Proper treatment may include administration of epinephrine and the implantation of an emergent temporary pacemaker. A permanent pacemaker may then be required once the etiology of the sinus arrest has been determined. Escape beats such as junctional or ventricular complexes as described above are not treated at this time. Increasing the heart rate is the treatment of choice. Once the heart rate is improved, these escape beats will not be necessary and they will cease. Causes of sinus arrest or pause are outlined in Table 7–2.

TABLE 7–2 Causes of Sinus Arrest	
Etiology	**Associated with:**
Diseased sinus node	**Fibrosis** Degeneration (**Idiopathic**)
Increased vagal tone	Valsalva maneuver Carotid sinus massage Carotid sinus sensitivity Vomiting
Medications	Digoxin (Lanoxin) Quinidine Procainamide Beta-blockers Calcium channel blockers Salicylate overdose
Disease processes	Coronary artery disease Hypoxia Myocardial ischemia Myocardial infarction (Inferior) Myocarditis Cardiomyopathy Hypertension Sick sinus syndrome Infectious processes
Electrolyte disturbances	Hyperkalemia

CLINICAL ALERT

Patients who are having prolonged or multiple recurrences of sinus arrest will not have a radial pulse during the time of the event. Observing the rhythm on the cardiac monitor while physically assessing the patient during the incident will assist the health care provider in identifying and properly treating the patient. This type of patient may also exhibit hypotension, mentation changes, cool, clammy skin, dizziness, blurred vision, lightheadedness, and/or a general feeling of weakness. Sometimes the health care provider needs to be a detective of sorts because the patient may be present for evaluation for other reasons including seizures, motor vehicle crashes, or falls. Including family members or significant others in the history taking portion of an assessment may provide insight into the event of which the patient is unaware.

Sinoatrial Blocks

Sinoatrial blocks are similar to sinus arrest and pause. Some authors relate difficulty in differentiating the two types of rhythms. One of the main differences between these dysrhythmias is the underlying problem. In sinus arrest or pause, there is a problem with automaticity, that is, the SA node fails to begin the process of electrical stimulation by simply not initiating an impulse. Sinoatrial blocks occur due to a problem with conductivity, that is, the impulse is there, but it cannot get through to the transitional cells to complete its task. In reality, it is difficult to discriminate between the two sinus problems.

There are four types of SA blocks. These subcategories are based on the length of the delay in conduction. In SA block, the impulse is being generated, but the EKG tracings and cardiac monitors do not display the actual SA node activity. Therefore, what is considered to be SA block type I cannot be detected by EKG. SA block type II is further subdivided into second-degree type I and second-degree type II. Second-degree type I SA block is noted when the P-P intervals of the preceding PQRST complexes become shorter and shorter before the actual beat is dropped (Fig. 7–6).

In second degree SA block type II there is no difference in the P-P intervals preceding the dropped complex. The measure of the area of the dropped complex between the two P waves is an exact multiple of the P-P intervals that are present in the underlying rhythm (Fig. 7–7).

In third-degree SA block the P-P intervals preceding the dropped complex are equal. The pause that occurs with this type of SA block is not an exact multiple of the P-P intervals. The greatest clue to this rhythm is that the pause

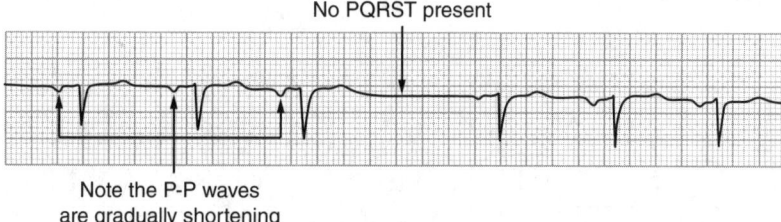

No PQRST present

Note the P-P waves
are gradually shortening

FIGURE 7-6 • **Second-degree SA block type I.** In second-degree SA block type I the complexes immediately preceding the dropped PQRST complex gradually shorten the P-P interval. The PQRST complex that is dropped would have occurred within this period of time between complex number 3 and 4.

itself ends with a sinus beat whereas sinus arrest will often end with either a junctional or ventricular escape beat (Fig. 7–8).

Etiologies, treatment, and concerns regarding SA block are the same as for sinus arrest. The major difference with these two dysrhythmias is that SA block is a problem of conductivity and sinus arrest or pause is a problem with automaticity. In SA block the impulses are being formed, but they are blocked from the rest of the tissue. With sinus arrest, no impulses are being generated.

CLINICAL ALERT

It is important to remember that the SA node blocks are different than the AV node blocks, which can cause emergent issues for patients. These will be discussed in Chapter 9.

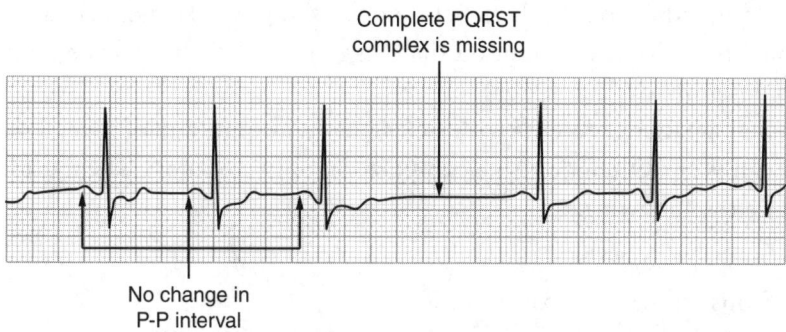

Complete PQRST
complex is missing

No change in
P-P interval

FIGURE 7-7 • **Second-degree SA block type II.** In second-degree SA block type II the preceding P-P intervals are the same length apart. The P-P interval in this strip is 21 small boxes. The blank interval is 42 small boxes in length. This correlates with the idea that the SA node is firing, but is blocked from progressing through. If it were there, it would appear at exactly the right time to be in line with the other P waves and subsequent QRST complexes.

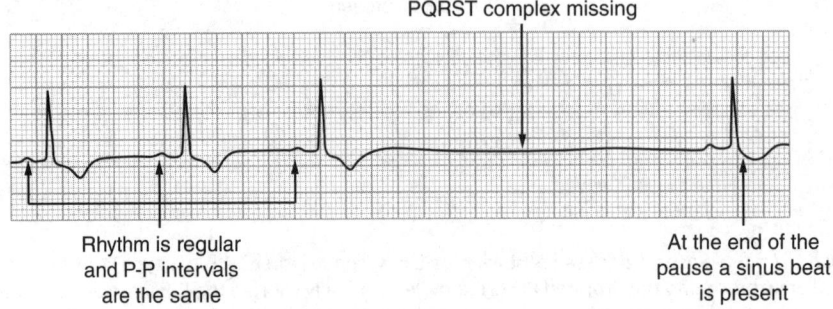

PQRST complex missing

Rhythm is regular
and P-P intervals
are the same

At the end of the
pause a sinus beat
is present

FIGURE 7–8 • **Third-degree SA block.** In third-degree SA block, the P-P intervals of the preceding complexes are the same. The loss of the PQRST complex ends with a sinus complex.

Sick Sinus Syndrome

Sick sinus syndrome is also known as *sinus nodal dysfunction* and *brady-tachy syndrome*. A combination of both conductivity and automaticity occur with this syndrome. It usually is present in older adults (>age 60) and can occur in children who have had open heart surgical procedures in which the SA node sustained damage. Although occurrences with complications from sick sinus syndrome can occur acutely, the disease itself develops over a period of time and becomes a chronic, progressive debilitating disease.

Destruction of the node itself from situations that lead toward fibrosis such as hypertension, cardiomyopathy, atherosclerosis, and the normal aging process can be the cause of this dysfunction. Other major etiologies include direct trauma to the SA node (pericarditis, open heart surgery, rheumatic fever that leads to rheumatic heart disease), problems with the autonomic nervous system, and medications such as beta-blockers, digoxin (Lanoxin), and calcium channel blockers. Any condition that triggers atrial tissue to become inflamed or to deteriorate is a potential source.

When a patient presents with sick sinus syndrome, any of several dysrhythmias can occur. Often there is a combination of two or more. The most frequent include the following:

- Sinus bradycardia
- Sinus arrest/Sinus pause
- Alternating Bradycardia/Tachycardia of sinus node etiology
- Atrial fibrillation/Atrial flutter

Since such a variety of rhythms can occur with this difficult diagnosis, it is impossible to note standard measurements or configurations for EKG tracings

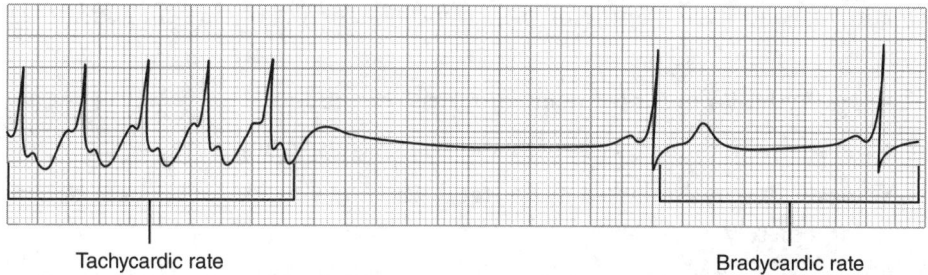

Tachycardic rate   Bradycardic rate

FIGURE 7−9 • Typical rhythm strip for sick sinus syndrome. This strip is representative of one way in which sick sinus syndrome may be manifested. A wide variety of cardiac monitor or EKG tracings can occur in this disease state.

or cardiac monitor strips. The alternating bradycardic and tachycardic rhythms are classic in this patient. Figure 7–9 is a typical strip for this patient.

Patients with this disorder may present with signs of heart failure including crackles in the lungs and an S_3 sound. They may also have a fluttering feeling in their chest, syncopal or near syncopal episodes, hypotension, chest pain, shortness of breath which worsens with exertion, blurred vision, and varying heart rates noted both on the cardiac monitor and by physically checking the radial pulse. Another interesting symptom that may occur is that the pulse does not increase with exercise and there is no other identified cause for this such as medications that the patient may be taking.

Asymptomatic patients may not require therapeutic regimens. Treatment for sick sinus syndrome is targeted at the underlying cause of the problem. If the patient is symptomatic, interventions should be provided that are directed at relief of these symptoms such as hypotension. Sometimes treating the tachyarrhythmia is counterproductive and can actually worsen the syndrome. Anticoagulants may be prescribed for the atrial fibrillation or flutter that represents the tachycardic portion of the disorder. The bradycardia may need to be treated with atropine or epinephrine. A temporary and subsequent permanent pacemaker is often used.

Conclusion

Sinus node dysrhythmias include sinus bradycardia, sinus tachycardia, sinus arrhythmia, sinus arrest and pauses, SA node blocks, and sick sinus syndrome. Each of these abnormal heart rhythms has its own distinguishing characteristics, symptoms, and treatment regimens. Often when patients are asymptomatic, no treatment is necessary. Some of the important aspects of this chapter are as follows:

- Dysrhythmias occur for many different reasons.
- Some dysrhythmias are benign and do not cause symptoms.
- Some dysrhythmias can be fatal if interventions are not begun immediately.
- Symptoms that patients may have include chest pain, palpitations, vomiting, anxiety, cold, clammy skin, arm and jaw pain, syncope, blurred vision, and sudden death.
- A perception of the heartbeat is called palpitations.
- Dysrhythmias are caused by disruptions of rate, regularity, originating impulse, or conduction of the impulse.
- The most common rhythm is normal sinus rhythm. All other rhythms are judged off of this rhythm.
- Sinus bradycardia is a slow heart rate that is below 60 beats per minute.
- All other aspects of the rhythm in sinus bradycardia are normal except for the rate.
- An inferior of posterior MI is associated with a bradycardic rhythm.
- Vagal stimulation will cause a slow heart rate.
- The vagus nerve is part of the parasympathetic nervous system.
- Coughing, straining, or vomiting can cause stimulation of the vagus nerve.
- Vagal stimulation is often performed on purpose to decrease fast heart rates.
- Atropine is one drug that can be used for symptomatic bradycardia.
- A pacemaker is a viable option for treatment of symptomatic bradycardia.
- An asymptomatic patent with sinus bradycardia often does not need treatment or may have a pacemaker placed on a scheduled, rather than emergent, basis.
- Bradycardia in an infant or child is an ominous sign.
- Sinus tachycardia occurs when the heart rate is over 100 beats per minute and all other parameters are normal.
- One of the most common causes of sinus tachycardia is anxiety.
- Some other etiologies of sinus tachycardia include hemorrhage, pain, hyperthyroidism, and pulmonary embolus.

- A patient with a very fast heart rate will have a weak and thready radial pulse.
- Sinus tachycardia can create a situation of decreased cardiac output.
- When cardiac output drops, this may be manifested by a low blood pressure and reduced peripheral oxygenation.
- Sinus tachycardia associated with an acute MI may be a sign of impending heart failure or cardiogenic shock.
- Patients with sinus tachycardia may need antianxiety medications, but also may require fluid replacement, cessation of bleeding, pain relief, temperature control, or the discontinuance of certain medications or street drugs.
- One of the first ways that children compensate for problems in the body is to increase the heart rate.
- Health care providers need to remember that even though children and infants normally have high heart rates, they should be cognizant of the fact that tachycardias do exist for these age groups and need to be recognized and treated seriously.
- Sinus arrhythmia is a normal cardiac response for children and for some adults up to age 30.
- Changes in heart rate associated with sinus arrhythmia are related to inspiration and expiration.
- Sinus arrhythmia has an irregular pattern. All other parameters are normal.
- Observe the cardiac monitor or the EKG tracing for a long period of time when interpreting the rhythm as sinus arrhythmia.
- Sinus arrest occurs when the SA node does not create an impulse.
- Sinus pause occurs when one to two complexes are lost. Sinus arrest is identified when there are three or more lost complexes in a row.
- Escape beats may occur from other cardiac tissue when sinus arrest occurs.
- Some patients with sinus pause or arrest may be asymptomatic.
- Other patients with sinus pause or arrest may have symptoms of light-headedness or syncopal episodes.
- An emergent or planned pacemaker may be necessary to treat patients with sinus arrest.
- Patients may present with other chief complaints such as falls or seizures when they are actually having episodes of sinus arrest or sinus pause.

- SA blocks exist but are difficult to interpret through the cardiac monitor or EKG tracing.
- Four SA blocks are listed in the literature, but SA block type I is not able to be distinguished from sinus arrest or pauses.
- The problem with sinus arrest or pauses has to do with a lack of automaticity.
- The problem with SA blocks is a lack of conductivity.
- Second-degree SA block type I is interpreted when there is a dropped complex and the previous beats have shorter and shorter P-P intervals.
- Second-degree SA block type II is seen when the P-P intervals are the same, but the period of time from the last complex before the dropped complex to the next complete complex is an exact multiple of the P-P interval.
- Third-degree SA block ends the dropped sinus beat period with a sinus beat.
- Sick sinus syndrome presents with a variety of dysrhythmias including sinus bradycardia, sinus arrest, sinus pause, atrial fibrillation, atrial flutter or an alternating bradycardia/tachycardia.
- Another name for sick sinus syndrome is brady-tachy syndrome.
- Sick sinus syndrome occurs due to destruction of the SA node.
- No standard measurements or configurations are manifested with sick sinus syndrome.
- Treating the cause of the problem is the main treatment regimen for sick sinus syndrome.
- Treating the tachyarrhythmia in sick sinus syndrome can be counterproductive.
- A pacemaker is the usual treatment of choice for sick sinus syndrome.

PRACTICE QUESTIONS

1. **A cause of dysrhythmias associated with sympathetic stimulation is:**

    A. pulmonary embolus.

    B. myocardial infarction.

    C. hyperthyroidism.

    D. tricyclic overdose.

2. **A palpitation would best be described as:**

   A. a feeling of impending doom.

   B. chest pain.

   C. diaphoresis.

   D. fluttering feeling in chest.

3. **In which of the following patients would a bradycardic rhythm most likely be a normal finding?**

   A. 3-year-old girl with strep throat

   B. 52-year-old male taking a beta-blocker

   C. 82-year-old female with a fractured hip

   D. 36-year-old male taking clindamycin (Cleocin)

4. **Sinus tachycardia can cause a patient to have a decreased cardiac output due to:**

   A. a decreased filling time.

   B. an increase in stroke volume.

   C. the slow heart rate.

   D. slower contraction of the ventricles.

5. **Children respond to illnesses by which of the following mechanisms?**

   A. Increase in stroke volume

   B. Strengthen ventricular contractions

   C. Accelerate heart rate

   D. Constriction of vessels

6. **Which of the following EKG characteristics would be present for an interpretation of sinus arrhythmia?**

   A. Irregular rhythm

   B. PR interval of 0.28 seconds

   C. P wave present—every other complex

   D. Rate—180 beats per minute

7. **A patient with prolonged periods of sinus arrest may need:**

   A. beta-blocker medications.

   B. a bolus dose of digoxin (Lanoxin).

   C. a temporary pacemaker.

   D. anticoagulant therapy.

8. **Which of the following characteristics would be present on the EKG tracing for an interpretation of SA arrest?**

   A. One to two dropped beats or complexes

   B. Regular rhythm

    C. Prolonged PR interval

    D. P wave present for each QRS present

9. Patients with either sinus arrest or SA node block may experience which of the following symptoms?

    A. Hypertension

    B. Syncope

    C. Fast heart rate

    D. Chills

10. SA node block occurs when there is a problem with:

    A. automaticity.

    B. contractility.

    C. reflexivity.

    D. conductivity.

11. Which of the following is another name for sick sinus syndrome?

    A. Sinus bradycardia

    B. Brady-tachy syndrome

    C. Sinus arrhythmia

    D. Sinus tachycardia

12. Which of the following would most likely be present with a diagnosis of sick sinus syndrome?

    A. Lack of increased pulse with exercise

    B. Hypertension with movement

    C. Temperature greater than 100.5°F (38°C)

    D. Double vision with halos around objects

13. Interpret this rhythm

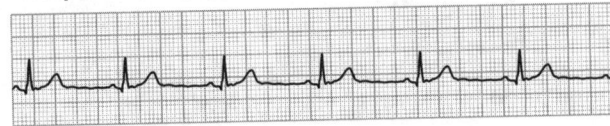

    A. Sinus tachycardia

    B. Sinus arrhythmia

    C. Sinus bradycardia

    D. Sinus pause

14. Interpret this rhythm

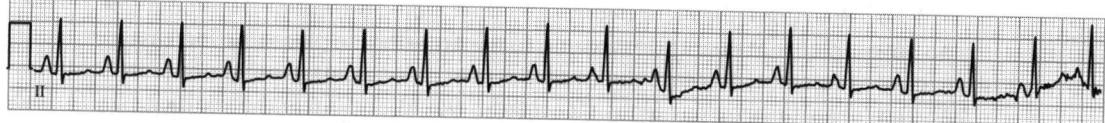

A. Sinus tachycardia
B. Sinus arrhythmia
C. Sinus bradycardia
D. Sinus pause

15. Interpret this rhythm

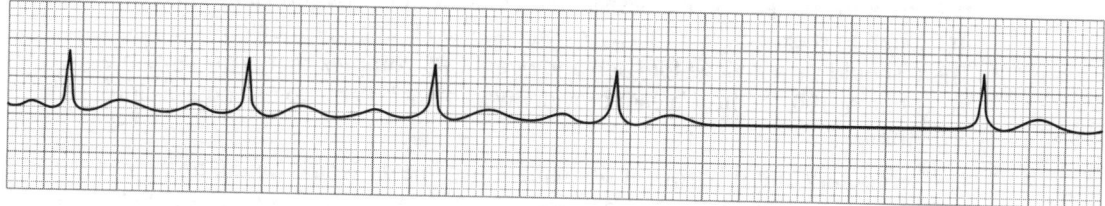

A. Sinus tachycardia
B. Sinus arrhythmia
C. Sinus bradycardia
D. Sinus pause

ANSWER KEY

1. **C.** Of the disease processes listed, hyperthyroidism is the one that deals with sympathetic stimulation which can cause major tachycardias. A pulmonary embolus would cause hypoxia which in turn would cause the tachycardia. A myocardial infarction would cause ischemia to a part of the heart which would cause the heart to beat faster and tricyclic overdose is a medication oriented cause that can cause tachycardia.

2. **D.** Most patients who have "palpitations" will relate a "fluttering feeling in my chest." The others listed are symptoms that might accompany a patient having cardiac problems, but would not explain the feeling of palpitations.

3. **B.** A patient taking a beta-blocker type of medication is at risk for not being able to increase their heart rate during periods of stress or other times when health care providers would expect the heart rate to be increased, that is, hypovolemia or dehydration. A child usually has a tachycardic rhythm until they become of an age when they near the normals for an adult (usually about age 12 or so). The antibiotic should not impact the heart rate and the hip fracture would only be accurate in this question if the patient were taking a beta-blocker.

4. **A.** When the heart rate increases, it decreases the time available for the ventricles to fill. This then correlates to a decrease in the cardiac output or the amount of blood available for the ventricles to send to the appropriate places. An increase in stroke volume would increase the cardiac output. A slow heart rate is not associated with sinus tachycardia. Sinus tachycardia would not cause the ventricles to contract more slowly.

5. **C.** Children attempt to increase their cardiac output and thus respond to stressors by accelerating their heart rate. They have a fixed stroke volume and the only thing left to do in order to increase cardiac output is to go into a tachycardia. This can be a normal compensatory response in ill children.

6. **A.** An irregular rhythm would be present in sinus arrhythmia due to the respiratory pattern of the patient. An increase in heart rate during inspiration and a decrease in expiration is expected in this dysrhythmia. The PR interval should not change. There should be a P wave for each and every QRS complex that is present. In a heart rate of 180, the health care provider would not be able to distinguish sinus arrhythmia.

7. **C.** A temporary and subsequent permanent pacemaker would be the treatment option of choice for a patient who is dealing with symptomatic sinus arrest. Beta-blockers and digoxin (Lanoxin) would decrease the pulse rate and potentially make it worse. Anticoagulant therapy would not be used for this dysrhythmia.

8. **D.** A P wave would precede each QRS complex that is present on a rhythm strip interpreted as sinus arrest. In sinus arrest greater than three dropped beats would be needed to diagnose this rhythm. One to two missed complexes are seen with sinus pause. The rhythm is irregular and there is no difference in the PR interval.

9. **B.** Syncope or near syncopal episodes can be associated with both sinus arrest and SA node block. The health care provider would not expect to see hypertension, tachycardia, or chills with these dysrhythmias.

10. **D.** SA node block is associated with a problem with conductivity. The SA node is firing, but the impulses are being blocked. In sinus arrest, the issue is with automaticity in which the SA node is not firing at all.

11. **B.** Another name for sick sinus syndrome is brady-tachy syndrome because both fast and slow heart rates are seen with this disorder.

12. **A.** One of the identifying characteristics associated with sick sinus syndrome is the inability for the heart to compensate during exercise with an increased pulse rate. The other symptoms would not be associated with this disease process.

13. **C.** This is a rhythm strip showing sinus bradycardia with a rate of 54. The rate is near normal but falls below the normal range of 60. All other aspects are normal.

14. **A.** This is an example of sinus tachycardia. All aspects are within normal range except the rate of 106 which is above the normal accepted rate of 100.

15. **D.** This rhythm shows sinus pause. Only one beat is missed and the complex that recovers the heart rate is junctional in nature because there is no P wave. If more than three complexes were missing, it would be called *sinus arrest*.

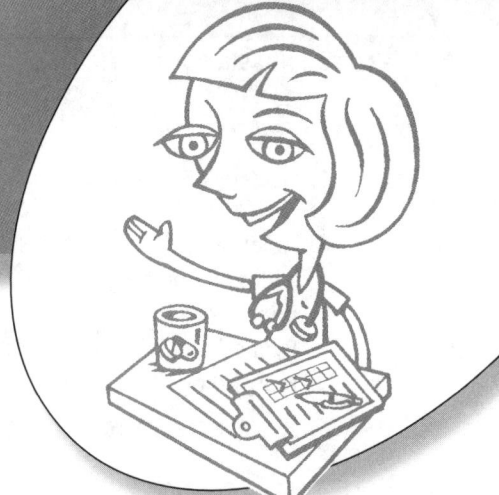

chapter **8**

Atrial/AV Nodal and Junctional Dysrhythmias

At the end of this chapter, the student will be able to:

1 List the atrial, AV nodal, and junctional dysrhythmias.

2 Distinguish the characteristics of each atrial, AV nodal, and junctional dysrhythmias.

3 Understand causes of atrial, AV nodal, and junctional dysrhythmias.

4 Define treatment regimens for atrial, AV nodal, and junctional dysrhythmias.

5 List health care provider responsibilities and special instructions/cautions for treatments of supraventricular tachycardias.

6 Describe symptoms that patients may experience with atrial, AV nodal, and junctional dysrhythmias.

Overview

In this chapter atrial/AV nodal and junctional rhythms will be discussed. Atrial/AV nodal rhythms are also known as supraventricular because they occur above the ventricles. Atrial rhythms arise from an area within the atria that is different than the SA node. AV nodal rhythms occur due to problems in conduction through the AV node. Junctional rhythms stem from the tissue surrounding the AV node and the bundle of His known as the AV junction. These abnormal electrical impulses generate altered complexes and cardiac contractions that may not be able to provide for the best cardiac output. Atrial kick, as discussed in Chapter 2, that provides a boost in blood volume of 10% to 30% during the last part of the atrial contraction is usually diminished in these dysrhythmias and therefore, impacts the end cardiac output for the patient. Atrial dysrhythmias are thought to occur from one of three separate disturbances. These were discussed in Chapter 3 and are reviewed below for the reader's convenience.

- Enhanced automaticity occurs in atrial tissue that does not normally function as an impulse generator. If the SA node is weakened and is not firing in a normal fashion, these foci will take over and create a new rhythm. Some of the causes of this reason for atrial dysrhythmias are hypocalcemia, hypokalemia, drug toxicity such as with digitalis compounds, hypoxia, acidosis, or something that might cause increased vagal tone. Remember that when the vagus nerve is stimulated, heart rate is decreased. Therefore, if the SA node has been given a command to decrease its automaticity, another site may choose to take over and cause new and varied rhythms to be produced.

- Reentry rhythms occur when an impulse is able to return through the circuit and restimulate tissue during the repolarization phase of the myocardium. This can happen due to a potential circuit in an accessory AV pathway, a blocked circuit (so it finds a different way to get around the block), or a delay in the conduction circuit. Disease processes such as an acute myocardial infarction, cardiomyopathy, hyperkalemia, ischemic cardiac tissue, coronary arterial disease, or some types of medications may be etiologies.

- Another name for triggered activity is "afterdepolarizations" and occurs during repolarization when cardiac cells are supposed to be silent or resting. A single impulse is created and it then stimulates tissue again or an escape type of pacemaker is triggered. This can create both atrial and ventricular dysrhythmias. This may produce one extra beat, extra beats that occur in "pairs," or three or more beats in a row called a run. A sustained rhythm developed from this triggered activity can also be generated. This may occur from such things as hypoxia, increase in release of epinephrine and norepinephrine in the body, injury to myocardial cells, ischemia to cardiac tissue, medications that might prolong the repolarization process (some antibiotics, antidepressants, heart medications, antipsychotics, etc.), and hypomagnesemia.

Atrial/AV Nodal Dysrhythmias

Premature Atrial Contraction

Any beat that appears out of the normal pattern and is "early," is considered to be a premature contraction or beat. It is easy to determine "prematurity" by using either calipers or a piece of paper to mark the QRS complexes. Find a point in the rhythm strip where there are two normal appearing sinus beats in a row. Make a mark on the piece of paper for each of these two QRS complexes. Move the piece of paper (or the calipers) so that the first mark on the piece of paper is on the second beat that was marked and note that the next beat falls exactly on the second mark on the piece of paper. Walk the piece of paper across the rhythm strip. The premature beat will fall out of the normal cadence of the regular sinus beats, that is, it will take place before the second mark on the piece of paper where a normal beat would be expected. If calipers are used, march the calipers across the rhythm strip in the same way and the premature beat will again be seen to fall short of the expected pace.

Premature beats occur from any tissue: atrial, AV junction, or ventricular. Premature atrial contractions or PACs, an atrial dysrhythmia, will be considered here. These may also be termed "premature atrial (or other location) complex" since many of them do not actually produce a contraction. These premature beats originating in the atrium are thought to occur as a consequence of altered automaticity or reentry problems.

Patients who have cardiac disease are at risk when PACs arise because they can be the forerunner of other atrial rhythms such as atrial fibrillation or atrial flutter. When associated with an acute myocardial infarction, they may indicate an impending episode of heart failure. Other causes of PACs include atrial enlargement, valvular disease, medication toxicities such as digitalis, electrolyte imbalances, or increased levels of thyroid hormone (hyperthyroidism).

> ### CLINICAL ALERT
>
> PACs can be considered to be a normal phenomenon and many "healthy" people can experience these. These extra beats can be prompted by the intake of certain items such as caffeine, nicotine, or alcohol and can also be generated during periods of fatigue or anxiety producing situations as well as disease processes such as infections or generalized fever. People who have these PACs may complain of "palpitations" or the feeling of a "skipped beat." PACs in patients who have non-diseased hearts are ordinarily not harmful.

A premature atrial contraction can be identified by a P wave that is both early in the cycle and has a different appearance than the other P waves in the rhythm strip. This P wave may have a notched formation, may be biphasic, or may look flat or pointed. The QRS that follows the premature P wave has the same configuration as the other QRS complexes that are present. There is also an incomplete or **noncompensatory pause** after the premature beat. A noncompensatory pause means that the distance between three normal beats compared to three beats that includes the premature beat is longer, that is, the three beats that include the premature beat is shorter. Figure 8–1 demonstrates the noncompensatory pause found with premature atrial contractions.

Characteristics of a PAC are given as follows (Fig. 8–2):

- **Regularity:** Irregular rhythm (underlying rhythm is regular)

- **Rate:** Can be normal, bradycardic, or tachycardic—more often is normal between 60 to 100 beats per minute

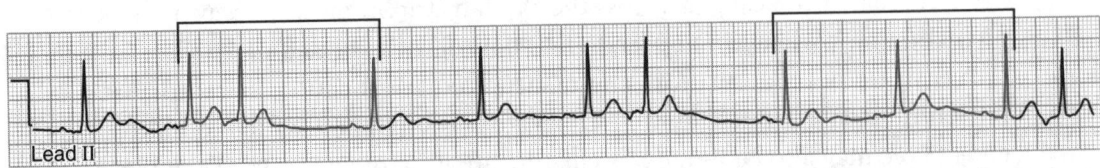

FIGURE 8–1 • Noncompensatory pause with PACs. In this lead II rhythm strip, the length of time between beats 2,3, and 4 (which includes the PAC as beat number 3),is 43 small boxes or 2.15 seconds. The length of time between three normal beats, that is, beats 8, 9, and 10 is 51 small boxes or 2.55 seconds. This is considered to be a noncompensatory pause because the time between three beats with the PAC is shorter than that noted between three normal beats.

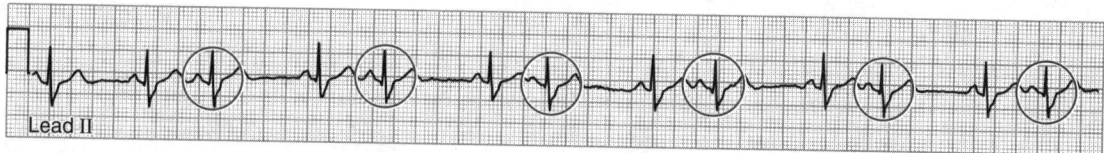

FIGURE 8–2 · Underlying normal sinus rhythm with PACs. Each of the circled complexes are PACs. This rhythm strip shows an underlying normal sinus rhythm with bigeminal PACs.

- **P wave:** Present for each QRS complex but is premature and can be of different configuration
- **PR interval:** May be normal—0.12 to 0.20 seconds or can be prolonged
- **QRS complex:** Less than 0.10 seconds in width—depends on the underlying rhythm
- **QT interval:** Normal
- **T wave:** Normal configuration and size
- **ST segment:** Normal configuration and size

Figure 8–2 demonstrates PACs that are occurring with an underlying normal sinus rhythm. Note that the PACs are arising after each normal beat. This is known as *bigeminy*. When these or other premature beats develop after every second beat, so that every third beat is premature, it is called *trigeminy*. Every fourth beat as a premature complex is *quadrigeminy*. When they occur otherwise, they are noted to be occasional. When premature beats occur together, they are said to "coupled" or "couplets". Three premature beats together would be called *tripling*.

Two other abnormalities that can occur with PACs are aberrantly conducted PACs and nonconducted PACs. If the PAC comes about very early in the cardiac cycle, it can be carried through the right bundle branch very slowly. This will cause a widened QRS complex which will not mimic the underlying rhythm. A nonconducted PAC means that the P wave occurred so early that it is actually buried within the T wave of the preceding complex and therefore was unable to complete conduction. The AV junction could not carry through another contraction or complex at that time.

Wandering Atrial Pacemaker

Wandering atrial pacemaker is also known by its abbreviation, WAP. A newer term is multiform atrial rhythm. When WAP occurs, the origination of the impulse changes from the SA node to another location or locations in the atria, or in the AV junction. This can also be known as a supraventricular rhythm because it occurs above the ventricles. Each impulse is conducted in a normal fashion through the ventricles; consequently, the duration of the QRS is the same. The P waves change their **morphology** each time the focus or origination of the impulse changes. In order to label a rhythm strip as wandering atrial pacemaker (multiform atrial rhythm) three or more distinct P waves are identified. P waves may be the same for at least two to three beats before the site travels to another location in the atria. The rate is usually normal or slow and may be a routine variant in normal, healthy young people, in athletic individuals, or in some patients during the sleep cycle. If the rate is higher than 100, this takes on a new classification called multifocal atrial tachycardia.

The rhythm strip will have the following features (Fig. 8–3):

- **Regularity:** May be slightly irregular due to different foci
- **Rate:** Usually normal or bradycardic
- **P wave:** Present for each QRS complex but at least three distinct P waves are seen per rhythm strip
- **PR interval:** Variable but usually remains below 0.20 seconds
- **QRS complex:** Less than 0.10 seconds in width
- **QT interval:** Normal or can vary
- **T wave:** Normal configuration and size
- **ST segment:** Normal configuration and size

CLINICAL ALERT

This is a dysrhythmia that is usually temporary. Because of this, the health care provider may see it on the cardiac monitor, but it may not manifest itself during the time the EKG tracing is taken. Be sure to print out rhythm strips that demonstrate this fleeting rhythm. Although it is not usually serious, in those patients who have cardiac disease, it bears watching and notification of the patient's medical provider. Patients may experience this if they have an increase in vagal or parasympathetic tone, some types of heart disease, or if they have developed digitalis toxicity.

Patients are usually unaware that this rhythm abnormality is taking place and no treatment is usually necessary. This dysrhythmia will usually assume a normal rhythm when the SA node is able to generate impulses at its normal firing rate again. Existing underlying disease processes or toxicity problems should be addressed as treatment.

Lead II

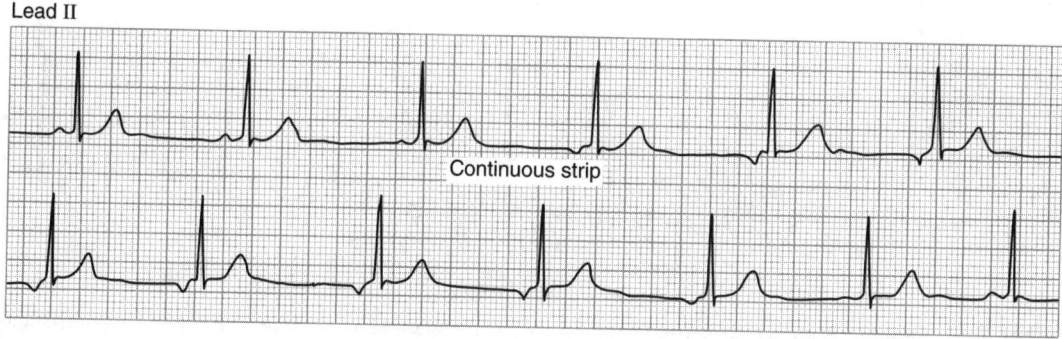

FIGURE 8–3 • Wandering atrial pacemaker/multiform atrial rhythm. Note the P waves on this rhythm strip. Each of these P waves are different and the R-R spacing is slightly irregular due to the different foci generating the impulse. This strip is a continuous strip and is sometimes documented as such in the chart by placing one strip on top of the other and noting on the information that it is a "continuous strip."

Multifocal Atrial Tachycardia

Wandering atrial pacemaker that presents with a rate greater than 100 beats per minute is labeled as multifocal atrial tachycardia (MAT), another supraventricular rhythm. Another name that might be used interchangeably with this is chaotic atrial tachycardia. As in wandering atrial pacemaker, the site that is generating the impulse for conduction is changing and therefore the P waves will have different configurations throughout the rhythm strip. One of the greatest identifying characteristics for this dysrhythmia is that although the rhythm is irregular and fast, there is a distinct P wave for each QRS complex.

The most common reason for this dysrhythmia is chronic obstructive pulmonary disease. Other causes include acute myocardial infarctions, hypoxia, sepsis, toxicities such as digitalis or theophylline, respiratory failure, electrolyte imbalances, and rheumatic heart diseases.

This is another dysrhythmia that usually will resolve once the underlying condition is diagnosed and treated appropriately. Therefore, the focus of treatment will include the overall picture of the patient and does not center on the dysrhythmia that the primary disorder has created. Medications may be ordered to control the rate.

Characteristics of multifocal atrial tachycardia include (Fig. 8–4):

- **Regularity:** Irregular
- **Rate:** Greater than 100 beats per minute (usually 100-200 beats per minute)
- **P wave:** Present for each QRS complex but at least three distinct P waves are seen per rhythm strip
- **PR interval:** Variable

Lead II

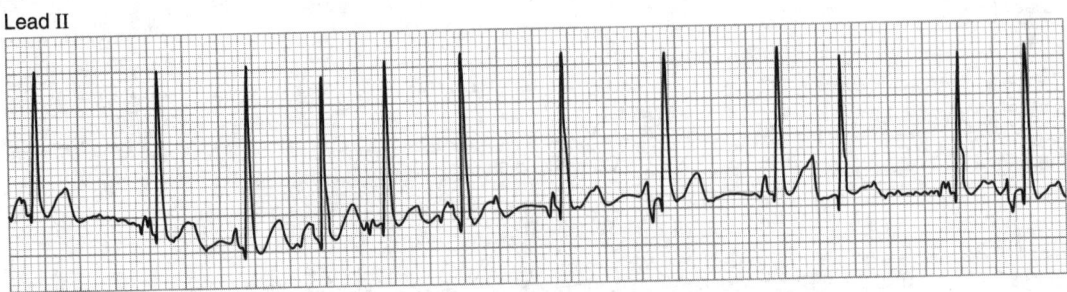

FIGURE 8–4 • Multifocal atrial tachycardia. Note that each QRS complex has a P wave. The P waves are of changing configurations.

- **QRS complex:** Less than 0.10 seconds in width
- **QT interval:** Can be difficult to determine
- **T wave:** Usually distorted
- **ST segment:** Usually distorted

CLINICAL ALERT

This dysrhythmia can sometimes be confused with atrial fibrillation. If the health care provider looks closely at the EKG tracing, multifocal atrial tachycardia will have visible P waves present for each QRS, which atrial fibrillation will not have.

Atrial Tachycardia

Both altered automaticity and triggered activity can cause atrial tachycardia, a form of a supraventricular tachycardia. When irritable tissue in the atria supersedes the SA node and fires at a high rate of speed—150 to 250 beats per minute—this action can shorten diastole reducing the atrial kick, ultimately shrinking cardiac output. This loss of cardiac output also places stress on heart tissue since coronary perfusion is decreased at the same time.

In generic atrial tachycardia each QRS complex is preceded by a P wave and the QRS complex is usually normal, however, the P wave will usually have a different type of configuration than if the SA node were the firing tissue. Short bursts of atrial tachycardia can be exhibited if three or more complexes are noted to represent a rate of 150 to 250 beats per minute. A sustained rhythm (lasting more than 30 seconds) may or may not arise (Fig. 8–5).

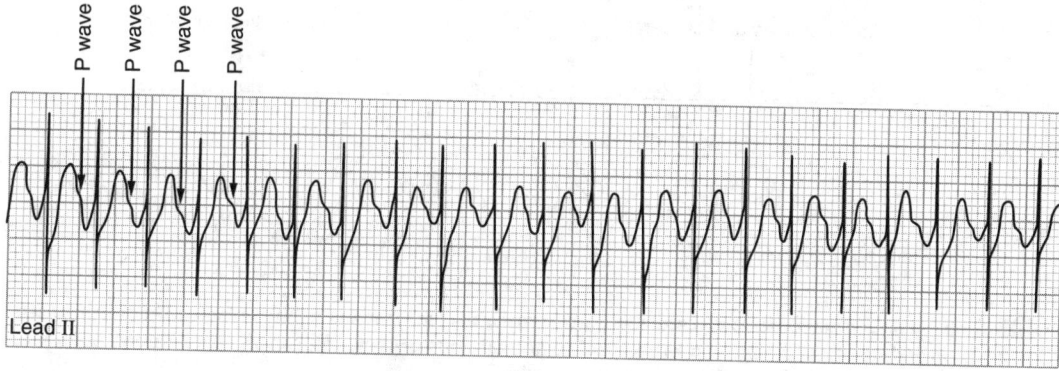

FIGURE 8–5 • **Atrial tachycardia.** In atrial tachycardia the rate is between 150-250 beats per minute. Each QRS has a P wave, but it is usually hidden within the T wave of the preceding complex. The rhythm is regular.

Characteristics of atrial tachycardia include:

- **Regularity:** Regular
- **Rate:** 150 to 250 beats per minute
- **P wave:** Present but the rate is so fast that they can be buried in the T wave of the previous beat—will have different configuration than normal SA node P wave
- **PR interval:** May vary
- **QRS complex:** Less than 0.10 seconds in width—may be aberrant
- **QT interval:** May be difficult to discern
- **T wave:** Usually distorted due to presence of P wave
- **ST segment:** Usually distorted

One form of atrial tachycardia is known as paroxysmal atrial tachycardia (PAT). This variety has a sudden beginning and ending and can be initiated by PACs. This can look closely like paroxysmal supraventricular tachycardia (PSVT), but may not respond to carotid massage as well as PSVT. A buildup to the increased rate and a slowdown period may be seen with the rhythm, PAT. In this type, a reentrant circuit may be present (Fig. 8–6).

Characteristics of paroxysmal atrial tachycardia include:

- **Regularity:** Regular
- **Rate:** 150 to 250 beats per minute for period of atrial tachycardia
- **P Wave:** Present—abnormal—may be buried in previous T wave
- **PR interval:** May vary
- **QRS complex:** Less than 0.10 seconds in width, but may be aberrant
- **QT interval:** May be difficult to determine

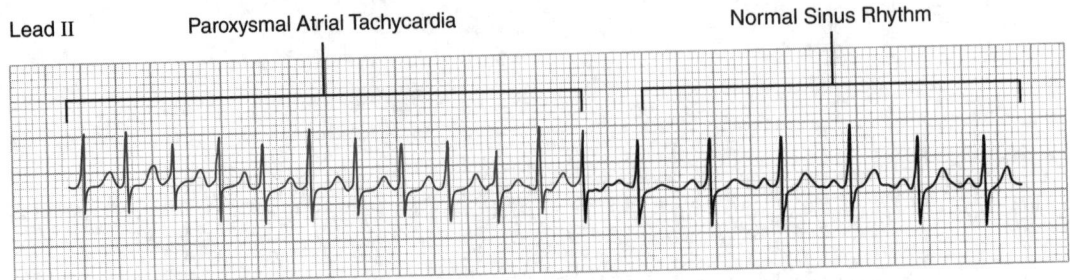

FIGURE 8–6 • Paroxysmal atrial tachycardia. In paroxysmal atrial tachycardia the beginning and ending may see a gradual build up and slowdown before converting back to normal sinus rhythm. This can also occur spontaneously. The P waves are buried in the T waves of the preceding complex.

- **T wave:** Usually distorted due to presence of P wave

- **ST segment:** Usually distorted

Another form of atrial tachycardia is atrial tachycardia with block. In this form the atria are firing at an increased rate of 150 to 250 beats per minute; however, the AV node protects the heart by not allowing each of these impulses to be conducted. The ventricular rate is slower and the block within the AV node can be constant or variable. Therefore, all three components—the atrial rate, the ventricular rate, and the block—can be regular, but separate. When regular blocks are present, the terms 2:1, 3:1, etc. may be used which denote that there are two atrial beats for each ventricular beat or three atrial beats for each ventricular beat that occurs. If the block is variable, that is, at times there are two atrial beats prior to a ventricular response and then three atrial beats with a ventricular response (this is only one example, any variety of variability can occur), then the rhythm is stated as atrial tachycardia with variable block. Multifocal atrial tachycardia (MAT) is also considered to be a form of atrial tachycardia (Figs. 8–7, 8–8, and 8–9).

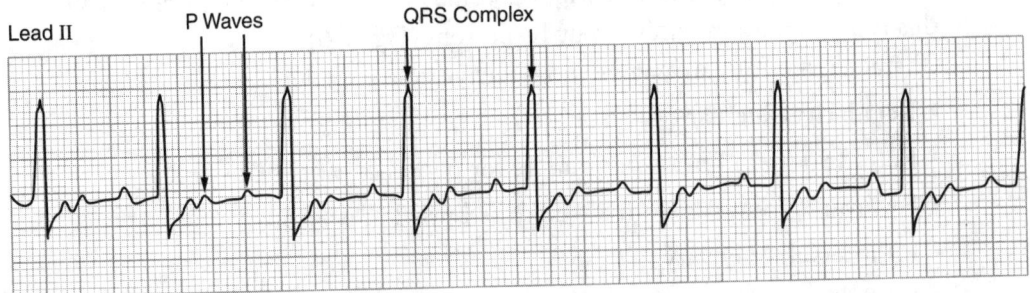

FIGURE 8–7 • Atrial tachycardia with 2:1 block. The atrial rate, the ventricular rate, and the block (2:1) are all regular. The AV node is blocking every other beat.

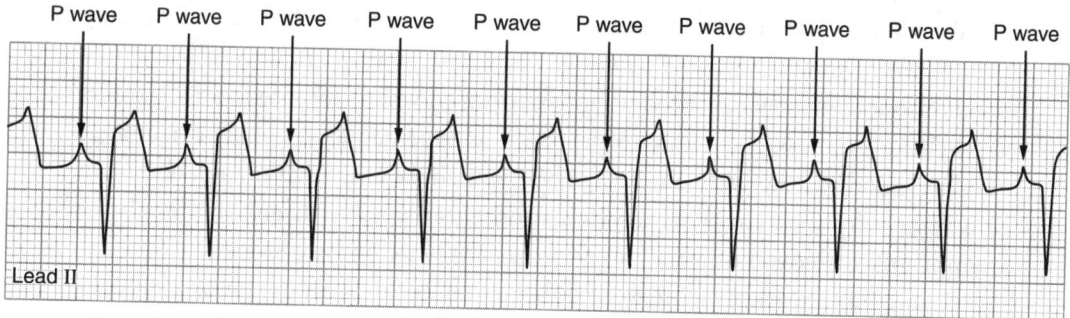

FIGURE 8−8 • Atrial tachycardia with 2:1 block. At times the P waves are hidden within the T wave or ST segment. Note the top of the T wave in each of these complexes. It has the same pointed type of appearance as the P waves before each QRS complex. Atrial rate is 180 beats per minute with a ventricular response of 90 beats per minute.

Characteristics of atrial tachycardia with block are:

- **Regularity:** Regular or irregular depending on block
- **Rate:** 150 to 250 beats per minute for period of atrial tachycardia
- **P wave:** Present—morphology may be abnormal— may be buried in previous T wave—more P waves than QRS complexes
- **PR interval:** 0.12 to 0.20 seconds
- **QRS complex:** Less than 0.10 seconds
- **QT interval:** May be difficult to determine
- **T wave:** Can be distorted due to presence of P wave
- **ST segment:** Usually distorted

CLINICAL ALERT

Interpreting EKGs can be a difficult process when attempting to determine rhythms that are fast. Health care providers will find throughout their practice that sometimes practitioners will not always agree with analyses of EKG tracings. The faster rhythms are difficult and do not always conform to "black and white" rules.

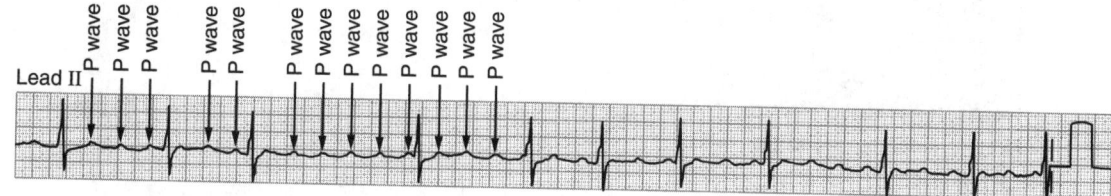

FIGURE 8−9 • Atrial tachycardia with variable block. Notice the variable number of P waves between each QRS complex. The P waves represent an atrial rate of 210 and the QRS complex displays a ventricular rate of 62.

Patients with atrial tachycardias may present with no symptoms or may complain of the feeling of "fluttering" associated with palpitations. They may feel dyspneic, have generalized weakness, blurred vision, hypotension, dizziness or lightheadedness, chest pain or pressure, or have had a syncopal or near syncopal episode. If the tachycardic episode was short, they will most likely have no symptoms or state that they felt momentarily ill with any of the above symptoms. Etiologies of atrial tachycardias are listed in Box 8–1.

Caring for individuals with atrial tachycardias depends on the patient's condition, the cause, and the type of tachycardia. Treating the cause is a vital intervention. It is important to know what medications the patient is taking, such as digitalis, as well as creating an environment in which the patient feels safe to acknowledge the intake of illicit drugs. Valsalva's technique and carotid sinus massage (to be discussed later) can be attempted, but does not usually work as well with these dysrhythmias. A momentary slowing of the heart rate may be seen with a subsequent return to the rhythm. Medications such as Adenocard (adenosine),

---

BOX 8–1   Etiologies of Atrial Tachycardias

- Pharmacologic Ingestions
  - Caffeine
  - Marijuana
  - Bath salts
  - Cocaine
  - Digitalis
  - Albuterol
  - Theophylline compounds
- Infectious processes
- Hyperthyroidism
- Acute myocardial infarction
- Cor Pulmonale
- Hypertension (systemic)
- Electrolyte abnormalities
- Stress
- Hypoxia
- Cardiomyopathy
- Wolff-Parkinson-White (WPW) syndrome
- Excessive catecholamines
- Valvular disease
- Sick Sinus Syndrome

Amiodarone, calcium channel blockers, or beta-blockers may be attempted. **Synchronized cardioversion**, atrial overdrive pacemaker, or catheter **ablation** may also be used when medications are not successful.

Paroxysmal Supraventricular Tachycardia

The term supraventricular simply means that the impulse generator is above the ventricles. Many types of dysrhythmias are labeled "supraventricular" including the atrial tachycardias listed above and both atrial fibrillation and atrial flutter. When P waves are not present, the term PSVT or paroxysmal supraventricular tachycardia can be used. Two types of PSVT are usually discussed and are known by the causative factor that generates their impulse formation and subsequent conductions. These are known as AV nodal reentrant tachycardia (AVNRT) and AV reentrant tachycardia (AVRT). In AVNRT a reentry problem occurs at the AV node. Two pathways are actually present—one fast and one slow. Two factors are present which allows for the extremely fast heart rate. These factors are the rate at which the impulse can be conducted through the pathway and the recovery time, known as the *refractory period*. One pathway conducts impulses rapidly but has a slower refractory period which allows for an extended recovery period. The second pathway, the slower one, takes a longer time to process the impulse and conduct it through the tissue, but has a shorter refractory time which allows for a more rapid recovery phase. When these two are working together, impulses are going through both areas, and a loop is formed where one side is in its recovery or refractory interval and the other is generating an impulse that is able to pass through. An open ended circuit is created and rapid, regular rhythms are created. These are usually narrow complex tachycardias.

In AVRT the reentry occurs due to a pathway that is not in the AV node or the bundle of His. This pathway is still above the ventricles; however, since it travels through a different passageway, it has a special term, **preexcitation**, associated with it. Preexcitation means that the ventricle is triggered earlier than expected because of the special conduit that has been created. This pathway is an **accessory pathway**. Sometimes an accessory pathway will actually connect back to the normal route of the AV node. If this happens it is called a **bypass tract**.

One very good example of this type of reentry supraventricular tachycardia is Wolff-Parkinson-White (WPW) syndrome. In this disease process, the pathway is created during fetal development by extra filaments of cardiac tissue that constructed a special bridge connecting the atria and the ventricles. This bridge is called the **bundle of Kent**.

CLINICAL ALERT

When the tachycardia, WPW is present, the identifying characteristics of this distinctive syndrome are not able to be recognized. These characteristics are noted on the normal EKG tracing prior to or after the tachydysrhythmia has terminated. See Table 8–1 for the distinguishing traits of this disorder. Another important aspect of this unique disease process is that it usually occurs in infants, young children, and adults up to the age of 35 years.

TABLE 8–1   Distinguishing Traits for Wolff-Parkinson-White (WPW) Syndrome

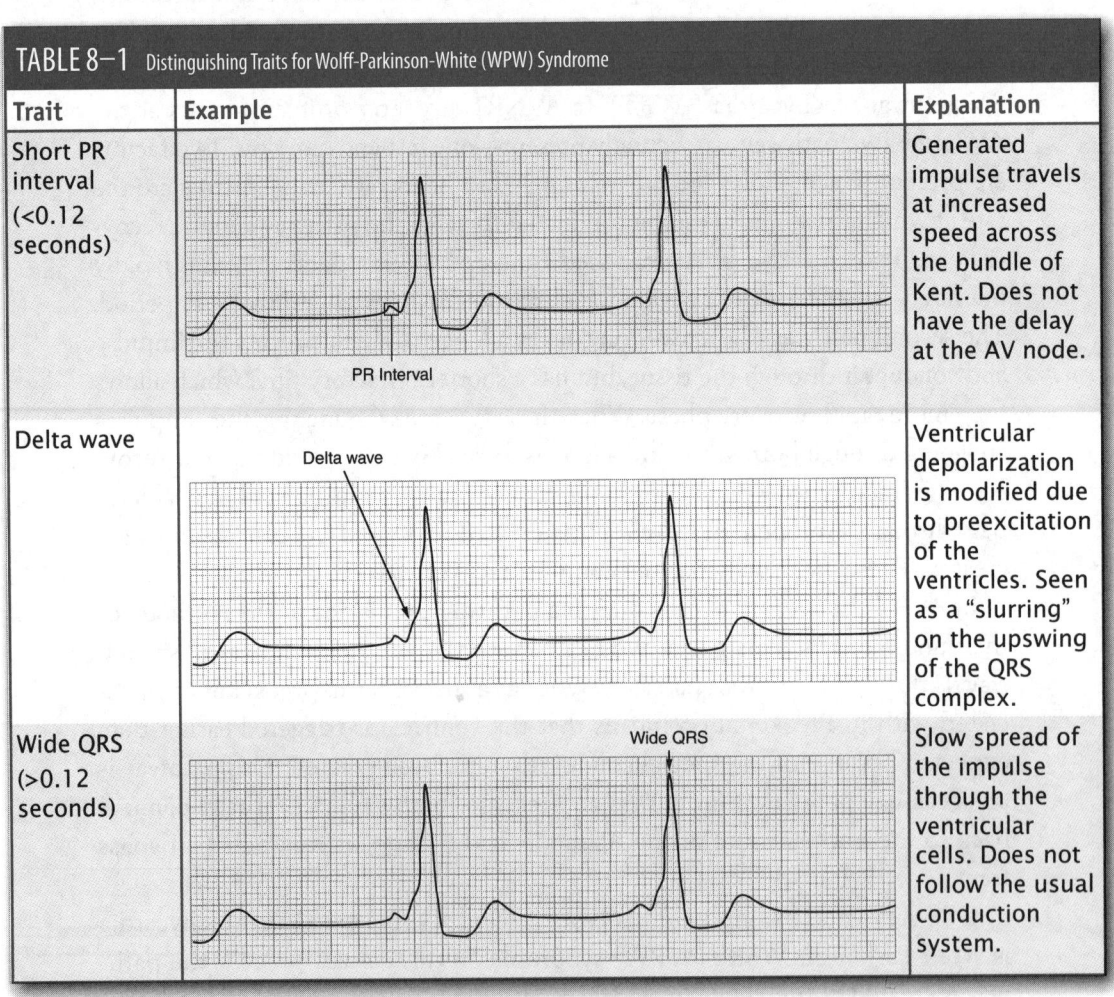

Trait	Example	Explanation
Short PR interval (<0.12 seconds)	PR Interval	Generated impulse travels at increased speed across the bundle of Kent. Does not have the delay at the AV node.
Delta wave	Delta wave	Ventricular depolarization is modified due to preexcitation of the ventricles. Seen as a "slurring" on the upswing of the QRS complex.
Wide QRS (>0.12 seconds)	Wide QRS	Slow spread of the impulse through the ventricular cells. Does not follow the usual conduction system.

Lead II

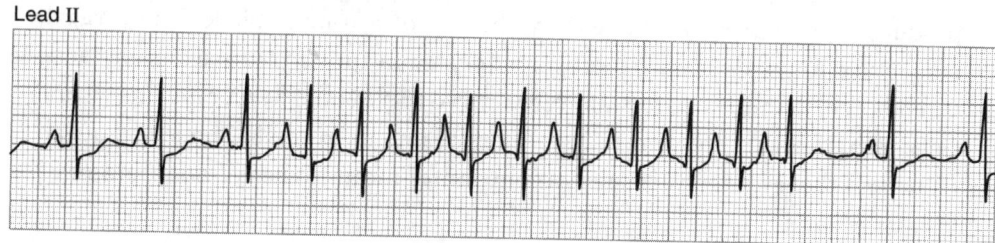

FIGURE 8–10 • **Paroxysmal supraventricular tachycardia.** Paroxysmal supraventricular tachycardia (PSVT) begins and ends suddenly. This tracing shows the abrupt beginning and ending.

When PSVT is present, the following characteristics will be present (Figs. 8–10 and 8–11):

- **Regularity:** Regular
- **Rate:** 150 to 250 beats per minute
- **P wave:** Undetectable—may be hidden within the QRS complex
- **PR interval:** Not measurable
- **QRS complex:** Less than 0.10 seconds
- **QT interval:** May be difficult to determine
- **T wave:** Can be distorted due to presence of P wave
- **ST segment:** May be depressed

Patients who present with PSVT are usually symptomatic. They may complain of dizziness, shortness of breath, chest discomfort, palpitations, lightheadedness, near syncope, syncopal episodes, anxiety, heart failure, decreased mentation, nausea, vomiting, and general weakness. The health care provider may be able to see the heart beats in the neck (carotid artery). Hypotension can also occur and is a good sign that the patient is not tolerating the fast rhythm.

Treatments for PSVT include Vagal maneuvers which include massaging the carotid artery, placing the patient's face in ice water or using ice to the face, Valsalva's maneuver, having the patient cough or hold their breath, or

Lead II

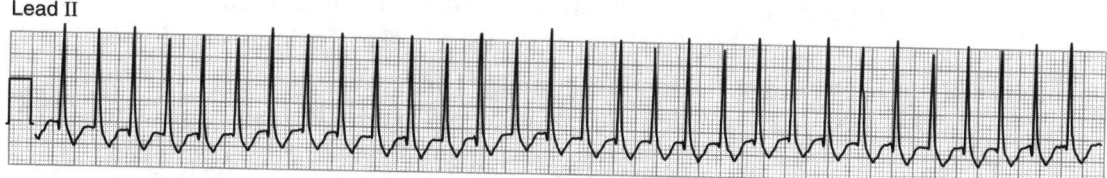

FIGURE 8–11 • **Sustained paroxysmal supraventricular tachycardia.** Paroxysmal supraventricular tachycardia can sustain for a lengthy period of time. Interventions will be necessary for this rhythm.

producing gagging in the patient by the use of a tongue blade. These vagal maneuvers stimulate the baroreceptors, located in the carotid arteries and aortic arch, which in turn incites the vagus nerve to slow the heart rate. The right-sided vagus nerve is thought to have more filaments in the SA node and atrial tissue and the leftsided vagus nerve contributes more to the AV node and ventricular muscle.

Other treatment options include the use of Adenocard (adenosine), diltiazem (Cardizem), synchronized cardioversion, and catheter ablation. See Table 8–2 for procedures, physiological responses, responsibilities for the health care provider, and special instructions/cautions to be observed for each of these treatment options.

> ### CLINICAL ALERT
>
> Do not use Adenosine (Adenocard) on patients with Wolff-Parkinson-White (WPW) syndrome. Any medication that slows the conduction through the AV node can actually speed up the use of the accessory pathway and cause an increase in the already high speed rate. Other medications to avoid include digitalis (Digoxin) and diltiazem (Cardizem).

Atrial Fibrillation

Atrial fibrillation, a common dysrhythmia, can be caused by either a reentry problem or the rapid firing of ectopic sites within the atrial tissue (altered automaticity). When this rhythm occurs, there is a loss of atrial kick and stroke volume, and cardiac output can suffer. The atria are not able to produce good quality contractions during this dysrhythmia. They are in a state of quivering or fibrillation and therefore, no discernible P waves are present in this rhythm. A wavy or straight line (fibrillatory waves or f waves) between R waves is seen which is very irregular. These waves may be large (coarse A fib) or small (fine A fib). The AV node protects the heart by blocking the hundreds of chaotic impulses which are rapidly firing at that time. Intermittent impulses are conducted through to the ventricles. The atrial rate can in fact rise as far as 400 to 600 beats per minute. The ventricular rate will vary dependent on the rate of block in the AV node. This rhythm can occur with WPW as well which can then progress to ventricular tachycardia. This is contingent on the refractoriness of the bundle of Kent as the impulses are directed through this passageway.

TABLE 8–2 Treatment Options for Supraventricular Tachycardias

		Treatment Options for Supraventricular Tachycardias	
Procedure	Physiological Response	Health Care Provider Responsibilities	Special Instructions/Cautions
Carotid massage	• Stimulation of baroreceptors with subsequent stimulation of vagus nerve	• This is a physician procedure. • Monitor patient before, during, and after procedure. • Patient should have oxygen applied as per institution policy, a patent intravenous line, and placement on cardiac monitor. • Resuscitative equipment should be at the bedside. • Be sure to document pre massage rhythm via cardiac monitoring strip or EKG tracing, patient response to rhythm, and vital signs. • Document time of start and completion of carotid massage. • Run continuous strip during massage. • Document return to normal sinus rhythm via notes, rhythm strip, new EKG tracing, patient response, and vital signs.	• Physician should listen for bruits prior to performing this procedure. • Watch closely for bradycardia or asystole as the massage is being performed. • Always make sure EKG is performed post conversion to NSR • Older adults should not have carotid massage performed due to possibility of the presence of atherosclerosis in the carotid artery that could cause a stroke during manipulation of the carotid artery. • Both carotid arteries should **never** be massaged at the same time.
Valsalva maneuver	• Stimulation of baroreceptors with subsequent stimulation of vagus nerve • (Increases intrathoracic pressure)	• This is a physician procedure. • The patient will be instructed to hold their breath and bear down as if they are having a bowel movement. • Another way to perform this is to have the patient attempt to blow through a small straw such as a coffee stirrer or a straw that is closed at the other end. • Obtain 12-lead EKG and cardiac monitor strip prior to this procedure. • Monitor patient before, during, and after procedure.	• Watch closely for conversion to normal sinus rhythm. Patient may convert to a bradycardia or asystole. • Perform EKG post conversion.

TABLE 8–2 Treatment Options for Supraventricular Tachycardias (*Continued*)

Treatment Options for Supraventricular Tachycardias

Procedure	Physiological Response	Health Care Provider Responsibilities	Special Instructions/Cautions
		• Patient should have oxygen applied as per institution policy, a patent intravenous line, and placement on cardiac monitor. • Resuscitative equipment should be at the bedside. • Be sure to document pre-maneuver rhythm via cardiac monitoring strip or EKG tracing, patient response to rhythm, and vital signs. • Document time of start and completion of Valsalva maneuver. • Run continuous strip during procedure. • Document return to normal sinus rhythm via notes, rhythm strip, new EKG tracing, patient response, and vital signs.	
Coughing, holding breath, gagging	• Stimulation of baroreceptors with subsequent stimulation of vagus nerve	Same as for Valsalva maneuver. Gagging usually performed by physician using tongue blade to stimulate gag reflex through contact with oropharynx.	• Same as for Valsalva maneuver.
Cold water	• Stimulation of baroreceptors with subsequent stimulation of vagus nerve	• This can be accomplished in a variety of ways : • Place ice water in a basin and have patient immerse their face in the basin. • Place a towel or cloth soaked in iced water over the face of the patient • Place a cold pack on the patient's face. • Place an iced glove or plastic bag on patient's face. • During this procedure follow the same instructions as for Valsalva maneuver.	• Same as for Valsalva maneuver.

| Adenosine (Adenocard) | • Slows the SA node
• Slows conduction in the AV node
• Impedes reentry pathways | • This procedure can be performed by a health care provider who is allowed via appropriate legal practice acts to administer this medication. Health care providers who are licensed to administer this medication may perform this procedure as outlined in institutional or organizational policies.
• The physician should be present in the room at the time of administration. (This may also be performed in a prehospital setting at which time the physician will not be present).
• Monitor patient before, during, and after procedure.
• Patient should have oxygen applied as per institution policy, a patent intravenous line in the right antecubital area, and placement on cardiac monitor.
• Resuscitative equipment should be at the bedside.
• Be sure to document pre medicated rhythm via cardiac monitoring strip or EKG tracing, patient response to rhythm, and vital signs.
• Document time of start and completion of administration of medication.
• Run continuous strip during administration of medication.
• Document return to normal sinus rhythm via notes, rhythm strip, new EKG tracing, patient response, and vital signs.
• Up to three doses can be used to attempt to return the heart rhythm to a normal baseline. The first dose is 6 mg. Subsequent doses are 12 mg. | • The preferred intravenous site is the right antecubital area. A large bore intravenous catheter is also preferred. This is due to the very short half-life (<10 seconds) of the medication. It must get to the heart very quickly.
• An intravenous wide open drip of the physician's choice should be running during administration.
• Use most proximal port in the intravenous tubing as possible.
• This medication must be administered as fast as possible (again due to short half-life).
• Two health care providers are necessary to administer this medication.
• One health care provider pushes the medication quickly as a bolus dose.
• As soon as the first health care provider has pushed the actual medication another health care provider must then administer 20-30 ml of normal saline as quickly as possible behind the bolus dose of the medication. |

(Continued)

TABLE 8–2 Treatment Options for Supraventricular Tachycardias (*Continued*)

Treatment Options for Supraventricular Tachycardias

Procedure	Physiological Response	Health Care Provider Responsibilities	Special Instructions/Cautions
		• If this medication does not work, Diltiazem (Cardizem) may be used. This medication is given as a bolus dose, however, given slowly with observations of heart rate and blood pressure during the administration and then as a drip.	• Each health care provider will utilize closely approximated ports in the intravenous tubing and will work in concert with each other in the administration of each bolus. • Make sure the fluids are infusing in a wide open manner during this procedure. • It is sometimes useful for the right arm (the one in which the intravenous line is running) to be raised immediately after the bolus doses have been provided. • Watch the cardiac monitor closely. • This medication usually causes a short period of asystole. Be prepared for this event. • After the asystole, normal sinus rhythm should resume, however, other rhythms could also occur. • Make sure to prepare the patient for symptoms they may experience during the period of asystole—breathlessness—chest pain—lightheadedness. Explain that this will be short lived.

- Reassure them that they are surrounded by health care providers, the physician is present and that it is expected. Do not hesitate to hold the patient's hand during this experience. It is quite frightening for the patient.
- If family is allowed in the room during this procedure, be sure to explain that "flat line" on the monitor is expected.
- Acquire a second EKG after conversion to a normal rhythm.
- Recheck vital signs immediately after conversion.
- This medication can cause flushing of the face, cough, and bronchospasm.
- This medication should **not** be used on patients who are severely asthmatic.
- Other patients who should be considered to be at high risk for the use of this medication are those with advanced coronary artery disease due to the potential of coronary vascular ischemia in diseased vessels.
- Do not administer this medication to patients with WPW. It will exacerbate the problem.

(Continued)

TABLE 8−2 Treatment Options for Supraventricular Tachycardias (*Continued*)

Treatment Options for Supraventricular Tachycardias

Procedure	Physiological Response	Health Care Provider Responsibilities	Special Instructions/Cautions
Synchronized cardioversion	• Interrupts atrial depolarization	• This procedure can be performed by a health care provider who is allowed via appropriate legal practice acts to administer this medication. Health care providers who are licensed to deliver synchronized cardioversion may perform this procedure as outlined in institutional or organizational policies. • The physician will be present during the performance of this procedure. • Monitor patient before, during, and after procedure. • Patient should have oxygen applied as per institution policy, a patent intravenous line, and placement on both cardiac monitor and defibrillator monitor. • Resuscitative equipment should be at the bedside. • Be sure to document preprocedure rhythm via cardiac monitoring strip or EKG tracing, patient response to rhythm, and vital signs. • Document time of delivered shocks and joules delivered. • Run continuous strip during delivery of shocks or immediately after. • Document return to normal sinus rhythm via notes, rhythm strip, new EKG tracing, patient response, and vital signs.	• Explain the procedure to the patient in detail. This is again a frightening procedure and requires much reassurance and compassion from the staff. • Remove any patches such as nitroglycerin patches etc. from the patient's chest. • Apply patches appropriately to the patient's chest as per institution policy and equipment instructions. • If paddles are going to be used make sure that appropriate gel or gel pads are present and appropriately positioned on the patient's chest. • **The "sync" (synchronization) button must be "on."** • The patient must be connected to the machine that will be delivering the shock. • The machine must be recognizing each R wave on the screen. • The gain may need to be adjusted on the machine for it to recognize each R wave. • A "blip" or some type of marker should be seen at the top of each R wave that is "flagging" each R wave. This is important in order for the machine to deliver the shock at the appropriate time.

		• Administer sedation as prescribed by the provider caring for the patient.
		• Set the appropriate joules to be delivered dependent on provider choice and rhythm presenting.
		• Charge the machine.
		• Make sure that no one is touching the patient—"All Clear—All Clear" or an accepted version of this.
		• When delivering the charge, the discharge button must be held until the charge is delivered (per equipment instructions). The charge is delivered at the top of one of the R waves.
		• If there are two buttons to deliver the charge, both must be held until delivery.
		• If handheld paddles are utilized, they must be held in place until delivery of the charge. (Synchronized cardioversion is different than defibrillation.)
		• If subsequent shocks are necessary, each of the above steps will need to be repeated including turning the sync button on each time.
		• Monitor and observe patient prior to admission.
Catheter ablation	• Delivery of high frequency current to destroy tissue	• Prepare the patient for admission to unit or electrophysiology laboratory.

> ## CLINICAL ALERT
>
> Heart rates can vary with atrial fibrillation. When the heart rate is under 100 beats per minute, it is said to be "controlled." Over 100 beats per minute constitutes an "uncontrolled" atrial fibrillation. Heart rates over 100 beats per minute are also classified as RVR or rapid ventricular response. Bradycardic rates can also be realized in this rhythm. When counting rates for this type of rhythm the rule of counting R waves in a 6-second strip is usually utilized due to the irregularity. This will provide an average of the rate. The small or large box method can be utilized as well. When this is performed, a range of the pulse rate is obtained. The health care provider will notice that often a wide range will be present with this method. It is not unusual to document "heart rate ranges from mid 70's to 120" or more specific numbers may be obtained using the box method between two complexes.

The cornerstone of characteristics for this rhythm is the irregularly irregular rhythm and the loss of the P wave. The features are as follows (Figs. 8–12 and 8–13):

- **Regularity:** Irregularly irregular
- **Rate:** Atrial—400 to 600 beats per minute. Ventricular—varies
- **P wave:** Undetectable
- **PR interval:** Not measurable
- **QRS complex:** Less than 0.10 seconds
- **QT interval:** Not measurable
- **T wave:** Undetectable
- **ST segment:** Can be depressed

Atrial fibrillation can occur in short episodes or can become a sustained rhythm. New onset atrial fibrillation is especially concerning. In older patients and those who have underlying cardiac disease, the loss of cardiac output associated with this rhythm, particularly with the faster rhythms, can place

Lead II

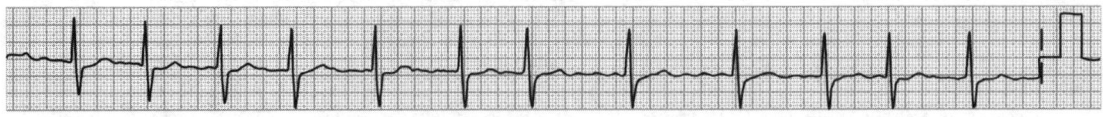

FIGURE 8–12 • Controlled atrial fibrillation. The average ventricular response in this rhythm strip is 78 beats per minute. Notice the irregularly irregular rhythm and the wavy line between QRS complexes.

Lead II

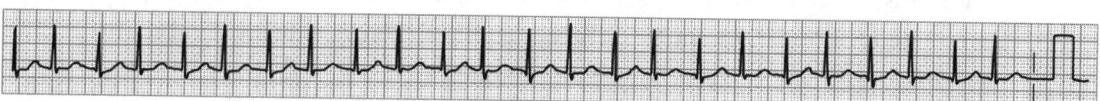

FIGURE 8–13 · Uncontrolled atrial fibrillation (RVR). The heart rate in this rhythm strip is an average of 145 beats per minute. Notice again the irregularly irregular rhythm. As ventricular rates increase, the irregularity is sometimes more difficult to see.

these populations of patients at high risk for complications. Box 8–2 includes several disease processes which can instigate atrial fibrillation.

On occasion normal healthy individuals will develop atrial fibrillation associated with elevated alcohol intake, stress, or increased caffeine intake. In these instances, the rhythm is usually temporary and responds easily to medications or spontaneously converts to a normal sinus rhythm.

BOX 8–2 Causes of Atrial Fibrillation

- Acute myocardial infarction
- Status post cardiac surgery
- Hypotension/hypertension
- Excessive alcohol intake
- Nicotine excess
- Stress
- Pulmonary embolism
- Aging
- Rheumatic heart disease
- Chronic obstructive pulmonary disease
- Electrolyte imbalances
- Sick sinus syndrome
- Heart failure
- Ischemic heart
- Wolff-Parkinson-White (WPW) syndrome
- Diabetes
- Caffeine intake
- Mitral valve problems (Insufficiency/stenosis)
- Hyperthyroidism
- Hypoglycemia
- Electrocution
- Infectious processes
- Coronary artery disease
- Pericarditis
- Hypoxia
- Congenital atrial septal defects

Symptoms associated with atrial fibrillation can include hypotension, palpitations, syncope or near syncope, lightheadedness, dizziness, shortness of breath, chest discomfort, or fatigue. Apical and radial pulses can vary. Some patients are asymptomatic.

CLINICAL ALERT

Health care providers should be aware that it is important to actually feel radial pulses in their patients even though machines are present to perform the function of pulse rates. An irregular radial pulse can alert the health care professional to an asymptomatic atrial fibrillation or encourage proper questioning of a patient who is unknowingly withholding information regarding symptoms.

Treating atrial fibrillation is dependent on the length of time the dysrhythmia has been present and the manner in which the patient is tolerating the abnormal rhythm. Treatment regimens consist of controlling the rate with medications such as diltiazem (Cardizem), prescribing anticoagulants, and the use of synchronized cardioversion in the face of a seriously symptomatic patient. Cardioversion can also be attempted in patients who are not responding to other treatment options. Best results for the patient are achieved with this option if the rhythm has not been present for long periods of time, especially for those who have experienced it less than 48 hours. Another treatment option may be that of catheter ablation in the electrophysiology setting.

CLINICAL ALERT

Patients who have atrial fibrillation (or flutter) are at risk for the development of thrombi in the atria since they are not fully contracting and emptying their chambers. This is a problematic factor in caring for someone who carries this rhythm normally as well as for the patient who suddenly develops it. Thrombi can break off from the wall of either atria and be propelled into either the systemic or pulmonary system at any time. These patients are at high risk for stroke due to this phenomenon. Long term atrial fibrillation requires the use of anticoagulants to decrease the possibility of this event. If synchronized cardioversion is used after 48 hours of the onset of this dysrhythmia, anticoagulant therapy is recommended if it is possible depending on the patient's condition. When the patient converts to a normal rhythm, the propulsion of a thrombus can occur at this time as the atria are able to contract in a better form.

Atrial Flutter

Atrial flutter, a reentry rhythm, occurs when there is one ectopic focus in the atrium that is sending multiple impulses. Again, the protective AV node only allows so many of these impulses through and there is a variance in the atrial and ventricular rates. The atrial rate typically ranges from 250 to 450 beats per minute and the ventricular rate will depend on the number of impulses allowed through the AV node. When interpreting this rhythm, the "conduction" will be addressed as a ratio of atrial beats to ventricular responses such as "2:1 conduction," or "4:1 conduction." At times the conduction will be variable and is recorded as such, that is, "variable conduction." It is appropriate to use the term "conduction" instead of "block" since the AV node is responding in a physiological manner, not a diseased state. A 1:1 conduction may be caused by the presence of an accessory pathway. In this situation the AV node is bypassed.

The chief identifying characteristic of this rhythm is the sawtooth pattern to the P waves. The isoelectric line is absent as these flutter waves occupy the entire period between QRS complexes. These waves are also known as F waves (capital F as opposed to lower case f for fibrillatory waves). Atrial flutter may be divided into two categories:

- *Type I* indicates a reentry problem where the inciting impulse loops around one particular area in the right atrium. This produces atrial rates ranging from 250 to 350 beats per minute.

- *Type II* is also known as "atypical." Patients will have very fast atrial heart rates ranging from 350 to 450 beats per minute and may develop atrial fibrillation. The mechanism of action has not been clearly defined.

Sometimes patients will move back and forth between atrial fibrillation and atrial flutter.

CLINICAL ALERT

When naming this rhythm it is often hard to distinguish a 2:1 or 1:1 conduction from other tachycardias. Look for the sawtooth pattern. The performance of vagal maneuvers by the physician or licensed practitioner may slow the rhythm enough to visualize the sawtooth design. Also, when vagal maneuvers are used, the rhythm will decelerate but will not convert with atrial flutter.

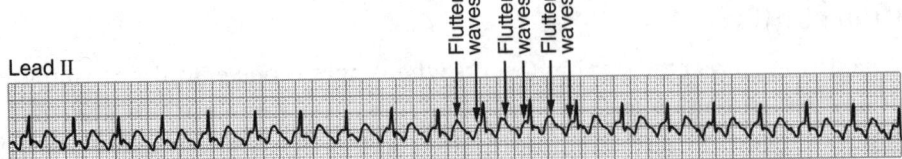

FIGURE 8–14 · Atrial flutter with 2:1 AV conduction. The sawtooth pattern is apparent and the second "P wave" is buried in the QRS complex. The atrial rate in this rhythm strip is 280 beats per minute and the ventricular rate is 140 beats per minute. Every other beat, or every second beat is allowed through the AV node. The R waves are regular.

The following are distinguishing traits for atrial flutter (Figs. 8–14 and 8–15).

- **Regularity:** Atrial regular—ventricular dependent on rate of AV conduction—will be regular or irregular with a variable conduction
- **Rate:** Atrial—250 to 450 beats per minute. Ventricular—varies
- **P wave:** Undetectable—sawtooth flutter waves
- **PR interval:** Not measurable
- **QRS complex:** Less than 0.10 seconds—buried flutter waves may broaden this
- **QT interval:** Not measurable
- **T wave:** Undetectable
- **ST segment:** Unidentifiable

Symptoms associated with atrial flutter are the same as atrial fibrillation. Causes are similar; however, atrial flutter does not usually occur in healthy hearts. It is common with valvular diseases and post cardiac surgery. Alcohol intoxication, pulmonary emboli, and situations which produce ischemia to cardiac tissue are also common etiologies. Treatment options are similar and concern for **mural thrombi** (atrial chamber clots) are the same.

Junctional Dysrhythmias

Junctional dysrhythmias originate in the AV junction. This encompasses the area surrounding the AV node and the beginning portion of the bundle of His

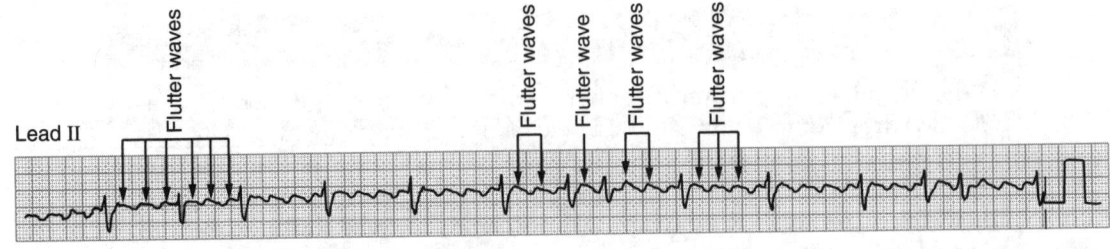

FIGURE 8–15 · Atrial flutter with variable conduction. Note the sawtooth pattern of the "P waves". The R waves are irregular in this rhythm since it is variable conduction.

before it bifurcates into the two bundle branches. The job of the AV node, itself, is to delay conduction through to the ventricles, creating a situation in which the atria are able to fully contract and fill the ventricles. Optimal cardiac output depends on this and other aspects of the cardiac cycle to perform their required duties in a systematic and efficient manner. When problems occur and the cycle is interrupted, stroke volume can suffer and cardiac output can fall.

The AV node does not initiate impulses. The AV junction, however, does have pacemaker cells present which can take over when the SA node is not functioning optimally. The impulse rate for the junctional area is 40 to 60 beats per minute. When impulses are generated in this area, depolarization will progress in a different manner. One situation which can occur is that in which the stimulus will proceed in a retrograde or backward direction causing the atria to depolarize first, but a P wave that is negative in deflection will be produced in a normally upright P wave lead such as lead II. (Some abnormalities in the atria may create a negative deflection in the P wave. The PR interval that is very short—<0.12 seconds—is the key to proper interpretation that this complex did indeed originate in the AV junction.) The second situation in which the ventricles are depolarized first produces a P wave that occurs after instead of prior to the QRS complex. The last situation which can come about is when both the atria and ventricles are depolarized at the same time generating a P wave that is buried within the QRS complex (Fig. 8–16).

Junctional Rhythm

Junctional rhythms (also known as junctional escape rhythms) can occur in which the P waves are presented as above. The intrinsic rate of the junctional pacemakers is 40 to 60 beats per minute (can be as high as 50-80 beats per minute in children).

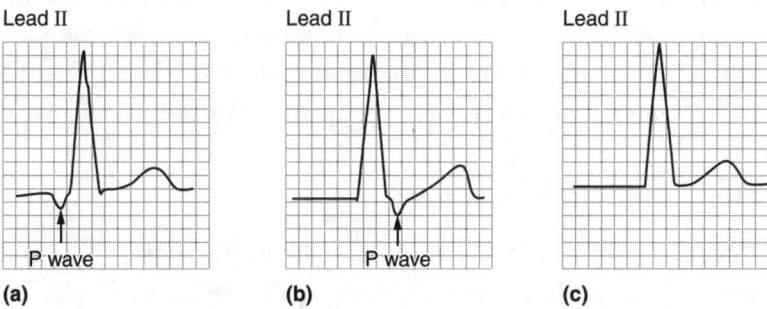

FIGURE 8–16 • **P wave formation in junctional tissue.** (a) Negative P wave in lead II. Atria depolarized first. (b) P wave appears after the QRS complex. Ventricles depolarized first. (c) P wave within in QRS complex. Both the atria and ventricles depolarized simultaneously.

Lead II

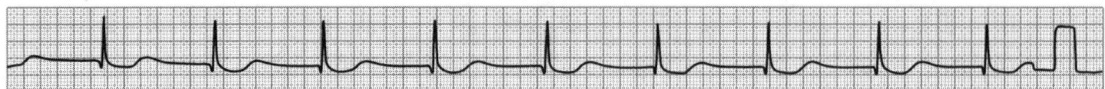

FIGURE 8–17 • **Junctional rhythm.** Note that there do not appear to be P waves present. They are most likely hidden in the QRS complex. The rate is 55 beats per minute.

P waves that occur before, after, or buried within the QRS complex and a slow heart rate are the identifying characteristics of a junctional rhythm. Rates below 40 beats per minute are considered to be junctional bradycardia. Junctional rhythms that have heart rates above 60 beats per minute are considered to be accelerated. These rates usually are within the parameters of 60 to 100 beats per minute. In this situation the bundle of His is experiencing enhanced automaticity.

The following are the basic factors present in a junctional rhythm (Fig. 8–17):

- **Regularity:** Regular
- **Rate:** 40 to 60 beats per minute (unless bradycardic or accelerated)
- **P wave:** Will either be negative deflection (in leads II, III, aVF), after QRS, or embedded in QRS
- **PR interval:** Less than 0.12 seconds if seen before QRS—no PR interval if seen after QRS or embedded in QRS
- **QRS complex:** Less than 0.10 seconds (unless aberrant conduction)
- **QT interval:** Usually normal
- **T wave:** Normal—may be distorted if P wave present after QRS
- **ST segment:** Normal—may be distorted if P wave present after QRS

Junctional rhythms occur when the SA node is not performing its function of impulse generator. This can happen as a response to sick sinus syndrome, hypoxia, digoxin toxicity, hypokalemia, inferior or posterior wall myocardial infarction, rheumatic heart disease, vagal stimulation (increased parasympathetic tone), or use of calcium-channel or beta-blockers. Symptoms of decreased cardiac output can take place. Treatment options for this rhythm include treating the cause and the use of atropine sulfate, dopamine, or epinephrine or the use of a pacemaker.

Premature Junctional Contraction

Just as a premature atrial contraction appears early in the context of the underlying rhythm, a premature junctional contraction (PJC) will do the same. The QRS will have similar morphology to the normal QRS complexes. The pause that occurs after the early beat is noncompensatory as described earlier in this chapter

Lead II

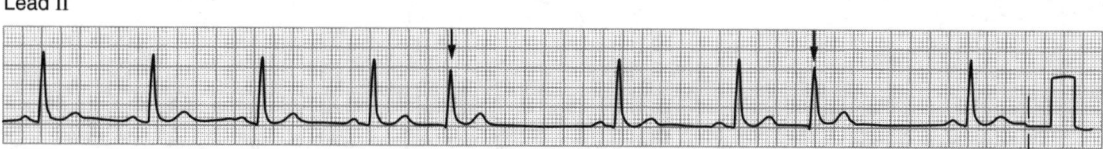

FIGURE 8–18 • **Normal sinus rhythm with premature junctional complexes.** Complexes number five and eight are premature junctional complexes. The P wave is embedded in the QRS complex. The underlying rhythm is normal sinus rhythm.

with the premature atrial contraction information (see Fig. 8–1). At times the QRS may be wide due to aberrant conduction through the ventricles. Most premature junctional beats are of normal width. This abnormality is the presence of one or more extra complexes and therefore the original or underlying rhythm is identified first with the addition of "occasional PJCs" or "multiple PJCs."

Characteristics of premature junctional contractions are (Fig. 8–18):

• **Regularity:** Underlying rhythm may be regular—PJC creates irregularity

• **Rate:** Depends on underlying rhythm

• **P wave:** Will either be negative deflection (in leads II, III, and aVF), after QRS, or embedded in QRS

• **PR interval:** Less than 0.12 seconds if seen before QRS—no PR interval if seen after QRS or embedded in QRS

• **QRS complex:** Less than 0.10 seconds (unless aberrant conduction)

• **QT interval:** Usually normal

• **T wave:** Normal—may be distorted if P wave present after QRS

• **ST segment:** Normal—may be distorted if P wave present after QRS

Similarities are present between PJCs and PACs regarding symptomatology and causes. Increased intake of caffeine, nicotine, and alcohol can bring on these extra beats as well as heart failure, fatigue, inferior myocardial infarction, valve diseases, hypoxia, coronary artery disease, post cardiac surgery, and digitalis toxicity. Treating the underlying cause is the most important therapeutic intervention. Watch the patient for signs of decreased cardiac output if the PJCs are extremely frequent.

Junctional Tachycardia

When at least three premature junctional contractions occur in a row with a heart rate that exceeds 100 beats per minute, it is considered to be a junctional tachycardia. In this condition, enhanced automaticity is behind the irritable focus

Lead II

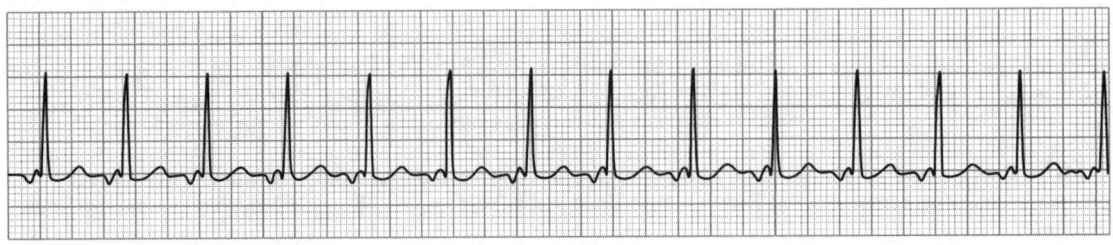

FIGURE 8–19 • **Junctional tachycardia.** Notice the inverted P waves in lead II. The rate is 115 beats per minute.

in the AV junction. Both paroxysmal and nonparoxysmal junctional tachycardia can present. Nonparoxysmal rates can range from 100 to 140 beats per minute and are usually triggered by an accelerated junctional rhythm that increasingly speeds up. Paroxysmal rates can exceed 140 beats per minute and are usually unexpectedly started by a premature junctional contraction. Once rates surpass 150 beats per minute, it is often difficult to establish the actual cardiac tissue responsible for the dysrhythmia.

Unique traits of this dysrhythmia are (Fig. 8–19):

- **Regularity:** Regular
- **Rate:** 100 to 180 beats per minute
- **P wave:** Will either be negative deflection (in leads II, III, and aVF), after QRS, or embedded in QRS
- **PR interval:** Less than 0.12 seconds if seen before QRS—no PR interval if seen after QRS or embedded in QRS
- **QRS complex:** Less than 0.10 seconds (unless aberrant conduction)
- **QT interval:** Usually normal
- **T wave:** Normal—may be distorted if P wave present after QRS or the rate is too fast
- **ST segment:** Normal—may be distorted if P wave present after QRS or the rate is too fast

Etiologies for junctional tachycardia consist of digoxin toxicity, inferior or posterior myocardial infarctions, heart failure, congenital heart disease processes, administration of theophylline based medications, or cardiac surgery (may cause AV junctional swelling). The patient may complain of lightheadedness, palpitations, anxiety, or chest pain/discomfort and may have changes associated with a decreased cardiac output such as hypotension. This can cause increased strain on a heart that is already in a stressed situation when accompanied by a myocardial infarction and can extend the size of the initial infarction. Treatments presented to treat tachycardias previously can be attempted with this tachycardia as well.

> ### CLINICAL ALERT
>
> When dysrhythmias occur due to digitalis toxicity, medications such as Digibind or DigiFab (digoxin immune fab) can be used to treat the process. Be aware that if the patient is showing signs of heart failure, these medications can precipitate an increase in the symptoms.

Conclusion

Dysrhythmias can occur from several different foci in the atrium and the AV nodal area. These can occur for a variety of reasons within the tissue and arise from many disease processes. Some of the key points of this chapter are:

- Atrial and AV nodal rhythms are also known as supraventricular.
- Atrial rhythms will have different foci in the atria than the SA node.
- End cardiac output is usually affected due to the loss of atrial kick with these rhythms.
- Atrial dysrhythmias arise from one of three causes: enhanced automaticity, reentry rhythms, and triggered activity.
- A premature atrial contraction (PAC) comes early in the rhythm cycle and looks like the other atrial beats.
- Premature contractions are also called premature complexes since not all of them always cause a contraction.
- A PAC may be a forerunner of another rhythm such as atrial fibrillation or atrial flutter.
- Causes of PACs include: atrial enlargement, valvular disease, medication toxicities, electrolyte imbalances, and hyperthyroidism as well as increased intake of caffeine or nicotine.
- Sometimes healthy individuals will have PACs without adverse effects.
- Patients will have the feeling of a skipped beat or palpitations with premature beats.
- A noncompensatory pause occurs after a PAC.

- When an extra or premature beat occurs after each regular beat, it is known as *bigeminy*.
- WAP is wandering atrial pacemaker and means that the origination of the impulse is changing from one place to the other.
- The morphology of the P waves changes in wandering atrial pacemaker depending on the impulse generating site.
- Wandering atrial pacemaker can be a normal variant for athletes or can occur during the sleep cycle.
- At least three distinct P waves are seen with WAP.
- Wandering atrial pacemaker at a rate greater than 100 beats per minute constitutes multifocal atrial tachycardia.
- Chronic obstructive pulmonary disease is one of the major causes of multifocal atrial tachycardia.
- Treatment for multifocal atrial tachycardia is to control the rate and resolve the underlying problem.
- Atrial tachycardia occurs at rates of 150 to 250 beats per minute.
- Atrial tachycardia has a regular rhythm.
- It may be difficult to see the P wave in atrial tachycardia due to it being lost or buried in the T wave.
- Paroxysmal atrial tachycardia (PAT) can occur with a sudden beginning and ending of the fast rhythm.
- PAT will not respond as well to vagal maneuvers as paroxysmal supraventricular tachycardia (PSVT).
- Atrial tachycardia with block occurs when the AV node protects the heart by blocking some of the fast impulses coming from the atria.
- Fast rhythms are often difficult to analyze and can therefore cause differences of opinion.
- P waves are not present in a supraventricular tachycardia.
- Two types of PSVT are AV nodal reentrant tachycardia (AVNRT) and AV reentrant tachycardia (AVRT).
- In AVNRT two pathways are present—one that is fast and one that is slow.
- The two factors present in AVNRT are the speed of the impulse and the refractory time of each pathway.
- A loop is formed in AVNRT.
- AVRT is a type of pre-excitation passageway.

- Wolff-Parkinson-White (WPW) syndrome is a form of AVRT.
- The impulse for Wolff-Parkinson-White (WPW) syndrome travels through the bundle of Kent.
- Important factors with Wolff-Parkinson-White (WPW) syndrome are short PR interval, presence of a delta wave, and a wide QRS.
- PSVT usually has rates of 150 to 250 beats per minute.
- Patients with PSVT are usually symptomatic.
- Hypotension can occur with PSVT.
- Treatments for PSVT can include vagal maneuvers, the use of Adenocard (adenosine), synchronized cardioversion, and catheter ablation.
- Do not use Adenocard (adenosine) on patients with Wolff-Parkinson-White (WPW) syndrome. This can speed up the heart rate.
- Carotid massage is a physician procedure.
- Bradycardia or asystole can occur with vagal maneuvers.
- Carotid massage should be used with great caution in the older patient.
- Adenocard (adenosine) must be given rapidly followed by the administration of a 20 to 30 mL bolus of normal saline (NS) and NS drip at a wide open rate.
- A short episode of asystole will precede the return of a normal sinus rhythm with Adenocard (adenosine).
- Always be sure to prepare the patient who is receiving administration of Adenocard (adenosine).
- With synchronized cardioversion the paddles must be held on to the chest and both buttons pushed until the energy load has been delivered.
- The "sync" button must be pushed prior to charging the paddles for the delivery of a synchronized shock.
- The machine being used to deliver the synchronized cardioversion energy must be recognizing each R wave prior to delivery of the shock.
- It is best to sedate patients who are receiving synchronized cardioversion.
- There are different amounts of joules delivered to different types of rhythms with synchronized cardioversion.
- In atrial fibrillation, the atria are firing so fast that the atria are quivering rather than actually contracting.
- The ventricular rate in atrial fibrillation is much lower than the atrial rate.
- The rhythm in atrial fibrillation is irregularly irregular.

- If a patient is displaying atrial fibrillation at ventricular rates greater than 100 beats per minute, they are said to be "uncontrolled."
- No P waves are discernible with atrial fibrillation.
- Mural thrombi can develop in patients who are experiencing sustained atrial fibrillation.
- Mural thrombi can be expelled into the pulmonary or systemic circulation and cause disease processes such as strokes.
- In atrial flutter, the P waves take on a distinct sawtooth pattern.
- Conduction through the AV node in atrial flutter will cause a 2:1, 3:1, or 4:1 conduction. This conduction can also be variable.
- The P waves in atrial flutter are called *flutter waves*.
- Two types of atrial flutter are: Type I—rates of 250 to 350 and Type II— rates of 350 to 450 beats per minute.
- Vagal maneuvers will not convert atrial flutter but may slow it down enough to visualize the sawtooth pattern.
- Junctional dysrhythmias originate in the AV junction.
- The AV node itself does not have pacemaker cells. The AV junction area does have pacemaker cells.
- In a junctional rhythm, the P wave will come either before the QRS, but will be very short and negative, come after the QRS, or be buried within the QRS.
- The intrinsic rate of the junctional tissue is 40 to 60 beats per minute in the adult patient.
- Junctional pacemaker cells come into play when the SA node is not functioning correctly.
- Premature junctional contractions come early in the cycle of the underlying rhythm—just like a premature atrial contraction.
- Many different disease processes can cause premature junctional contractions as well as intake of caffeine, nicotine, or alcohol.
- Three premature junctional contractions in a row can constitute junctional tachycardia.
- With junctional tachycardia rates can surpass 150 beats per minute.
- The use of Digibind or DigFab, used to treat digitalis toxicity, can precipitate an exacerbation of heart failure.

PRACTICE QUESTIONS

1. Which of the following is a true statement regarding premature atrial complexes?
   A. A full compensatory pause occurs after a premature atrial complex.
   B. Increased intake of caffeine can be a cause of a premature atrial complex.
   C. No P wave is present with premature atrial complexes.
   D. Premature atrial complexes do not occur in healthy individuals.

2. A premature beat that occurs after every regular beat in a rhythm strip is known as:
   A. bigeminy.
   B. trigeminy.
   C. quadrigeminy.
   D. occasional.

3. Which of the following would constitute a characteristic of wandering atrial pacemaker?
   A. Rates are greater than 100 beats per minute
   B. T waves are distorted
   C. At least three distinct P waves are noted
   D. PR interval is lengthened

4. The MOST common reason for patients to have multifocal atrial tachycardia is:
   A. increased caffeine intake.
   B. digitalis toxicity.
   C. acute myocardial infarction.
   D. chronic obstructive pulmonary disease.

5. Which of the following will help the health care provider distinguish between atrial fibrillation and multifocal atrial tachycardia?
   A. The baseline heart rate
   B. The regularity of the rhythm
   C. The presence of P waves
   D. Wide QRS complexes

6. When a block is noted in the AV conduction with atrial tachycardia with block, the health care professional realizes this occurs because the AV node is:
   A. in a diseased state.
   B. not able to function.
   C. protecting the heart.
   D. working as the SA node.

7. In AV nodal reentrant tachycardia, a type of supraventricular tachycardia, the reentry problem occurs at the:

   A. SA node.
   B. AV node.
   C. bundle of Kent.
   D. bundles of HIS.

8. Wolff- Parkinson-White (WPW) syndrome is a type of:

   A. AV reentrant tachycardia.
   B. AV nodal reentrant tachycardia.
   C. atrial fibrillation.
   D. atrial flutter.

9. Which of the following is characteristic of Wolff-Parkinson-White (WPW) syndrome?

   A. Narrow QRS complex
   B. Presence of Osborn wave
   C. Prolonged QT interval
   D. Short PR interval

10. Carotid massage works through the action of:

    A. increasing intrathoracic pressure.
    B. stimulation of baroreceptors.
    C. impeding reentrant pathways.
    D. interrupting atrial depolarization.

11. Which of the following dysrhythmias should the health care provider be alert for, when carotid massage or Valsalva maneuver is used as a treatment option for paroxysmal supraventricular tachycardia?

    A. Bradycardia
    B. Atrial flutter
    C. Ventricular tachycardia
    D. AV block

12. Which of the following is a true statement regarding the use of Adenocard (adenosine)?

    A. A large left-sided wrist vein should be used to administer this medication.
    B. This medication can cause the patient to experience a burst of ventricular tachycardia.
    C. This is a good medication to be used with patients who have underlying Wolff-Parkinson-White (WPW) Syndrome.
    D. This medication must be administered as quickly as possible followed immediately by a normal saline bolus.

13. **When using synchronized cardioversion to treat supraventricular tachycardia, the machine must be marking each:**

    A. P wave

    B. Q wave

    C. R wave

    D. T wave

14. **Atrial fibrillation will be recognized on the rhythm strip by the:**

    A. increased QT intervals.

    B. wavy line between QRS complexes.

    C. regularity of the QRS complexes.

    D. increased PR interval.

15. **P waves in junctional rhythms may appear:**

    A. notched.

    B. biphasic.

    C. wavy.

    D. absent.

16. **Fast heart rates can cause:**

    A. increased stroke volume.

    B. decreased cardiac output.

    C. increased ventricular emptying.

    D. decreased atrial conductivity.

17. **In the following rhythm strip what is the rate of atrial to ventricular conduction?**

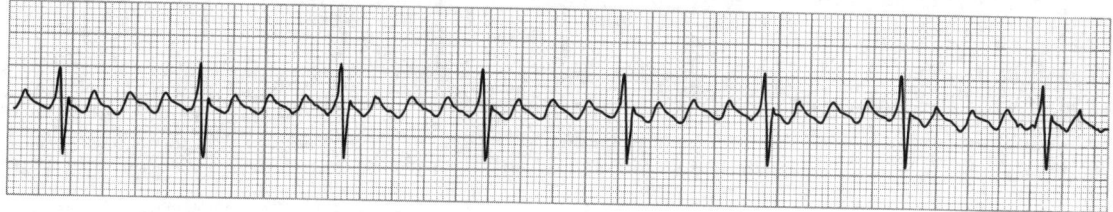

    A. 2:1

    B. 3:1

    C. 4:1

    D. Variable

18. **Identify the following dysrhythmia:**

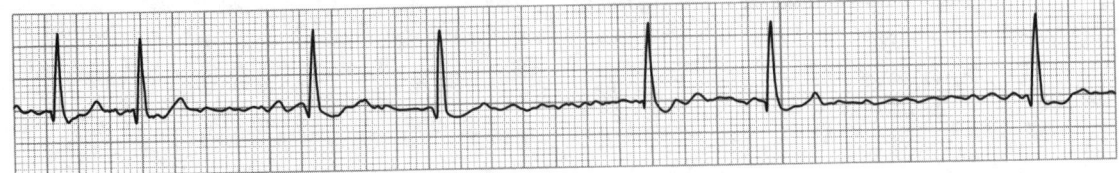

    A. Atrial flutter

    B. Junctional tachycardia

    C. Multiple PACs

    D. Atrial fibrillation

19. **What is the fifth complex in the following dysrhythmia?**

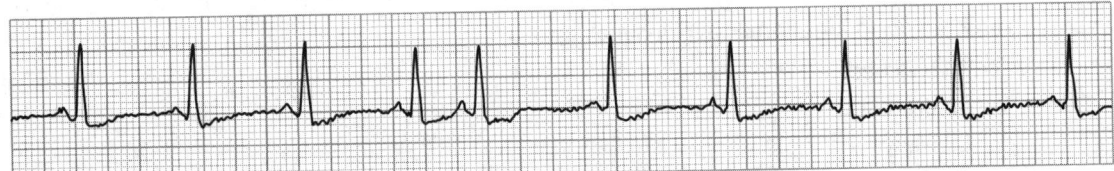

    A. Premature junctional complex

    B. Normal sinus beat

    C. Premature atrial complex

    D. WPW complex

20. **Which of the following treatment options would be appropriate for the rhythm:**

Lead II

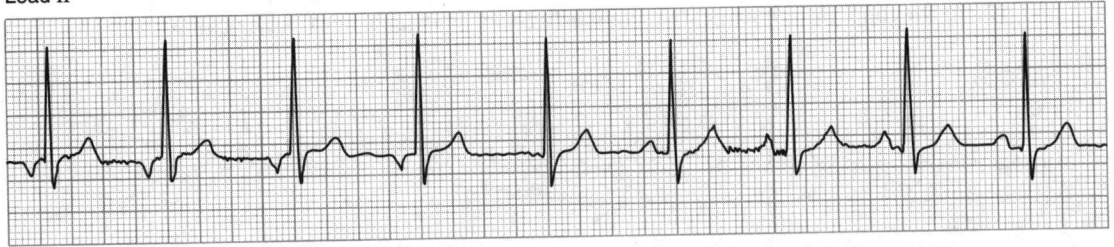

    A. Observe patient

    B. Administer atropine

    C. Synchronized cardioversion

    D. Administer adenosine (Adenocard)

ANSWER KEY

1. **B.** Premature atrial contractions can occur with the increased intake of caffeine, nicotine, or alcohol and can occur in normal, healthy individuals. The pause that arises after a PAC is a noncompensatory pause. The presence of normal P waves is a characteristic of premature atrial contractions.

2. **A.** When every other beat is a premature beat, the rhythm is known as *bigeminy*. Every third beat is *trigeminy* and every fourth beat is *quadrigeminy*. The term "occasional" is used when these occur every fifth beat or more.

3. **C.** The identifying factor in wandering atrial pacemaker is that there are at least three distinct P waves noted within the rhythm strip. Rates vary with this rhythm, but are usually normal or bradycardic. The T waves and PR intervals are usually normal.

4. **D.** The most common reason for multifocal atrial tachycardia (MAT) is chronic obstructive pulmonary disease.

5. **C.** Multifocal atrial tachycardia will have P waves that are of different configurations. This is a rapid type of wandering atrial pacemaker. Atrial fibrillation does not have distinguishable P waves. The rate in MAT is rapid and in uncontrolled atrial fibrillation the rate is also rapid. Both have irregular rhythms and the QRS complex is usually normal in both.

6. **C.** The AV node acts as a protector for the heart when rapid sinus or atrial rates take place.

7. **B.** AVNRT, AV nodal reentrant tachycardia, a type of supraventricular tachycardia, occurs as a result of a problem at the AV node when there are two pathways present—one fast and one slow. AVRT, AV reentrant tachycardia, involves the bundle of Kent, an accessory pathway or bridge.

8. **A.** Wolff-Parkinson-White (WPW) syndrome is associated with accessory pathways that occur in AVRT, AV reentrant tachycardia. This pathway is the bundle of Kent.

9. **D.** The three characteristics of Wolff-Parkinson-White (WPW) syndrome are: shortened PR interval, widened QRS complex, and the presence of delta waves.

10. **B.** Carotid massage, a type of vagal maneuver, works through the stimulation of the baroreceptors which are located in the carotid bodies and the aortic arch. Valsalva maneuver causes an increase in intrathoracic pressure. Adenocard (adenosine) impedes reentrant pathways and synchronized cardioversion interrupts atrial depolarization.

11. **A.** Carotid massage and Valsalva maneuvers can cause bradycardias and asystole.

12. **D.** Adenocard (adenosine) has an extremely short half-life and must be given as quickly as possible in order to work. A right-sided large gauge antecubital vein is the best intravenous access. Adenocard (adenosine) can cause a period of asystole for the patient and it should not be used to treat patients who have underlying Wolff-Parkinson-White (WPW) syndrome.

13. **C.** The machine being used to perform synchronized cardioversion must be marking each R wave prior to delivery of energy.

14. **B.** Atrial fibrillation will have f waves or a fibrillatory wave which is a wavy line between each QRS complex. There are no P waves so there is no PR interval to count. One of the highlights of atrial fibrillation is the irregularly irregular rhythm. The QT intervals are not impacted.

15. **D.** P waves in junctional rhythms are either negative deflections (in leads II, III, and aVF), after the QRS, or embedded in the QRS at which point they will be "absent."

16. **B.** Fast heart rates can cause a decrease in the cardiac output because there is not enough time for the chambers to fill adequately and there is often a loss of atrial kick.

17. **C.** In this rhythm strip, there are four P sawtooth waves for each one QRS complex. The first sawtooth wave is embedded in the ST segment of the prior QRS complex.

18. **D.** This rhythm is atrial fibrillation. The rhythm is irregularly irregular and there are not distinguishable P waves. The wavy or straight line represents the quivering atrium.

19. **C.** The fifth beat in this rhythm is a premature atrial contraction. Note the P wave prior to the QRS. The underlying rhythm is normal sinus rhythm.

20. **A.** This is wandering atrial pacemaker (WAP). These patients are not usually aware of any abnormality and the treatment option is to observe the patient. Atropine would be used for symptomatic bradycardias and synchronized cardioversion and the administration of Adenocard (adenosine) would be used for symptomatic tachycardias.

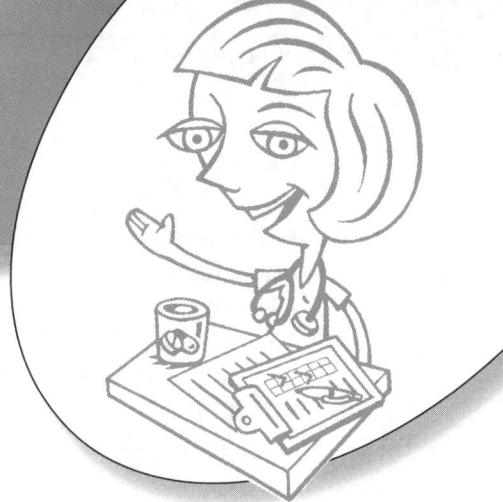

chapter 9

Ventricular Dysrhythmias and AV Nodal Blocks

LEARNING OBJECTIVES

At the end of this chapter, the student will be able to:

❶ Identify ventricular dysrhythmias and atrioventricular blocks through EKG characteristics.

❷ Understand etiologies of specific ventricular dysrhythmias and atrioventricular blocks.

❸ List causes of specific ventricular dysrhythmias and atrioventricular blocks.

❹ Discuss general treatment options for ventricular dysrhythmias and atrioventricular blocks.

❺ Understand the difference between synchronized cardioversion and defibrillation.

Overview

The ventricles are not effective pacemakers for the heart. The rate is inherently slow (20-40 beats per minute) and the contractions do not provide an efficient cardiac output. Atrial kick is absent which can decrease the cardiac output by as much as 30%. The ventricles may step in to take over the role of pacemaker if the SA node is not functional or if the impulse generated from the SA node is blocked in some way. At times the rate of the impulses is very slow and the ventricles will attempt to protect the heart through **escape beats**. Another reason for the ventricles to take over is when there is an irritable focus in the ventricles which can occur if an area becomes ischemic or injured.

Ventricular complexes have specific morphologic characteristics. The QRS portion of a ventricular beat is wide due to the longer conduction time. During a normal contraction, the ventricles will beat synchronously. In ventricular rhythms the normal pathway is disrupted and the ventricles can respond at different times. Therefore the QRS complex is larger than normal and carries an unusual or aberrant shape. Repolarization also occurs abnormally and the T wave will occur in the opposite direction of the QRS complex. P waves are not present (Fig. 9–1).

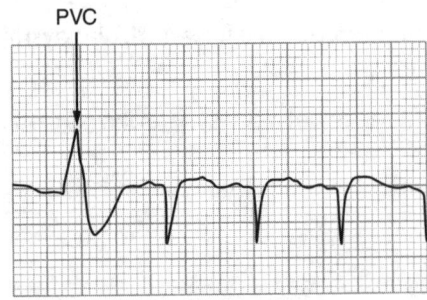

PVC

FIGURE 9–1 • Ventricular beat. The ventricular beat has no P wave, is wide in appearance, and the T wave will deflect in the opposite direction.

Ventricular dysrhythmias can occur due to reentry problems, enhanced automaticity, or triggered activity. Each of these abnormalities in conduction has been addressed in the previous chapter.

Atrioventricular dysrhythmias will also be discussed. These occur due to blocks at the atrioventricular (AV) junction. Both ventricular dysrhythmias and atrioventricular blocks can create serious outcomes for patients. More discussion on AV blocks will be presented in this chapter.

Ventricular Dysrhythmias

Premature Ventricular Contraction

A **premature ventricular contraction (PVC)** (or "complex" since they do not always create a true contraction) occurs when there is an ectopic focus in the ventricles that produces a complex. This irritable site produces a beat that occurs earlier than expected in the cardiac cycle on the cardiac monitor or 12-lead EKG. These extra beats normally create a full compensatory pause. To determine this compensatory pause, count the distance between three normal beats on the rhythm strip. Then measure the number of blocks between three beats that includes the PVC. To accomplish this either count the blocks, use calipers or a piece of paper with a mark placed at the first and third complexes. If a full compensatory pause is present, the distances will be the same. This means that the third beat (the normal beat) comes in within the cycle at the same time that it would have if the PVC were not present. Premature atrial complexes will usually have a noncompensatory or incomplete pause (Fig. 9–2). A PVC that occurs within the cycle but does not have a full compensatory pause is called "**interpolated.**" This means it fits in between two normal complexes but does not interfere with the underlying rhythm (Fig. 9–3).

Fusion beats can also appear. These beats represent simultaneous firing of both a supraventricular and a ventricular impulse. This complex will not look like a ventricular beat or any of the normal beats that appear on the EKG tracing or cardiac monitor (Fig. 9–4).

Characteristics of PVCs are:

- **Regularity:** Irregular rhythm (underlying rhythm can be regular)
- **Rate:** Can be normal, bradycardic, or tachycardic—dependent on underlying rhythm
- **P wave:** No P waves are noted with the PVC—may be present in the underlying rhythm

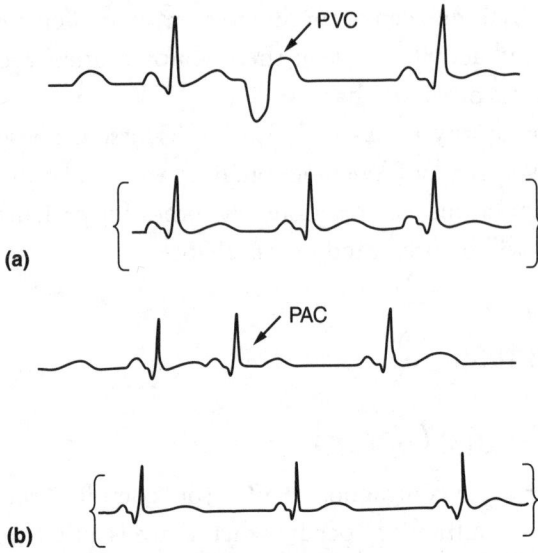

FIGURE 9–2 • Full and incomplete compensatory pauses. (a) Full compensatory pauses usually follow a premature ventricular contraction (PVC). (b) Premature atrial contractions (PAC) usually will have an incomplete compensatory (noncompensatory) pause.

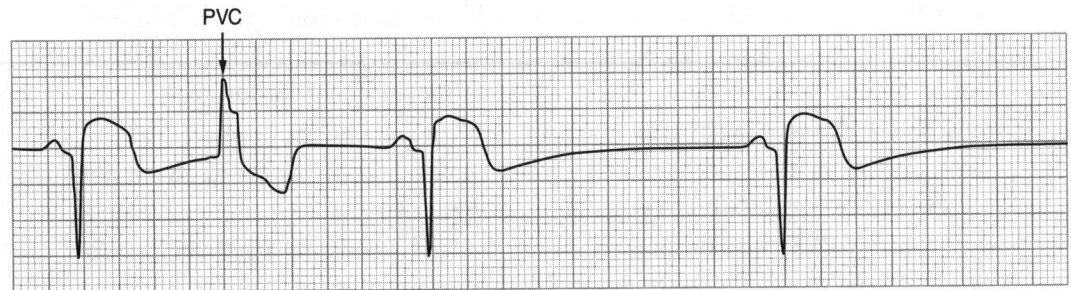

FIGURE 9–3 • Interpolated PVC. Note that the PVC (beat number 2) is exactly between the two normal beats. There is not a full compensatory pause.

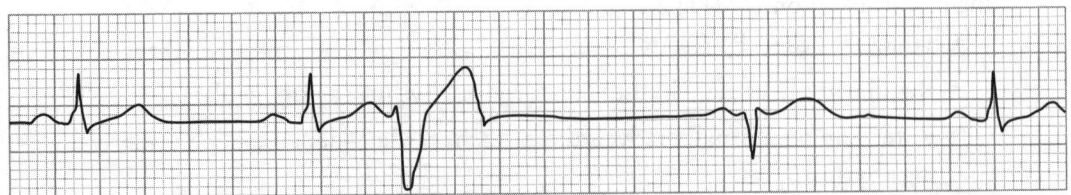

FIGURE 9–4 • Fusion beat. In this rhythm strip, the third beat is a premature ventricular contraction (PVC) and the fourth beat is a fusion beat.

Lead II

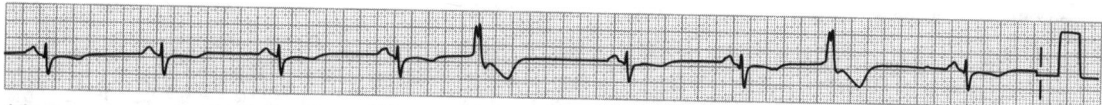

(a)

Lead II

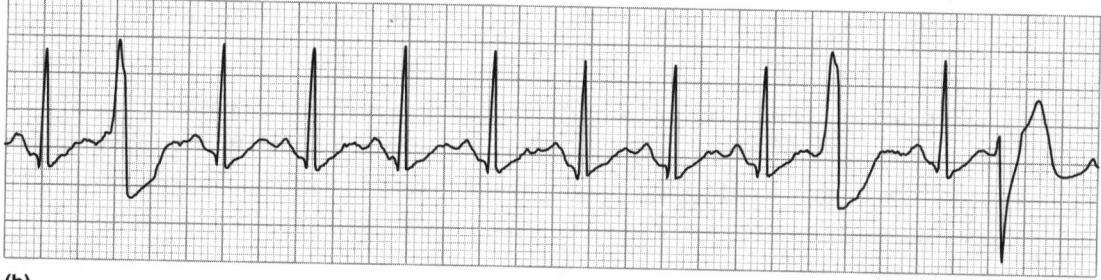

(b)

FIGURE 9–5 • **Unifocal and multifocal PVCs.** (a) Beats 5 and 8 are of the same shape and size. These are unifocal PVCs. (b) Notice that beats 10 and 12 are both PVCs but have different shapes and sizes, thus multifocal. Beat number 2 is also a PVC. Notice in both the full compensatory pauses.

- **PR interval:** Not present for PVC
- **QRS complex:** Usually greater than 0.12 seconds—wide and bizarre
- **QT interval:** Prolonged
- **T wave:** Appears as an opposite deflection of the QRS
- **ST segment:** Difficult due to the bizarre presentation of the QRS

CLINICAL ALERT

PVCs can be unifocal or multifocal. Another term for each of these is "uniform" or "multiform". Uniform PVCs look alike and arise from the same ectopic site. Multiform means that they have different configurations. It can signify diverse ectopic sites; however, all multiform PVCs do not always have different foci. A single ectopic site can produce multiform PVCs. When identifying rhythm strips the underlying rhythm is classified first with the PVCs mentioned second, that is, "normal sinus rhythm with frequent multifocal PVCs" or "atrial fibrillation with occasional unifocal PVCs" (Fig. 9.5).

Comparable to premature atrial contractions (PACs) and premature junctional contractions (PJCs), PVCs can occur as bigeminy (every other beat), trigeminy (every third beat), and quadrigeminy (every fourth beat). PVCs can also occur as a pairing or couplet—two PVCs together—or as tripling—three

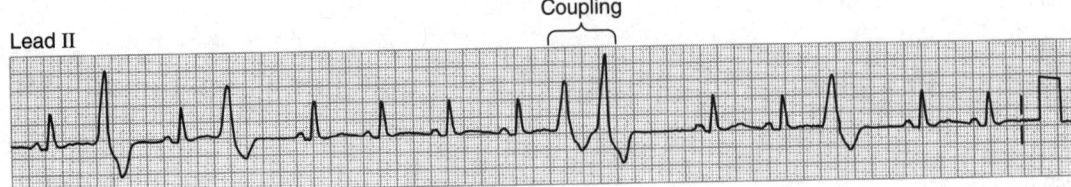

FIGURE 9–6 • **Premature ventricular coupling.** When two PVCs appear together, this is known as "coupling."

PVCs together. When three or more PVCs occur in a row, this is considered to be a short run or burst of ventricular tachycardia. When couplets or tripling occurs, this is considered to be a red flag that the ventricular tissue is very irritable and it may be a precursor to sustained ventricular tachycardia or ventricular fibrillation (Fig. 9–6).

The R-on-T phenomenon can also come about with a single PVC. When the PVC is initiated so early in the cycle that it falls on the T wave of the preceding complex, the repolarization process occurring at the end of the T wave is unable to complete and ventricular tachycardia or ventricular fibrillation can occur (Fig. 9–7).

PVCs can occur as protective measures as well. When the heart rates are slow and the risk is present that the heart is not experiencing sufficient numbers of contractions to supply adequate cardiac output, a ventricular beat can arise to "rescue" the heart. These ventricular beats are late in the cycle rather than early. While they may not provide as good a contraction as a normal beat, it is an attempt to help the heart rate. Do not administer medications to the patient that would destroy these escape beats. The proper treatment for these is to deal with the underlying slow rhythm so that the escape beats are not needed (Fig. 9–8). Another interesting beat that can occur is an aberrantly conducted complex. Impulses that are generated above the ventricles can follow a deviant pathway creating a QRS complex that looks similar to a PVC. These aberrant beats will have a P wave associated with them.

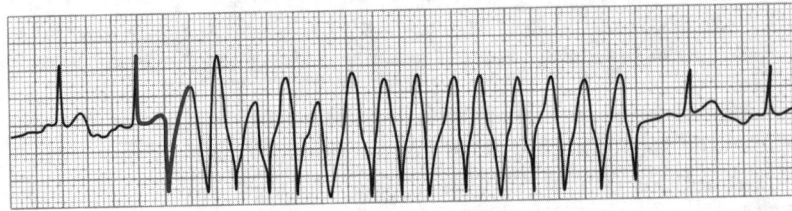

FIGURE 9–7 • **R-on-T phenomenon.** When a PVC falls on the T wave of the preceding normal beat, ventricular tachycardia can occur.

Escape Beat

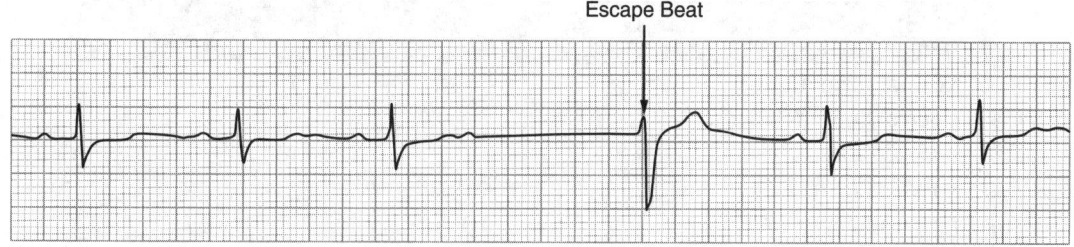

FIGURE 9–8 • Escape beat. Escape beats occur late in the cycle and appear wide and bizarre, just like a premature ventricular contraction (PVC).

CLINICAL ALERT

PVCs can occur for a variety of reasons. See Box 9–1 for etiologies. Sometimes individuals have PVCs that are simply "normal" for them. It is not considered necessary to treat all PVCs. The health care provider should talk to the patient to help determine if these extra beats are common for them. Patients are not always great historians or may not understand their past history or reasons for medications. Looking at the list of present medications the patient is taking may help to establish whether the PVCs are part of the patient's past history or not. Also old records can assist in this process as well as communication with the patient's primary care physician. Take into consideration symptoms or the lack of symptoms that the patient may be having. Always treat the patient, not the machines! If the patient is in the process of having an acute myocardial infarction and multiple PVCs are present, it may be in the best interests of the patient to treat these. Again, correlate the patient's presentation with laboratory values and EKG information before deciding if PVCs need to be treated or not.

Also be sure to check the patient's actual radial pulse with the number seen on the cardiac monitor. PVCs are not always perfusing. Just because they are seen on the screen does not mean that they are actually "working." This is especially important with the escape beats noted above.

Patients who are symptomatic with premature ventricular contractions will complain with "palpitations" or a feeling that the heart is "flip-flopping in my chest." They may describe it as "skipping beats" or a feeling that their heart is stopping (due to the long compensatory pause). Patients may have chest pain or discomfort associated with shortness of breath. Basic treatment for premature ventricular contractions is to treat the underlying cause and provide supportive therapy such as oxygen and pain relief. For symptomatic or concerning PVCs, medications that might be used are lidocaine and amiodarone (Cordarone).

BOX 9–1   Causes of Premature Ventricular Contractions

- Normal for patient
- Electrolyte imbalances
  - Hypokalemia
  - Hyperkalemia
  - Hypomagnesemia
  - Hypocalcemia
- Anxiety
- Stress
- Exercise
- Metabolic acidosis
- Cardiac ischemia
- Myocardial infarction
- Tricyclic overdose
- Street drug ingestion
  - Cocaine
  - Amphetamines
  - Ecstasy
- Digitalis toxicity
- Stimulant use of
  - Alcohol
  - Caffeine
  - Nicotine
- Ephedrine use
- Hypoxia
- Heart failure
- Myocarditis

Idioventricular Rhythm

When the heart is attempting to prevent ventricular standstill, escape beats as described above can occur. Three or more ventricular escape beats in a row is considered to be idioventricular rhythm or IVR. Ventricular tissue takes control when the SA and AV nodes are incapable of producing impulses or the impulses are too slow. At times the impulses are present but they are blocked from conduction. Some of the causes of this dysrhythmia are myocardial infarction or ischemia, digitalis toxicity, the use of beta-blocker medication, and metabolic disfunctions. Pacemaker malfunctions can also be an etiologic factor in this rhythm.

The QRS complexes in this rhythm are very wide and bizarre appearing and the rate is 20 to 40 beats per minute. No P waves are present. Patients in this rhythm may be unresponsive or may complain of dizziness, weakness, light-headedness, confusion, or syncope. The decrease in cardiac output will cause hypotension and weak radial pulses.

> ## CLINICAL ALERT
>
> If the patient does not have pulses, a situation called **pulseless electrical activity (PEA)** can occur. With this particular problem, any rhythm can be seen on the cardiac monitor or 12-lead EKG, but there is no contraction response. IVR is a common theme with pulseless electrical activity. While providing supportive cardiopulmonary resuscitation, the underlying cause must be determined and corrected to save the patient. Two mnemonics are used to remember treatable causes of PEA. These are: PATCH-4-MD and the 5 H's and T's. See Table 9–1 for a listing of these potential etiologies.

The following are characteristics of idioventricular rhythm (Fig. 9–9):

- **Regularity:** Regular rhythm
- **Rate:** 20 to 40 beats per minute
- **P wave:** No P waves are noted
- **PR interval:** Not present
- **QRS complex:** Usually greater than 0.12 seconds—wide and bizarre
- **QT interval:** Prolonged

TABLE 9–1 Causes of Pulseless Electrical Activity

PATCH-4-MD	5 H's and 5 T's	
• **P**ulmonary Embolus	• **H**ypovolemia	• **T**amponade (cardiac)
• **A**cidosis	• **H**ypoxia	• **T**ension pneumothorax
• **T**ension Pneumothorax	• **H**ypo/Hyperthermia	• **T**hrombosis (pulmonary)
• **C**ardiac Tamponade	• **H**ypo/Hyperkalemia	• **T**hrombosis (cardiac)
• **H**ypovolemia	• **H**ydrogen ion (acidosis)	• **T**ablets/toxins (overdose)
• **H**ypoxia		
• **H**ypothermia/Hyperthermia		
• **H**ypokalemia/Hyperkalemia		
• **M**yocardial infarction		
• **D**rug overdose		

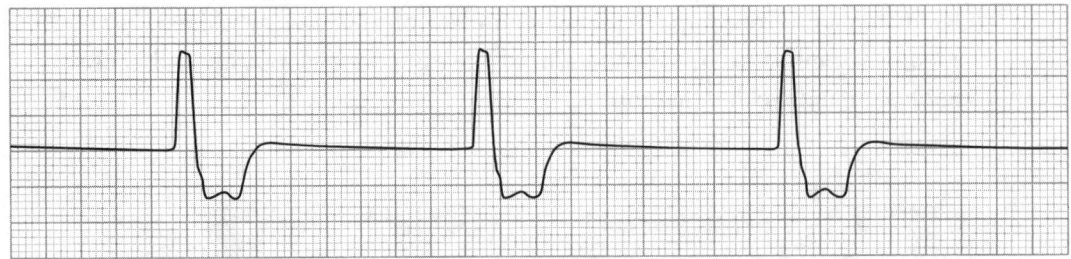

FIGURE 9–9 • **Idioventricular rhythm.** This rhythm strip shows an idioventricular rhythm with a rate of 35 beats per minute.

- **T wave:** Appears as an opposite deflection of the QRS
- **ST segment:** Difficult due to the bizarre presentation of the QRS

This dangerous dysrhythmia is often the precursor to asystole in dying patients. Atropine may be prescribed in an attempt to increase the heart rate. Do not treat this rhythm with lidocaine or other medications that might suppress its activity. A pacemaker is usually necessary for these patients. In this emergency situation, a **transcutaneous pacemaker** is the first choice until a temporary or permanent **transvenous pacemaker** can be placed.

Transcutaneous pacing is also known as external pacing. This is a life-saving procedure. If this is necessary, make sure that the patient is receiving appropriate oxygen and has a patent intravenous line. Record the rhythm via a 12-lead EKG and a rhythm strip from the cardiac monitor. The health care provider needs to be familiar with the monitor/defibrillator/pacing machine that is utilized for this process. Provide support to the patient and family. Pacing pads are placed on the patient according to the machine's provided instructions. Avoid areas that might be open such as cuts, abrasions, sores, wounds, or abscesses. Do not place the pads over pacemaker or implanted intravenous access sites that the patient may already have in place. The pads will then need to be attached to the monitor/pacing unit by the appropriate cable. Turn power on.

The provider will prescribe a particular pacing rate to begin—usually between 60 to 80 beats per minute. At this point the health care provider can start the pacing option on the machine. The mA (milliamperes) will then need to be set. This is the amount of electrical stimulating current that must be utilized to create a pacing spike before each QRS complex. Gradually increase the mA until capture is recognized. This application of electrical current to the skin can cause a considerable amount of pain for the patient. Be sure to provide analgesia for this process if necessary. Watch for facial grimacing, coughing, chest wall movement, or complaints of pain from the patient.

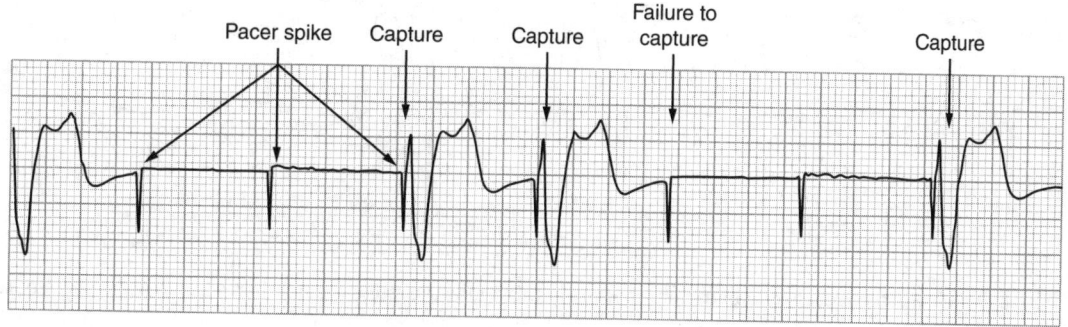

FIGURE 9–10 • **Capture and failure to capture with transcutaneous pacemaker.** Electrical capture on the rhythm strip is noted by a QRS complex following a pacer spike.

Both electrical and mechanical capture must be assessed. Check the machine for electrical capture. This will be indicated by a pacer spike or blip before each QRS complex. Mechanical capture is measured by palpable pulses and a blood pressure on the patient. Level of consciousness is another good measure of positive mechanical capture. Document patient response and cardiac monitor tracing (Fig. 9–10).

Accelerated Idioventricular Rhythm

Accelerated idioventricular rhythm is also known by the initials, AIVR. This occurs when the rate of idioventricular rhythm (IVR) is over the rate of 40. This rate can reach as high as 100 to 120. Fusion beats may be seen at the beginning and end of this rhythm which usually lasts for short periods.

Causes of this rhythm include acute myocardial infarction, digitalis toxicity, subarachnoid hemorrhage, cardiomyopathy, cocaine ingestion, or heart disease associated with systemic hypertension. This is a very common dysrhythmia when patients are reperfusing after administration of thrombolytics for myocardial infarctions.

Patients may complain of dizziness or lightheadedness or become hemodynamically unstable due to the decrease in cardiac output. When the atria are not participating in the creation of cardiac output, atrial kick is lost. A pacemaker may be necessary for this dysrhythmia if it persists, but it is usually an atrial pacemaker in an attempt to suppress this rhythm and allow the SA node to come back into play. Many times no treatment is necessary and it will spontaneously resolve.

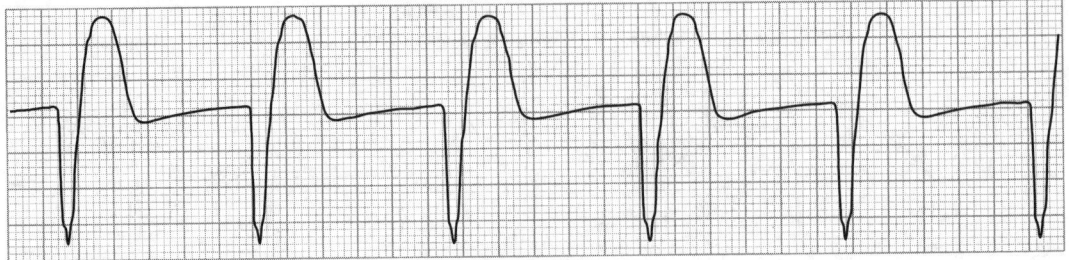

FIGURE 9–11 • Accelerated idioventricular rhythm. In this figure, the rate is greater than 40 at 56 beats per minute.

Characteristics of AIVR (Fig. 9–11):

- **Regularity:** Regular rhythm
- **Rate:** 41 to 120 beats per minute
- **P wave:** No P waves are noted
- **PR interval:** Not present
- **QRS complex:** Usually greater than 0.12 seconds—wide and bizarre
- **QT interval:** Prolonged
- **T wave:** Appears as an opposite deflection of the QRS
- **ST segment:** Difficult due to the bizarre presentation of the QRS

Ventricular Tachycardia

Ventricular tachycardia (VT) is also known as V-Tach. This is defined as three or more PVCs in a row with an increased rate of over 100 beats per minute. Short bursts of VT can occur or a sustained rhythm lasting greater than 30 seconds can take place. This is a life-threatening dysrhythmia in its own right and often a prodrome for ventricular fibrillation.

VT is divided into monomorphic and polymorphic types. Monomorphic VT carries QRS complexes which have the same shape and height. This uniformity is the identifying characteristic for the monomorphic type. In the polymorphic classification, two categories are present. These are separated dependent on the length of the QT interval. Normal QT interval is the first type of polymorphic VT. The second subtype is recognized by the prolonged QT interval. A further subclassification can be distinguished by whether the prolonged QT was congenital or acquired. Another term for congenital is **idiopathic** and the term associated with acquired is iatrogenic. (Table 9–2). Idiopathic reasons for this dysrhythmia are imperfections within the sodium and potassium channels which cause abnormalities of the electrical conduction system.

TABLE 9–2 Classification of Ventricular Tachycardia			
Ventricular Tachycardia			
Monomorphic VT	**Polymorphic VT**		
	Normal QT interval	Prolonged QT interval (LQTS)	
		Acquired (Iatrogenic)	Congenital (Idiopathic)

Mechanically, the heart is normal, but genetic problems cause disruption in the functionality of the electrical system. These genetic mutations can occur when an individual inherits a variant gene from one parent or when they inherit variations from both parents. Some research has been done in determining if there is a correlation between this congenital problem and sudden infant death syndrome (SIDS). **Iatrogenic** causes are those involved with medications that can prolong the QT interval. There are over 50 medications that can cause a prolonged QT including some of those used to treat infections, diabetes, psychiatric problems, anxiety, high cholesterol, allergies, and cardiac problems.

When polymorphic ventricular tachycardia occurs with a prolonged QT interval, it is known as *torsades de pointes* (TdP). In this situation, the QRS complexes that are present are of varying shapes, widths, and amplitude. The name of this special VT stands for "twisting of the points." This classification of polymorphic VT is also known as long QT syndrome (LQTS).

Factors that are present with ventricular tachycardia are listed as follows (Figs. 9–12 and 9–13):

- **Regularity:** Regular rhythm with monomorphic/or can be irregular with polymorphic
- **Rate:** 101 to 250 beats per minute (monomorphic), 150 to 300 beats per minute (polymorphic)
- **P wave:** No P waves are noted
- **PR interval:** Not present

Lead II

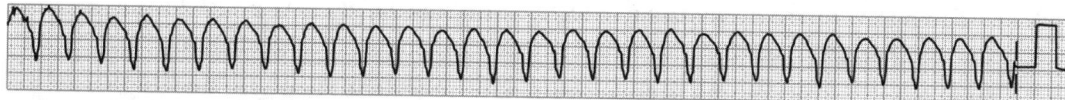

FIGURE 9–12 • Monomorphic ventricular tachycardia. This is ventricular tachycardia with a monomorphic configuration. Note the wide complexes. The rate is 185.

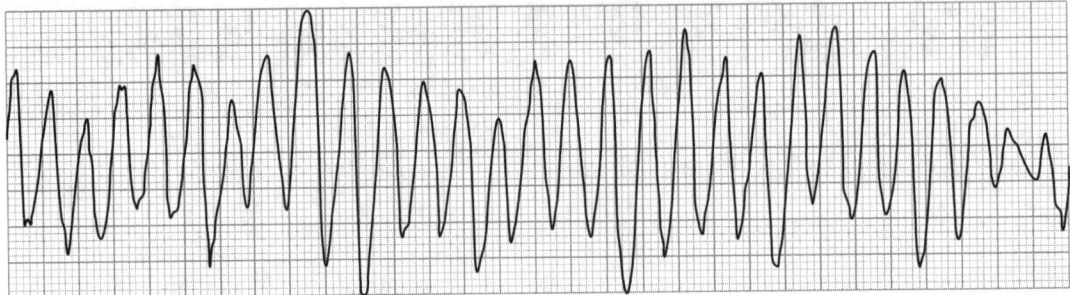

FIGURE 9-13 • Polymorphic ventricular tachycardia. This is an example of polymorphic ventricular tachycardia. Another name for polymorphic ventricular tachycardia that occurs in the presence of a long QT interval is torsades de pointes (TdP). It is important to have an EKG with regular beats on it to determine if the QT interval is prolonged or not.

- **QRS complex:** Greater than 0.12 seconds—wide and bizarre (variations in size, height, shape with polymorphic)
- **QT interval:** Unmeasurable
- **T wave:** Appears as an opposite deflection of the QRS
- **ST segment:** Difficult due to the bizarre presentation of the QRS

CLINICAL ALERT

Treatment for VT is dependent on whether monomorphic or polymorphic VT is present, the length of the QT interval, and the patient's response. Patients who have ventricular tachycardia can be pulseless and apneic or may maintain a pulse and respiratory effort. If patients are hemodynamically stable, alert, and oriented during monomorphic VT, apply oxygen, obtain a patent intravenous line, and prepare for the administration of antiarrhythmics such as amiodarone (Cordarone), procainamide (Pronestyl), or sotalol (Betapace). If they become unstable, synchronized cardioversion is the treatment of choice. Patients can be considered to be unstable when they have symptoms such as chest pain, shortness of breath, mental status changes, and hypotension. Those who are pulseless and apneic, require immediate defibrillation. Patients with polymorphic VT should receive defibrillation.

Patients who are in ventricular tachycardia can have chest pain, dizziness, altered mentation, shortness of breath, and hypotension. They can also have rapid onset of syncope and sudden death. It is important to determine whether the patient has a prolonged QT interval or not when treating these patients. If possible, an EKG or cardiac monitor tracing before the onset of the VT can help in assessing this. This is important when medications are prescribed post treatment. For those patients who are in torsades de pointes, magnesium is the drug of choice. Potassium chloride can also be used in this circumstance. Amiodarone, which might be used for VT, is inappropriate for torsades de pointes. This drug can actually prolong the QT interval and create a decline in the treatment of the VT rhythm. Search for electrolyte disturbances and correct these as well as remove medications which the patient may have been taking, that can prolong the QT interval. Overdrive pacing can also be performed which will help to eliminate or stop the triggering cause. The patient may also require the implantation of a cardioverter-defibrillator.

Some causes of VT include the following:

- Myocardial infarction
- Cardiomyopathy
- Overdoses of medications such as tricyclics or digitalis
- Street drugs such as cocaine
- Valve diseases
- Blunt cardiac injury
- Electrolyte imbalances
- Acid–base imbalances

LQTS should be suspected in young people who have syncopal episodes, especially if it occurs during activities, outbreaks of anger, loud noises, and tense situations. Family histories should be explored for instances of sudden death. LQTS should be suspected in children who present in cardiac arrest with no other explainable cause.

CLINICAL ALERT

Wide QRS tachycardia should be assumed to be VT until proven otherwise. It is often difficult to distinguish between VT and supraventricular tachycardia that has an intraventricular conduction defect.

Ventricular Fibrillation

Ventricular fibrillation (VF) can appear as either coarse or fine. This is a chaotic pattern that does not support cardiac output. Impulses from multiple foci in the ventricles create a situation in which no depolarization exists. In this

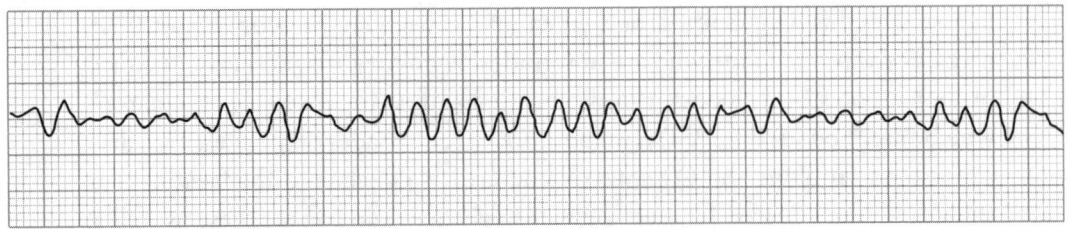

FIGURE 9–14 • Coarse ventricular fibrillation. Note the large, coarse features of the fibrillatory waves.

life-threatening dysrhythmia, the patient is unresponsive with no respiratory effort and absent pulses. The quivering heart is in a fibrillatory pattern that has no discernible waves or complexes.

There are many etiologies for ventricular fibrillation. These include (but are not limited to) the following:

- Ventricular tachycardia
- Myocardial infarction
- Electrolyte imbalances
- Electrocution
- Heart failure
- Acid–base imbalances
- Drug overdoses
- Hypoxia
- Medications including some antiarrhythmics

Features that are present on the EKG tracing are as follows (Figs. 9–14 and 9–15):

- **Regularity:** Chaotic—irregular
- **Rate:** Unable to discern
- **P wave:** Not present

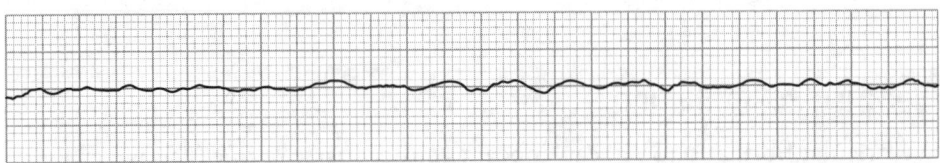

FIGURE 9–15 • Fine ventricular fibrillation. Small fibrillatory waves are an indication of fine ventricular fibrillation. These can sometimes be so small that they are misinterpreted as asystole.

- **PR interval:** Not present
- **QRS complex:** Not present
- **QT interval:** Not present
- **T wave:** Not present
- **ST segment:** Not present

CLINICAL ALERT

Several things can mimic the pattern of ventricular fibrillation on the cardiac monitor. Artifact, electrical interference, loss of patches, and movement of the patient having tremors or seizures can create a pattern similar to that of VF. Be sure to check the patient. Patients who are awake, alert, breathing, and speaking are not in ventricular fibrillation.

Treatment for ventricular fibrillation is included in algorithms taught in cardiac life support classes. Immediate defibrillation is the treatment of choice. Time is very important when dealing with this dysrhythmia. Provide basic cardiopulmonary resuscitation until the defibrillator or automatic external defibrillator (AED) is available. Defibrillation utilizes the same machine as when synchronized cardioversion is provided, however, the sync button is not utilized. The shock provided should cause the heart to stop (asystole), giving it an opportunity to restart with a normal pattern. Place patches or paddles as displayed on the instructions per the machine instructions. It is not necessary to have the patient on the machine monitor for this (as is done with synchronized cardioversion). Be sure to announce "all clear" or accepted phrase before delivering the shock. It is important to protect the health care providers who are assisting in the care of the patient. No one should be touching the patient when the electrical current is delivered.

Asystole

Asystole is present when the EKG tracing or cardiac monitor shows a flat or nearly flat line. No electrical activity is present and the patient should be unresponsive and apneic. Some of the etiologies that can cause an asystolic rhythm are myocardial infarction, pulmonary embolus, lightening injuries, extended hypoxia, electrolyte imbalances, street drug toxicities, and acid–base disturbances and can also be the immediate transient response to the ending of a tachycardic rhythm that has been treated with medications such as Adenocard (adenosine), synchronized cardioversion, or defibrillation. Refer also to the causes that are listed in pulseless electrical activity.

> ### CLINICAL ALERT
>
> When asystole is suspected on the monitor, it is essential to check the patient and to recheck the rhythm in a second lead. Fine ventricular fibrillation can mimic asystole. The patient may have pulled leads off accidentally or equipment failure may be the cause of the flat line on the monitor.

Asystole can also occur as ventricular standstill (P wave asystole). In this rhythm, P waves are present, but no ventricular activity is present. The following are the features of asystole (Figs. 9–16 and 9–17):

- **Regularity:** Unable to note—can have regular P waves in ventricular standstill
- **Rate:** Not discernible—slow atrial activity may be noted with ventricular standstill
- **P wave:** Not present—may be seen with ventricular standstill
- **PR interval:** Not present
- **QRS complex:** Not present
- **QT interval:** Not present
- **T wave:** Not present
- **ST segment:** Not present

Treat the patient in asystole with immediate cardiopulmonary resuscitation. Follow guidelines from cardiac life support classes regarding medications and treatment of potential causes.

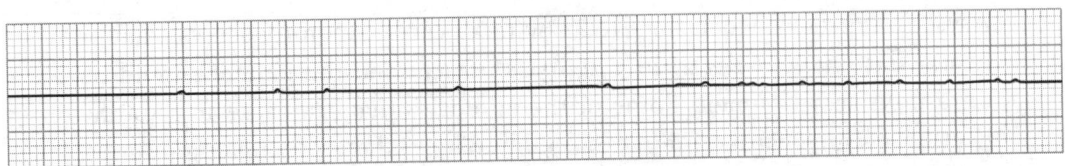

FIGURE 9–16 • **Asystole.** Asystole is indicated by a straight line or "flat line" on the cardiac monitor or EKG tracing. Be sure to verify this in another lead.

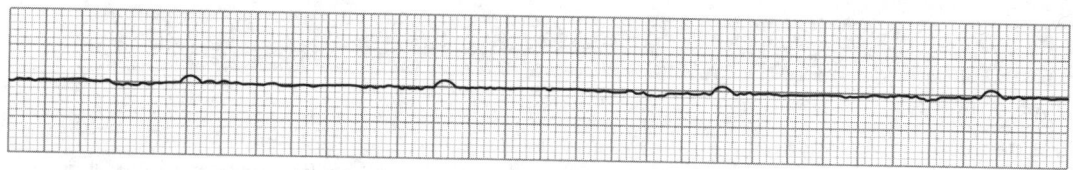

FIGURE 9–17 • Ventricular standstill. Note the P waves as the SA node is electrically sending out a signal. No ventricular response is noted.

AV Nodal Blocks

When a delay in conduction occurs within the AV node, the bundle of His, or the bundle branches, an AV nodal block is produced. Conducted impulses through this area are slower (the depolarization and repolarization process is lengthened) therefore, making this an area of opportunity for blockage of those impulses to take place. Three incomplete blocks and one complete block are involved in the descriptions of this problem within the cardiac conduction system. Each of these blocks has specific characteristics that make up the EKG features that are seen. The blocks are divided into first degree, second degree, and third degree. Second-degree blocks have two subcategories. Third-degree block is also known as complete heart block. Table 9–3 lists the types of blocks, the locations of the associated blocked areas, and the conduction that is found with each type. Patients can often tolerate these blocks and the consequences of each block revolve around the degree of the block, the rate of ventricular or junctional response, and the manner in which the patient reacts to the slowed heart rate. At other times the blocks can represent an emergent condition that must be responded to immediately.

First-Degree AV Block

First-degree AV block represents a delay or pause that occurs as the impulse attempts to cross the AV node. This can occur in some healthy individuals who are athletic (related to an increase in vagal tone) or may occur as a normal deviation during sleep when heart rates reduce. It can also occur when certain medications are taken that can increase the refractory period, such as digoxin, calcium antagonists, and beta-blockers. Other medications that may place the patient at risk for this block are quinidine (Quinaglute), procainamide (Pronestyl), sotalol (Betapace), and amiodarone (Cordarone). It can also be present with deterioration of the conduction system, a myocardial infarction (especially inferior), electrolyte disturbances (hypokalemia or hypomagnesemia),

TABLE 9–3 Atrioventricular Blocks

Type of Block	Location	Graphic Representation	Conduction
First degree	AV Node		• Delay in conduction • PR interval prolonged
Second degree type I	AV node		• Some conduction occurs • PR intervals progressively prolong until beat is dropped
Second degree type II	Bundle of His or Bundle Branches		• Some conduction occurs • PR intervals are constant and occasional or frequent beats are dropped
Third degree	AV Node or Bundle of His or Bundle Branches		• No conduction from P waves • No association between P waves and QRS complexes • No PR intervals

Lead II

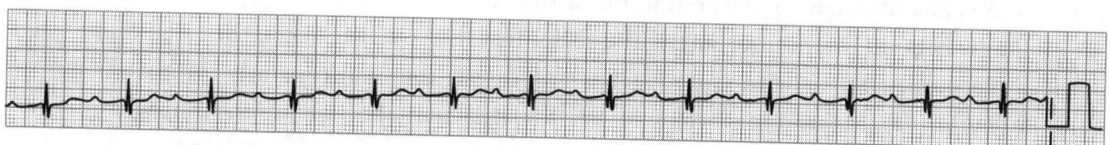

FIGURE 9–18 • **First-degree AV block.** Note that the PR interval in this tracing is 0.36 seconds. This would be read as "normal sinus rhythm with first-degree AV block".

endocarditis, and myocarditis and can be a posttreatment sequelae after catheter ablation for tachydysrhythmias.

Specific EKG tracing or cardiac monitor changes involve a lengthened or prolonged PR interval. This indicates the delay in conduction. When interpreting this rhythm, the underlying rhythm is recognized first with a notation for the first-degree block—"normal sinus rhythm with first-degree block" (Fig. 9–18).

Characteristics of first-degree block are:

- **Regularity:** Dependent on underlying rhythm
- **Rate:** Dependent on underlying rhythm
- **P wave:** Present for each QRS
- **PR interval:** Prolonged—greater than 0.20 seconds
- **QRS complex:** Present and dependent on underlying rhythm
- **QT interval:** Normal
- **T wave:** Normal
- **ST segment:** Normal

Most patients who are experiencing this dysrhythmia are asymptomatic. It does bear watchful observation since it can lead to further degrees of block, especially when it is present in a patient with a myocardial infarction.

Second-Degree AV Block Type I

Second-degree AV block type I is also known as Wenckebach (so named for Dr. Wenckebach, a Dutch internist, who noted changes in the jugular pulse with the two forms of second-degree block before the advent of the electrocardiogram). The term "Mobitz" is also used with second-degree blocks since Dr. Mobitz, a German cardiologist, was able to describe the characteristics of the subclassifications of second-degree AV block on the EKG tracing. The term "Mobitz type I" is used for the changes that occur with "Type I."

In this dysrhythmia, there is a progressive lengthening of the PR interval until a QRS complex is dropped. The abnormality occurs in the AV node. Just as R-R intervals have been measured in other rhythms, in AV blocks, the P-P intervals now become very important. If the P-P intervals are plotted on either a card or piece of paper or with calipers, it is noted that they fall regularly within the rhythm. This is also important to assist in the evaluation of the rhythm when considering a nonconducted PAC. If it were associated with a nonconducted PAC, the P wave would occur early in the cycle. In second-degree blocks, the P waves look alike as they are all coming from the SA node. The problem occurs as it attempts to conduct through the AV node. After the progressive prolongation of the P wave and the QRS complex is dropped, the series begins again until another beat is dropped. In order to identify this dysrhythmia, a rhythm strip must be explored. This cannot be recognized with only two to three beats on the 12-lead EKG. It can be suspected as the PR interval is seen to lengthen; however, to visualize the dropped beat a longer strip must be investigated. A pattern is usually set so that the dropped beat will occur in a recurring arrangement, that is, every third beat dropped, every fourth beat dropped, etc.

EKG characteristics of this rhythm are (Fig. 9–19):

- **Regularity:** Atrial regular, ventricular irregular (due to dropped beat)
- **Rate:** Dependent on underlying rhythm—atrial rate is greater
- **P wave:** Similar in size and configuration each time
- **PR interval:** Gradual prolongation until QRS complex is dropped
- **QRS complex:** Not present for each P wave— normal in width
- **QT interval:** Normal
- **T wave:** Normal
- **ST segment:** Normal

CLINICAL ALERT

Though patients can be asymptomatic with Wenckebach or Mobitz type I, some may require treatment. Slow rates associated with a drop in blood pressure or lightheadedness may require the use of a pacemaker.

Lead II

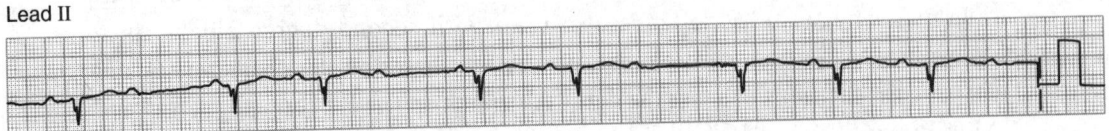

FIGURE 9–19 • Second-degree AV block Mobitz type I/Wenckebach. On this rhythm strip, note the first two P waves. The second P wave does not have a QRS associated with it. The third and fourth P waves have QRS complexes, but the PR interval of each is lengthening each time. The 5th and 8th P waves again do not have a QRS complex.

Causes of second-degree AV block, Mobitz type I (Wenckebach) include certain medications, an increase in parasympathetic activity, cardiac tissue ischemia or an inferior myocardial infarction or right ventricular infarct. Be especially observant for the patient who is experiencing this associated with infarctions as they can then elevate the seriousness of the degree of block.

Second-Degree AV Block Type II

Type II second-degree AV block, also known as Mobitz type II, occurs due to a delay in conduction at the level of the bundle of His or the bundle branches. While Mobitz type I is dependent on the progressive lengthening of the PR interval, in Mobitz type II, the PR intervals are constant. Dropped beats occur throughout the rhythm strip. The P waves will again plot out at regular intervals. The ventricular rate is typically slow and irregular and is lower than the atrial rate. When the ratio of atrial beats (P wave) to ventricular beats (QRS complex) is 2:1 (two atrial beats to one ventricular beat), the ventricular rate will be regular. A situation can occur in which there are more than two beats that are dropped in succession. This is indicative of a high grade AV block and is considered more dangerous than the normal pattern of Mobitz type II. This rhythm can be a precursor to third-degree or complete heart block.

Factors that are present for second-degree AV block, Mobitz type II are (Fig. 9–20):

- **Regularity:** Atrial regular, ventricular irregular (due to dropped beat)—may be regular with a 2:1 ratio

- **Rate:** Ventricular rate slow—atrial rate is greater

- **P wave:** Similar in size and configuration each time

- **PR interval:** Normal for each P wave except for the dropped beats—may be prolonged slightly, but will be constant

- **QRS complex:** Not present for each P wave—usually wider—greater than 0.10 seconds

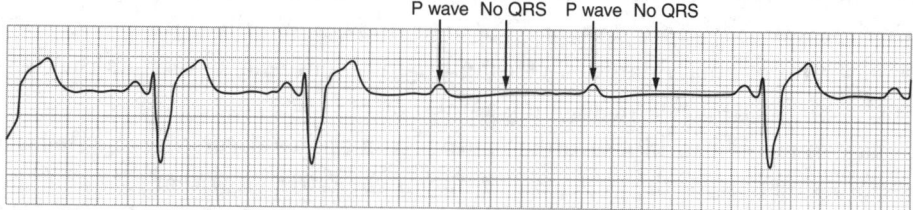

FIGURE 9–20 • **Second-degree AV block Mobitz type II.** In this rhythm strip the P waves will plot out regularly. The QRS complexes will not be regular due to the dropped beats. When this happens, provide the rate in a range – "20 to 60 beats per minute". Note the constant PR interval.

- **QT interval:** Normal
- **T wave:** Normal
- **ST segment:** Normal

CLINICAL ALERT

Mobitz type II can move rapidly into complete heart block. Observe the patient closely and prepare for emergent pacemaker insertion if this occurs. Atropine is not used in this dysrhythmia. This will cause the SA node to fire faster and can trigger more problems for the patient.

This type of second-degree heart block can be caused by an anterior myocardial infarction. Organic cardiac diseases such as myocarditis, endocarditis, and rheumatic fever can also cause this dysrhythmia. Sarcoidosis, Hodgkin's lymphoma, rheumatoid arthritis, and lupus have also been noted to cause this type of AV block. Medications that may contribute to this dysrhythmia are: digoxin, calcium channel blockers, beta-blockers, and sodium channel blockers.

Patients can be stable during episodes of second-degree AV block Mobitz type II. If this is the case, observe closely. If the patient is unstable including hypotension, chest pain, lightheadedness, and syncope, prepare for pacing.

Third-Degree AV Block

In third-degree or complete heart block, the atrial impulses are totally blocked. No conduction is passing through. This can happen at any level within the AV node, the bundle of His, or the bundle branches. The QRS complexes that occur can be generated from either junctional or ventricular tissue. Because of this, the QRS complexes may be narrow or wide. The cause of the block determines the level at which the block is occurring. For instance, an inferior myocardial infarction causing a complete heart block usually happens above the bundle of His. When the ventricles are responsible for the QRS complexes, the rhythm is usually more unstable. The rate is lower and the QRS is wider. An anterior myocardial infarction causing this problem usually recruits the ventricles for assistance in maintaining a pulse rate.

In complete heart block, cardiac output is not at an effective level. This is a serious situation for the patient. Not only is the rate so low that it affects the cardiac output, but atrial kick is also lost. The asynchrony between the atria and the ventricles is seen on the EKG tracing or cardiac monitor as a complete loss of association of the P waves and QRS complexes.

Lead II

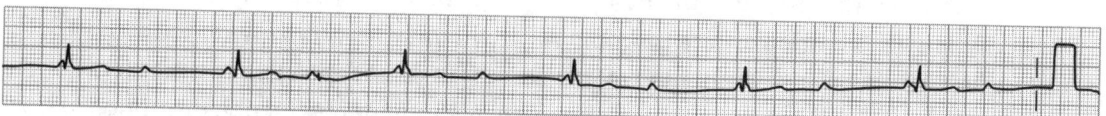

FIGURE 9–21 • Complete heart block/third-degree heart block. Note that both the P waves and the R waves march out across the rhythm in uniform and regular fashion. Even though there appears to be P waves before some of the QRS complexes, they are buried within the QRS. Use a paper with marks on or calipers to note how they march.

The following are characteristics of third-degree heart block (Fig. 9–21):

- **Regularity:** Atrial regular, ventricular regular—independent of each other
- **Rate:** Ventricular rate slow—atrial rate is greater
- **P wave:** Similar in size and configuration each time
- **PR interval:** None present
- **QRS complex:** May be narrow wide depending on site of generated impulse
- **QT interval:** May be elongated
- **T wave:** Normal
- **ST segment:** Normal

CLINICAL ALERT

If the rate is extremely slow, there may be "extra beats" that are escape beats. They will look like premature beats but will occur later in the cycle. It is important to not suppress these beats as they are attempting to help with cardiac output.

Patients with complete heart block can be asymptomatic. They may even remain hemodynamically stable. They will still require a pacemaker and should have close monitoring, but the pacemaker can be done on an elective basis rather than emergent. Others who are symptomatic with dizziness, dyspnea, change in mentation, chest pain, lightheadedness, hypotension, pallor, sweating, and syncope should be treated with transcutaneous pacing. A temporary pacer will need to be inserted until it is determined if the patient will require a permanent pacemaker. If it occurs with an anterior myocardial infarction, chances are that a permanent pacemaker will be necessary. Complete heart block associated with an inferior myocardial infarction may resolve and not involve a permanent pacemaker.

Another rhythm that might occur is complete AV dissociation. In this rhythm, the ventricular rate is simply faster and may be very close to the atrial rate. Consider this rhythm if the rate is faster. This can happen due to a problem with the SA node or an increased impulse generation or conduction disruption in the AV node.

Conclusion

Ventricular dysrhythmias and atrioventricular blocks can present serious issues for the patient experiencing them. Sometimes the patient will have no symptoms; however, the potential for deterioration is always present with these issues. The health care provider must be ready to intervene immediately when these occur. Some of the highlights of these dysrhythmias are:

- When ventricular rhythms occur, atrial kick is lost which can decrease cardiac output by 30%.
- The SA node can cease to function or blocks can occur as the impulse attempts to be conducted through the AV node and beyond.
- At times ventricular rhythms occur due to irritable tissue in the ventricles.
- Ventricular beats are wide, have aberrant shapes, and no P waves associated with them.
- PVCs do not always produce a "beat" or participate in perfusion. It is important to check the pulse on these patients.
- PVCs should have full compensatory pause unless they are considered to be interpolated.
- A fusion beat can occur that is a combination of a regular beat and a premature ventricular contraction.
- PVCs can be unifocal or multifocal.
- PVCs can occur as bigeminal, trigeminal, or quadrigeminal. They may also couple together. Three PVCs together constitutes a short burst of ventricular tachycardia.
- An escape beat occurs when a PVC attempts to come to the rescue of a slow rate. These beats will be late rather than premature in the cycle.
- PVCs can be normal for the patient or they can occur due to medications the patient may be taking. An acute myocardial infarction as well as other possible diagnoses can cause these.

- Three or more escape beats together can create an idioventricular rhythm.
- Idioventricular rhythms will cause a decrease in cardiac output and the consequences of that as demonstrated by hypotension, weak radial pulses, dizziness, lightheadedness, confusion, or syncope.
- PEA or pulseless electrical activity can occur with any rhythm, but can commonly occur with idioventricular rhythms.
- There are several etiologies for PEA. The mnemonic to remember these is PATCH-4-MD or the 5 H's and 5 T's.
- Idioventricular rhythm can be a precursor to asystole for patients.
- Transcutaneous pacing is a life saving procedure in which the patient receives electrical impulses through the skin.
- The mA on the transcutaneous pacer is the amount of electricity that must be delivered in order for the patient to attain and maintain "capture." This can be uncomfortable for the patient.
- When the rate of an idioventricular rhythm is over 40 beats per minute, it is known as accelerated idioventricular rhythm.
- Accelerated idioventricular rhythms can occur with several diagnoses such as acute myocardial infarction, subarachnoid hemorrhage, and cocaine ingestion. It is also known to occur transiently with reperfusion after the administration of thrombolytics.
- Ventricular tachycardia can be monomorphic or polymorphic.
- Polymorphic ventricular tachycardia can occur due to a prolonged QT interval or it can be present with a normal QT interval. This can be acquired or congenital.
- Patients in VT can be awake with a pulse or can be unresponsive and pulseless. Treatment depends on how the patient is responding.
- For those patients who are pulseless, immediate defibrillation is necessary.
- Torsades de pointes occurs when a long QT interval is the cause of polymorphic ventricular tachycardia.
- Long QT syndrome can be the cause of syncopal episodes in young people. It can lead to cardiac arrest. This must be diagnosed with an EKG tracing that is performed when the patient is not in VT.
- Ventricular fibrillation can be either coarse or fine.
- Fine VF can be misdiagnosed as asystole.

- Immediate defibrillation must be performed for VF.
- Asystole occurs when there is no electrical or mechanical activity present. It is represented by a flat line on the EKG tracing.
- Immediate CPR must be established with asystole.
- AV nodal blocks occur when there is a delay or block in conduction through the AV node, the bundle of His, or the bundle branches.
- First-degree AV block is represented by a prolonged PR interval on the EKG tracing or cardiac monitor. This is simply a delay in conduction.
- Many medications can cause first-degree AV block and other AV blocks.
- Usually no treatment is necessary for first-degree AV block.
- Second-degree AV block is divided into Mobitz type I (also known as Wenckebach) and Mobitz type II.
- Mobitz type I (Wenckebach) is seen on the EKG strip as a progressive prolongation of the PR interval until a beat is dropped.
- Mobitz type II is seen as dropped beats that occur on the EKG tracing but with consistent PR intervals.
- Both second-degree AV block, Mobitz type I, and Mobitz type II can require treatment and careful observation of the patient, but the patient may also be asymptomatic.
- Third-degree or complete heart block is recognized on the EKG tracing or cardiac monitor as a slow rate that has no relationship between the atrial beats and ventricular complexes.
- Patients with third-degree or complete AV block will require a pacemaker. Some may need it more emergently than others.

PRACTICE QUESTIONS

1. **Ventricular beats will have which of the following characteristics?**
   A. Prolonged PR interval
   B. Widened QRS complex
   C. T wave and QRS in same direction
   D. P waves will precede each beat

2. **Which of the following is a true statement regarding a premature ventricular contraction?**
   A. A P wave will always precede a premature ventricular contraction.
   B. A premature ventricular contraction will have a full compensatory pause.

C. A premature ventricular contraction will have a narrow QRS complex.

D. Fusion beats always accompany premature ventricular contractions.

3. **Which of the following is a correct statement regarding an escape beat?**

A. Escape beats occur early in the cardiac cycle.

B. Escape beats are present in an attempt to rescue the patient.

C. Escape beats should be treated by eradicating them.

D. Escape beats provide excellent cardiac output.

4. **Which of the following would be an appropriate medication to treat multiple premature ventricular contractions?**

A. Atropine sulfate

B. Epinephrine

C. Amiodarone (Cordarone)

D. Digitalis (Lanoxin)

5. **Which of the following rates would most likely be associated with an idioventricular rhythm?**

A. 28 beats per minute

B. 60 beats per minute

C. 82 beats per minute

D. 210 beats per minute

6. **Which of the following is considered to be a possible cause of pulseless electrical activity?**

A. Nicotine abuse

B. Pulmonary embolus

C. Hyponatremia

D. Arterial occlusion

7. **Which of the following would indicate mechanical capture when using a transcutaneous pacemaker on a patient?**

A. Pacer spike seen before each QRS complex

B. Chest wall movement on the patient

C. Coughing with each paced beat

D. Presence of blood pressure

8. **Which of the following is a rhythm in which *torsades de pointes* could be present?**

A. Monomorphic ventricular tachycardia

B. Ventricular Fibrillation

C. Ventricular Standstill

D. Polymorphic ventricular tachycardia

9. Which of the following should be performed on a patient with pulseless ventricular fibrillation?

   A. Administration of atropine sulfate
   B. Synchronized cardioversion
   C. Immediate defibrillation
   D. Administration of digitalis

10. Which of the following patients would be LEAST likely to have long QT syndrome?

    A. 12-year-old with syncope
    B. 6-month-old with SIDS
    C. 37-year-old with cocaine use
    D. 82-year-old with sudden death

11. When providing a defibrillatory shock to a patient who has coarse ventricular fibrillation, which of the following should occur?

    A. Short period of asystole
    B. Intermittent atrial fibrillation
    C. Change to ventricular tachycardia
    D. Conversion to third-degree AV block

12. A Mobitz type I block is also known as:

    A. First-degree AV block
    B. Wenckebach
    C. Third-degree AV block
    D. Second-degree AV block type II

13. In which of the following atrioventricular blocks would the health care provider expect the PR interval to be a constant 0.32 seconds with no dropped beats?

    A. First-degree AV block
    B. Second-degree AV block type II
    C. Wenckebach
    D. Third-degree AV block

14. At which part of the electrical conduction system is the block occurring when second-degree AV block Mobitz type I takes place?

    A. SA node
    B. AV node
    C. Bundle of His
    D. Bundle branches

15. Identify the following dysrhythmia:

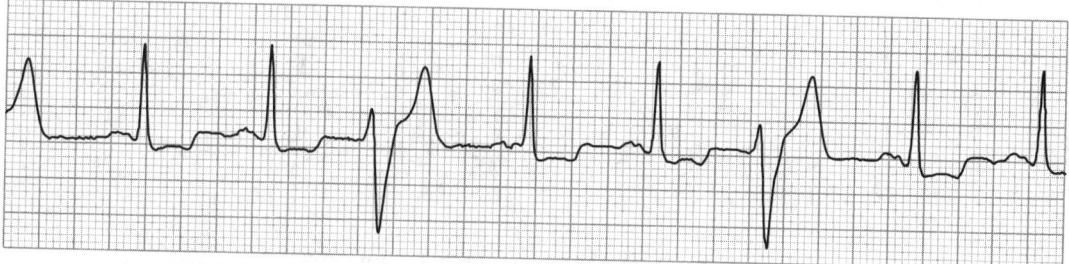

    A. Normal sinus rhythm with unifocal trigeminy
    B. Normal sinus rhythm with multifocal bigeminy
    C. Normal sinus rhythm with unifocal quadrigeminy
    D. Normal sinus rhythm with multifocal trigeminy

16. Identify the following dysrhythmia:

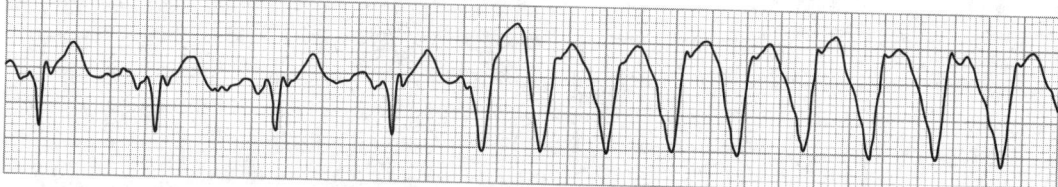

    A. Onset of polymorphic ventricular tachycardia
    B. Onset of monomorphic ventricular tachycardia
    C. Onset of coarse ventricular fibrillation
    D. Onset of accelerated idioventricular

17. Identify the following dysrhythmia:

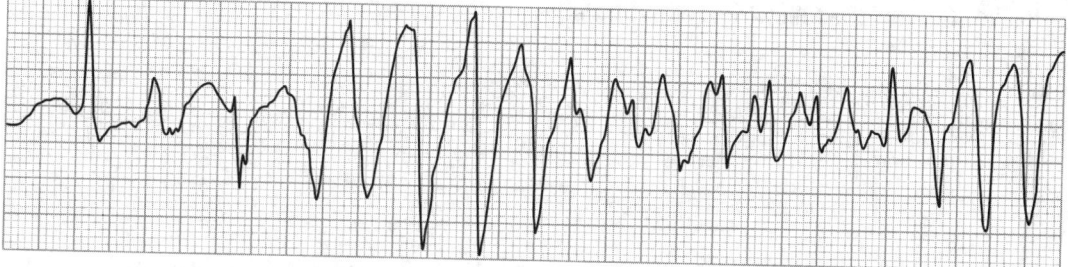

    A. Onset of polymorphic ventricular tachycardia
    B. Onset of coarse ventricular fibrillation
    C. Onset of monomorphic ventricular tachycardia
    D. Onset of accelerated idioventricular

18. Identify the following dysrhythmia:

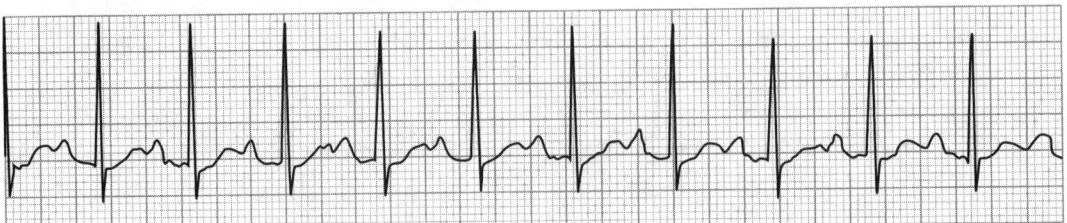

    A. Sinus tachycardia with second-degree AV block type I

    B. Normal sinus rhythm with second-degree AV block type II

    C. Sinus tachycardia with first-degree AV block

    D. Sinus bradycardia with third-degree AV block

19. Identify the following dysrhythmia:

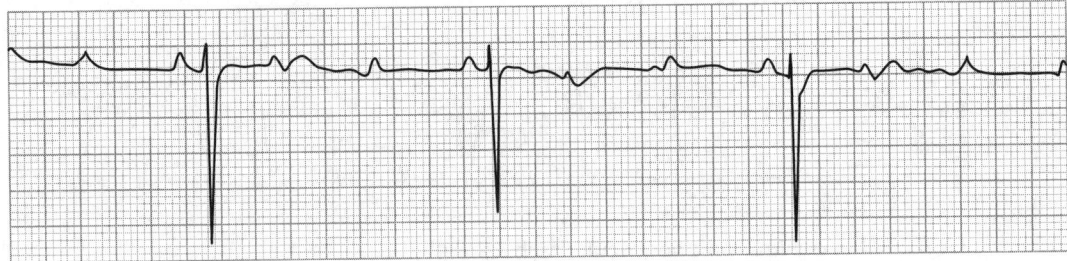

    A. First-degree AV block

    B. Second-degree AV block type I

    C. Second-degree AV block type II

    D. Third-degree AV block

20. Identify the following dysrhythmia:

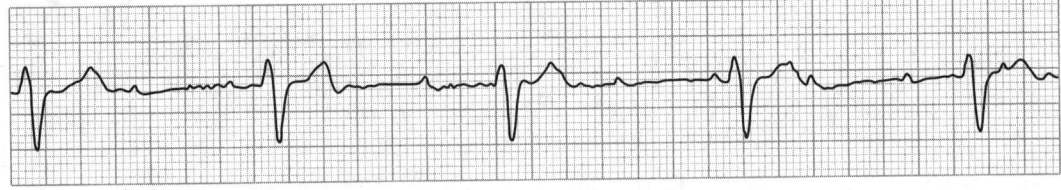

    A. First-degree AV block

    B. Second-degree AV block type I

    C. Second-degree AV block type II

    D. Third-degree AV block

ANSWER KEY

1. **B.** Ventricular beats will have wide QRS morphologies. The T wave will deflect in the opposite direction. No P wave is present; therefore, no PR interval is measurable.

2. **B.** Full compensatory pauses occur with PVCs as opposed to PACs which do not have this. P waves are not present and these complexes are wide and bizarre. Fusion beats can be present but are not necessarily present every time.

3. **B.** Escape beats are present in an attempt to help rescue the patient from a dangerously slow rhythm. These beats occur late in the cycle and medications to extinguish these beats should not be given. They do not supply as good cardiac output as a regular beat.

4. **C.** Amiodarone (Cordarone) would be the appropriate medication used to treat problems with multiple premature ventricular contractions. Lidocaine could also be used. Atropine and epinephrine would speed up the rate and this would not be desired at this time. Digitalis could be one of the causes of PVCs and would not do anything to suppress these extra beats.

5. **A.** The inherent rate for an idioventricular rhythm would be 20 to 40 beats per minute.

6. **B.** A pulmonary embolus, along with others listed in the mnemonic PATCH-4-MD and the 5 H's and 5 T's can cause pulseless electrical activity. The abuse of nicotine, hyponatremia, and arterial occlusion would not be potential causes of PEA.

7. **D.** Mechanical capture with a transcutaneous pacer would be indicated by the presence of palpable pulses and a blood pressure. The presence of a pacer spike prior to each QRS complex would indicate electrical capture. Movement of the chest wall and coughing with each paced beat would indicate that the patient might need to be sedated or the mA turned down if possible.

8. **D.** Torsades de pointes is a rhythm associated with a polymorphic ventricular tachycardia. It stands for "twisting of the points" and is present with long QT syndrome.

9. **C.** Pulseless ventricular tachycardia must be cared for in the same way that ventricular fibrillation is handled. This requires the use of immediate defibrillation. Synchronous cardioversion cannot be used on either pulseless ventricular tachycardia or ventricular fibrillation. Atropine and digitalis would be inappropriate medications to use.

10. **D.** A young person with syncope is a red flag for the possibility of a congenital long QT syndrome. Studies have been performed as to the possibility that SIDS deaths might be associated with a prolonged QT interval. The use of cocaine is another potential cause of long QT syndrome. An elderly patient with sudden death would be the least likely of those listed to have a long QT syndrome.

11. **A.** Immediately after defibrillation a short run of asystole is most often seen which then allows the heart to reset itself and return in a normal sinus rhythm.

12. **B.** Second-degree AV block, Mobitz type I is known as Wenckebach.

13. **A.** First-degree AV block is identified by a constant, prolonged PR interval. Second-degree AV block type I (Wenckebach) would have a progressively prolonging PR interval until a beat is dropped. Second-degree AV block type II would have constant normal PR when present. Third-degree block would not have a PR interval that was measurable.

14. **B.** Second-degree AV block type I (Wenckebach) is identified as having a block at the AV node. The SA node is not implicated in the diagnosis of an AV block. A block at the bundle of His or in the bundle branches could create either a second-degree AV block type II or a third-degree AV block (complete block).

15. **A.** This rhythm strip shows normal sinus rhythm with PVCs that are unifocal in morphology every third beat—unifocal trigeminy. Multifocal would mean the PVCs should show different morphologies. Bigeminy would have a PVC occurring every other beat. Quadrigeminy would present as a PVC every fourth beat.

16. **B.** This rhythm strip shows the onset of monomorphic ventricular tachycardia. Ventricular fibrillation is labeled either coarse or fine but not monomorphic or polymorphic. The rate is too high for accelerated idioventricular.

17. **A.** Polymorphic ventricular tachycardia is seen when the points of the QRS complexes are bizarre and not of the same height or width.

18. **C.** The underlying rhythm in this strip is sinus tachycardia. The PR interval is prolonged and there is a P wave for each QRS indicating a first-degree AV block. The underlying rhythm is not normal sinus rhythm or bradycardic. Second-degree AV block type I would have a progressively prolonged PR interval and second-degree AV block type II would have a constant normal PR interval.

19. **C.** This rhythm strip denotes a second-degree AV block type II. There is a 3:1 conduction rate which means there are three atrial beats for each one QRS complex.

20. **D.** In this rhythm strip there is no direct association between the P waves and the QRS complexes. Each is beating independently of the other. The ventricular rate is 45 beats per minute.

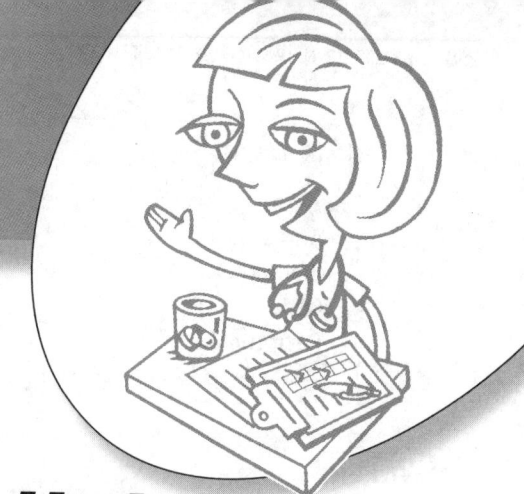

chapter 10

Acute Myocardial Infarction Patterns

LEARNING OBJECTIVES

At the end of this chapter, the student will be able to:

① Relate coronary pathophysiology to types of myocardial infarctions (MIs).

② Explain the difference between angina, ST segment elevation myocardial infarction (STEMI), and non-ST segment elevation myocardial infarction (NSTEMI) presentations of chest pain.

③ Understand common dysrhythmias associated with the different types of MIs.

④ Distinguish types of MIs based on changes in particular leads on the 12-lead EKG.

⑤ Identify the different EKG changes relevant to ischemia, injury, and infarction.

⑥ List symptomatology, diagnostic markers, and treatment options for patients experiencing an acute myocardial infarction (AMI).

KEY WORDS

Angioplasty

Biomarkers

Ostia

Reciprocal

Reperfusion

Stokes-Adams

Thrombolytic

Overview

An acute myocardial infarction (AMI) occurs due to the occlusion of a coronary artery with a thrombus formation. This event causes necrosis of cardiac tissue and can predispose the patient to the development of multiple dysrhythmias and death. The blood supply to the myocardium is accomplished through arteries that lie on the outside of the heart supplying the various areas of the myocardium. Plaques develop below the intima, the innermost layer of vessels, which then rupture through this layer developing a narrowed passage for the blood supply. Once the plaque is present inside the vessel, a clot forms at the site. This thrombus formation is the critical pathology that creates a situation for ischemia, injury, and necrosis in that particular part of the heart.

Pathophysiology of Acute Myocardial Infarction

Coronary Artery Supply

Two major arteries supply the heart with its own blood supply. These are the left and right coronary arteries. These arteries arise from the aortic valve through **ostia** or openings around the cusps. Each of these arteries then have branches that help to encircle the heart, providing oxygen rich blood to this important organ (Fig. 10–1).

Even though the make up of the coronary artery circulation is similar in all patients, there are congenital modifications that do occur. The terms "left dominant" and "right dominant" have to do with the origin of the posterior descending artery (PDA). When this arises from the circumflex branch (LCX) of the left coronary artery (LCA), the patient is said to be "left dominant." When the PDA develops from the right coronary artery (RCA), it is then known as "right dominant." Other alterations also occur, such as the source of the sinus node artery. This can arise from the RCA or the circumflex. In the majority of patients, this branch comes off of the RCA. These deviations are important

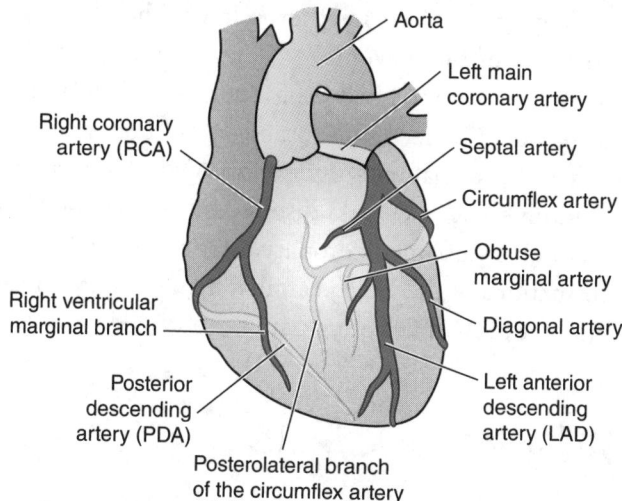

FIGURE 10–1 • Coronary arteries. The right and left coronary arteries are the main vessels to supply the heart. Each of these then have branches that help to encircle the heart. (*From Aehlert, B. ECG's Made Easy, 4e. Mosby JEMS, 2011.*)

when looking at potential problems that occur when patients develop blockages in certain vessels. Each of these arteries supplies not only different portions of the heart wall, but also distinctive areas within the heart such as the SA and AV node. For instance, when the RCA is obstructed, patients will most often have difficulty with the SA and AV node. See Table 10–1 for an explanation of the common areas supplied by each of the major arteries.

TABLE 10–1 Major Coronary Arteries and Areas Supplied

Coronary Artery	Areas Supplied
Left Anterior Descending (LAD) (from left coronary artery)	• Right ventricle • Left ventricle • Interventricular septum (anterior 2/3)
Circumflex (CX) (from left coronary artery)	• Left ventricle (anterior, lateral, and posterior) • Left atrium
Right coronary artery (RCA)	• Right atrium • SA node • AV node
Right marginal branch (of the RCA)	• Right atrium (lateral aspect) • Right ventricle (lateral aspect)
Posterior descending artery (PDA) (from the RCA) (also known as the posterior interventricular branch)	• Right ventricle (posterior aspect) • Left ventricle (posterior aspect) • Interventricular septum (posterior aspect)

The usual etiology for an AMI is atherosclerotic heart disease. However, there are other reasons for these events to occur. Coronary artery spasms, congenital anomalies, trauma, use of illicit drugs such as cocaine, hyperthyroidism, anemia, aortic dissection, GI bleed syndromes, and carbon monoxide poisoning are a few of the reasons for patients to develop AMIs. Children can also have MIs. Marfan's syndrome and Kawasaki disease can predispose children to this disease process, as well as inflamed coronary arteries, nephrotic syndrome, and congenital malformations of the LCA. Familial high cholesterol can also influence the development of AMI in young patients.

Acute Coronary Syndrome

Acute coronary syndromes include several aspects of the process of occlusion and possible necrosis of cardiac tissue. The three subcategories of this disease pattern are:

- Unstable Angina
- Non-ST segment elevation myocardial infarction (NSTEMI)
- ST segment elevation myocardial infarction (STEMI)

Unstable Angina

Angina causes chest pain when there is a decrease in the amount of oxygen available for the heart to function. This can happen because there is an increase in the demand for oxygen (exercise, stress, physical activity) or there is a decrease in the amount of oxygen available (hypoxia). One form of angina is considered to be "stable." This is when discomfort is noted during exercise, physical activity, or some type of stressful situation. This increase in demand for oxygen is relieved by rest or the use of nitroglycerin. The episodes are very short—from 2 to 15 minutes.

Unstable angina is present when one of three factors exists:

- Chest pain and associated symptoms occur during rest or with minimal physical exertion. This usually lasts for more than 20 to 30 minutes.
- Symptoms that are of new onset but occur due to extremely minimal physical exertion.
- Stable angina symptoms that are now occurring more frequently, are more severe, and lasting for greater periods of time.

Patients with unstable angina are often in a preinfarction stage. Treatment is necessary to prevent them from subsequently infarcting. Follow up studies are important for these patients to properly diagnose and treat this disorder.

Another form of unstable angina is called *Prinzmetal's angina*. Another term for this is variant angina. Though some patients may have associated atherosclerosis, many do not have this aspect of myocardial vessel disease. In this presentation, coronary arteries spasm thus causing a decrease in the blood supply to the myocardium. An interesting aspect of this type of angina is that it almost always occurs at rest with the prime time for symptomatic pathology occurring between midnight and 8 o'clock in the morning. For these patients, ST segments may be elevated during the time of pain and will return to baseline when the pain has resolved. Episodes may be short but can cause dysrhythmias including ventricular tachycardia and fibrillation leading to sudden death.

CLINICAL ALERT

When patients present with complaints of "not feeling well," they may not be able to identify that chest discomfort is a part of their distress. Oftentimes, when asked if they are having chest pain, they will quickly reply "no." However, on further questioning, the health care provider may be able to ascertain that chest "heaviness" or "tightness" is present that the patient does not qualify as "pain." Always make sure that these inquiries are made. It is part of the health care professionals "job" to help the patient to verbalize these difficult symptoms. Be sure to let them know that heaviness and tightness in the chest area is indeed pain. The health care professional and the patient must be able to "speak the same language" when it comes to symptoms.

Non-ST Segment Elevation Myocardial Infarction

The name defines it when a patient is diagnosed with non-ST segment myocardial infarction (NSTEMI). This simply means that the ST elevation that is seen with an ST segment elevation myocardial infarction (STEMI) is not present. Some EKG changes that can occur with the NSTEMI are: 1. Transient ST segment depression and 2. T wave inversion that is 1 mm or more. These changes should be seen in at least two contiguous leads. The chief identifying characteristic for this event is that the **biomarkers** will be increased indicating a leakage of enzymes from damaged cardiac tissue. These EKG changes may occur with unstable angina, but, the biomarkers are not elevated in unstable angina. The frequency of this type of AMI has increased.

ST Segment Elevation Myocardial Infarction

As the name implies, these myocardial infarctions carry the classic ST segment elevation in the leads associated with the damaged myocardium. Biomarkers will also be elevated in this type of AMI. Most of these patients will eventually produce the Q wave, which marks actual necrosis. These patients are candidates for thrombolytic therapy and percutaneous transthoracic coronary angiography and subsequent interventions.

EKG Changes

T Wave Changes

The outermost part of the area of infarction involves an area of ischemia or decreased oxygen supply to a particular part of the heart. The T wave is associated with this area. In the early stages of an MI, the T waves can become hyperacute, meaning they are tall and peaked. This then changes to the depressed or inverted T wave which can be present for extended periods of time. This can occur alone or concurrently with the ST segment elevation (Figs. 10–2, 10–3, and 10–4).

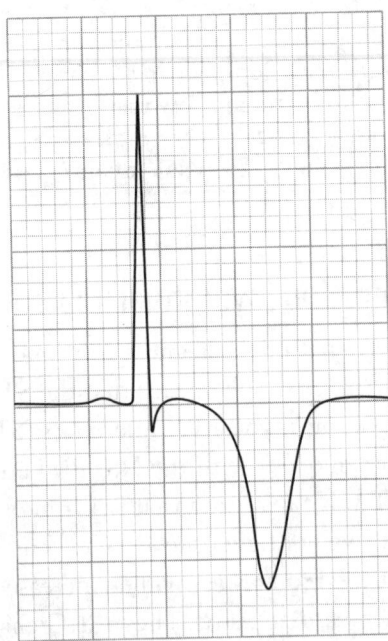

FIGURE 10–2 • T wave inversion . T wave inversion is depicted as the negative deflection (below the isoelectric line) in leads that normally should have a positive direction (above the isoelectric line).

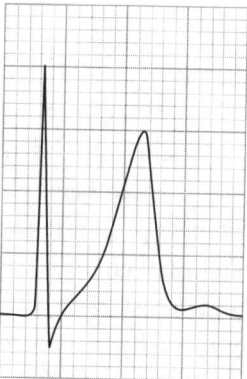

FIGURE 10–3 • **Hyperacute T wave.** Tall, peaked T waves can occur early in the transformation of the myocardial infarction, before T wave depression occurs.

CLINICAL ALERT

It is important to compare the EKG in question with old EKGs. Changes may or may not be occurring. If suspected changes are the same as they were "6 months ago," they may or may not be important in diagnosing the patient with ischemia at "this particular time." Also, some patients may actually have inverted T waves that they normally carry. In this case, the T wave may become "normal." This is called *pseudonormalization*. The only way to determine this phenomenon is to judge the electrocardiograms side by side.

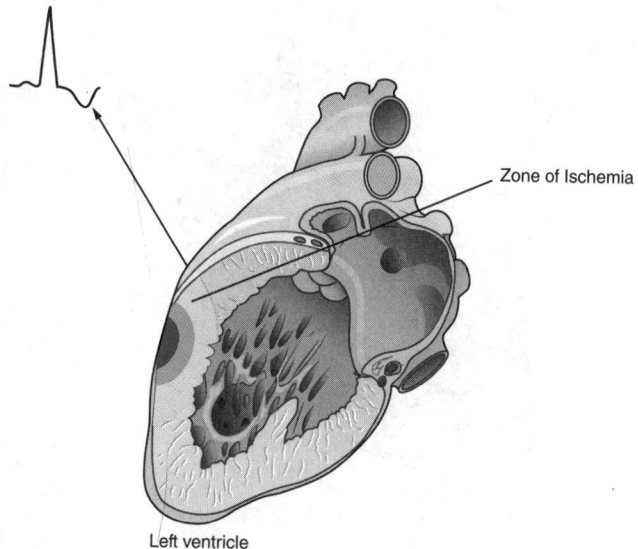

FIGURE 10–4 • **Zone of ischemia.** The area of ischemia is the outermost layer of the area of infarction. (*From Aehlert, B. ECG's Made Easy, 4e. Mosby JEMS, 2011.*)

ST Segment Elevation

ST segment elevation, noted in two contiguous leads, which means the leads look at the same area of the heart, occurs as an indicator of injury. The middle area, lying between the zone of ischemia and the zone of infarction, is the region revealed by this change in the EKG (Fig. 10–5).

This ST elevation, seen in patients presenting with STEMI, will be observed in the patient evolving to infarction. When ST segment elevation is noted on the EKG, it is not an indicator of necrosis of myocardium. ST changes can occur and stay elevated (>1 mm) for several hours before actual infarction takes place. This is reversible at this time.

These can return to baseline after a period of time or can be a factor in **reperfusion** of myocardium when **thrombolytic** therapy or **angioplasty** is performed. ST segment elevation is an indicator for reperfusion interventions.

This ST segment elevation can occur with other circumstances as well, such as pericarditis, hyperkalemia, a pulmonary embolism, or hypothermia. ST segments that tend to stay elevated for prolonged periods of time could signify an aneurysm that has formed in a ventricle. When elevated ST segments are present, they will vary as to the morphology, but the configuration will usually appear as an upward swing in the ST segment as it merges with T wave (Fig. 10–6).

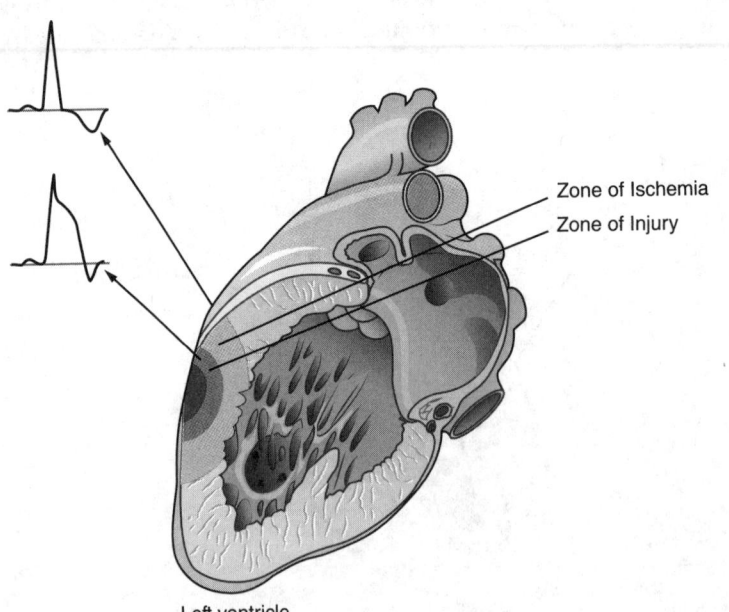

Zone of Ischemia
Zone of Injury

Left ventricle

FIGURE 10–5 • **Zone of injury.** The zone of injury lies between the zones of ischemia and infarction. This is shown in the elevation of the ST segment. (*Modified From Aehlert, B. ECG's Made Easy, 4e. Mosby JEMS, 2011.*)

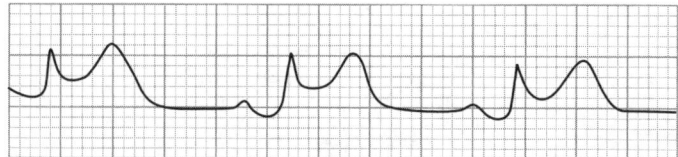

FIGURE 10–6 • ST segment elevation. ST segment elevation is present to indicate an area of injury to the myocardium. (*Modified From Aehlert, B. ECG's Made Easy, 4e. Mosby JEMS, 2011.*)

CLINICAL ALERT

ST segment depression can occur in some MIs, when the leads in which it is present are directly opposite to the true area of infarction. This depression is known as "**reciprocal**" ST changes. A reciprocal change is actually a mirror image; therefore, these will occur in the opposite leads from where the actual injury is occurring. As an example, if an anterior MI occurs, reciprocal changes will be seen in the inferior leads.

Pathologic Q Wave

The Q wave is seen when necrosis actually occurs in the area. This is the last layer of the zones (Fig. 10–7). When necrosis occurs, no depolarization is able to take place. The absence of conduction correlates with a deep negative

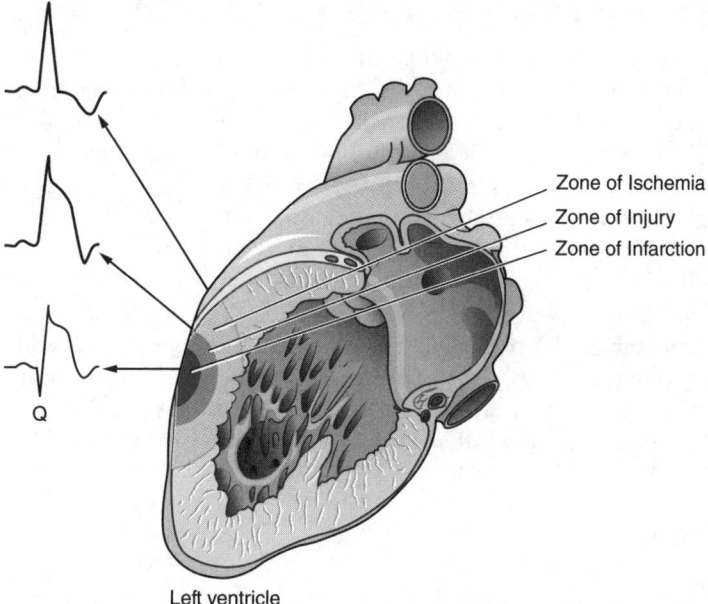

Zone of Ischemia
Zone of Injury
Zone of Infarction

Q

Left ventricle

FIGURE 10–7 • Zone of infarction. The zone of infarction is the necrotic portion of the heart wall. (*Modified From Aehlert, B. ECG's Made Easy, 4e. Mosby JEMS, 2011.*)

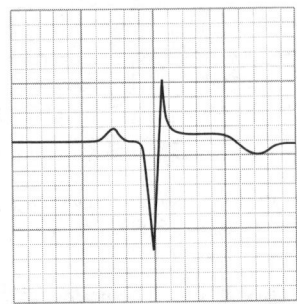

FIGURE 10–8 • Pathologic Q wave. This Q wave is wide and deep. It is greater than 0.04 seconds in width and deeper than one third the overall R wave in the QRS complex.

deflection (below the isoelectric line) on the EKG tracing. The infarction is now in an irreversible stage.

Q waves are said to be "pathologic" when they are greater than 0.04 seconds in duration (wider) or the Q wave is one third the overall R wave height (deeper) (Fig. 10–8). ST segments are usually no longer elevated by the time the Q waves become present in the leads associated with the area of infarction. Q waves can occur within hours of the development of the AMI or may take longer to form. This is something that can remain on the EKG for the patient's lifetime and is evidence of the infarction forever. This is called a "Q wave" MI.

> ### CLINICAL ALERT
>
> Lead aVR normally has a deep and negatively deflected Q wave. It should not be analyzed for the presence of a myocardial infarction. It can be used to help determine that the leads have been correctly placed on the patient. If the negative deflections are not noted, the leads should be rechecked. It could also mean a major change in axis. Children can have normal "pathologic—appearing" Q waves in certain leads including II, III, aVF, V_5, and V_6. If "pathologic" Q waves are present in this population in other leads, it could reflect cardiac disease processes. Other changes that may be normal for the infant or child are T wave inversion in leads V_1, V_2, and V_3 and long QT intervals in infants under the age of 6 months. Another aspect that is different when attempting to identify the presence of a myocardial infarction is a left bundle branch block. When this is present, it is difficult to recognize any of the normal changes that are typically noted with an AMI.

Areas of Infarction

When analyzing the 12-lead EKG, it is easy to determine the areas that are involved in an acute ST segment elevation myocardial infarction. As explained in Chapter 4, different leads look at distinct areas of the heart. When leads are contiguous, that is, particular leads look at specific parts of the heart and changes are seen in two or more "contiguous" leads, this is a key aspect of identifying AMIs and marking its location. Contiguous does not mean that they follow one another in succession rather they look at the same aspect of the heart. Consequently, when categorizing myocardial infarctions, two or more leads are listed which meet the criteria for the precise site of ischemia, injury, or infarction.

It is important to remember that some individuals do have variances in their heart anatomy, so it must be recognized that some variations might exist. However, for the majority of the population, there are particular conclusions that can be drawn for each area. In general, the anatomic areas of infarction are: inferior, anterior, lateral, septal, and posterior. Depending on the vessel occluded, combinations of these can also occur such as an anterolateral or an inferoposterior MI. It is also important to understand that when the health care practitioner is determining the site of an infarction, two separate entities are involved, they are:

- The artery and its branches that are expected to be supplying the area.

- The leads that actually "look" at the area.

Table 10–2 describes the artery involved, the leads depicting the area, and common dysrhythmias associated with each type of MI.

CLINICAL ALERT

Not every MI is going to present as a "pure" type of infarct. Reading EKGs for this problem is not always "black and white." There are many variances that can occur and individuals can have infarctions in two places in the heart. Therefore, "classic" pictures are not always visualized.

Anterior Myocardial Infarction

Leads indicating a blockage in the anterior portion of the heart are V_1, V_2, V_3, and V_4 (Fig. 10–9). The left coronary artery (LCA) and the left anterior descending artery (LAD) are implicated in an anterior MI. When it occurs in the left main coronary artery, this is often known as the "widow maker." The left coronary artery also feeds the circumflex. An anterolateral MI which would include blockage to the LAD and the circumflex would include leads I, aVL, V_3, V_4, V_5, and V_6. An anteroseptal MI, which indicates damage to the septum, would include the leads V_1 and V_2. Reciprocal changes would be seen in the inferior leads, II, III, and aVF.

TABLE 10–2 Types of Myocardial Infarctions

Type of Myocardial Infarction	Coronary Artery Involved	Leads	Common Dysrhythmias
Anterior	Left coronary artery and left anterior descending (LAD)	V_1, V_2, V_3, V_4	Atrial fibrillation Atrial flutter Tachydysrhythmias PVCs Second-degree AV blocks
Lateral	Circumflex	I, aVL, V_5, V_6	PVCs
Septal	Left anterior descending (LAD)	V_1, V_2	Second-degree and Third-degree AV blocks
Inferior	Right coronary artery (RCA)	II, III, aVF	Sinus bradycardia Sinus arrest First-degree and Second-degree AV Blocks PVCs
Right ventricular infarct	Marginal branch of right coronary artery	V_4R, V_5R, V_6R	Atrial flutter Atrial fibrillation AV blocks PACs
Posterior	Right coronary artery and circumflex	V_7, V_8, V_9	SA and AV node blocks

An anterior MI causes major malfunction of the left ventricle leading to left-sided heart failure, decreased cardiac output, and hypotension. Cardiogenic shock is often present. Oxygenated blood is normally delivered to the left ventricle, the septum, and the bundle branches from this location. A variety of dysrhythmias can occur with an anterior MI including atrial fibrillation, atrial flutter, tachydysrhythmias, premature ventricular contractions (PVCs) (due to irritability), and second-degree blocks. Bundle branch blocks are also prevalent. Poor R wave progression may also be present.

Lateral Myocardial Infarction

A lateral MI involves blockage in the circumflex artery. Changes are seen in leads I, aVL, V_5, and V_6 (Fig. 10–10). This may occur with either an anterior or inferior myocardial infarction. Dysrhythmias linked to this area are AV blocks and PVCs. Reciprocal changes will be seen in the inferior leads II, III, and aVF.

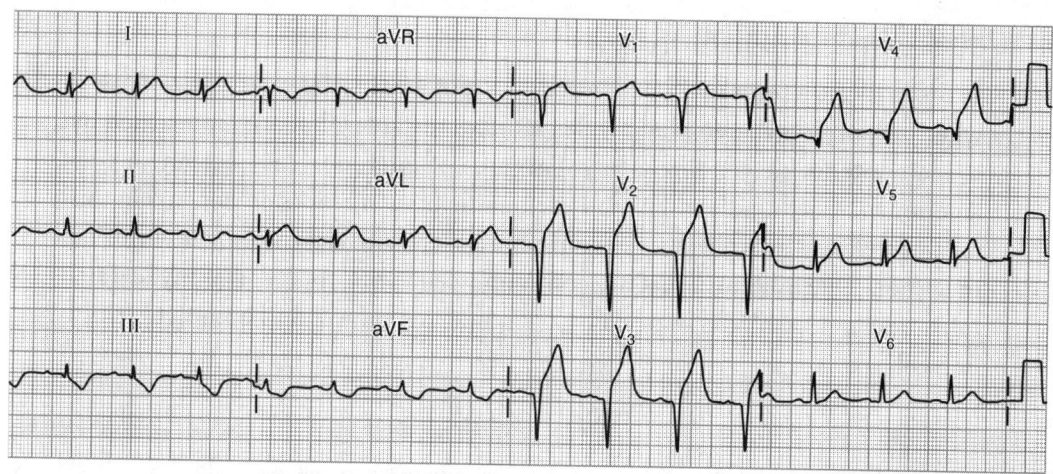

FIGURE 10–9 • **Anterior-lateral myocardial infarction.** This EKG shows ST segment elevation in leads V_1, V_2, V_3, V_4, and V_5. There is also ST elevation in leads I and aVL consistent with lateral injury. Reciprocal changes are seen in the inferior leads II, III, and aVF.

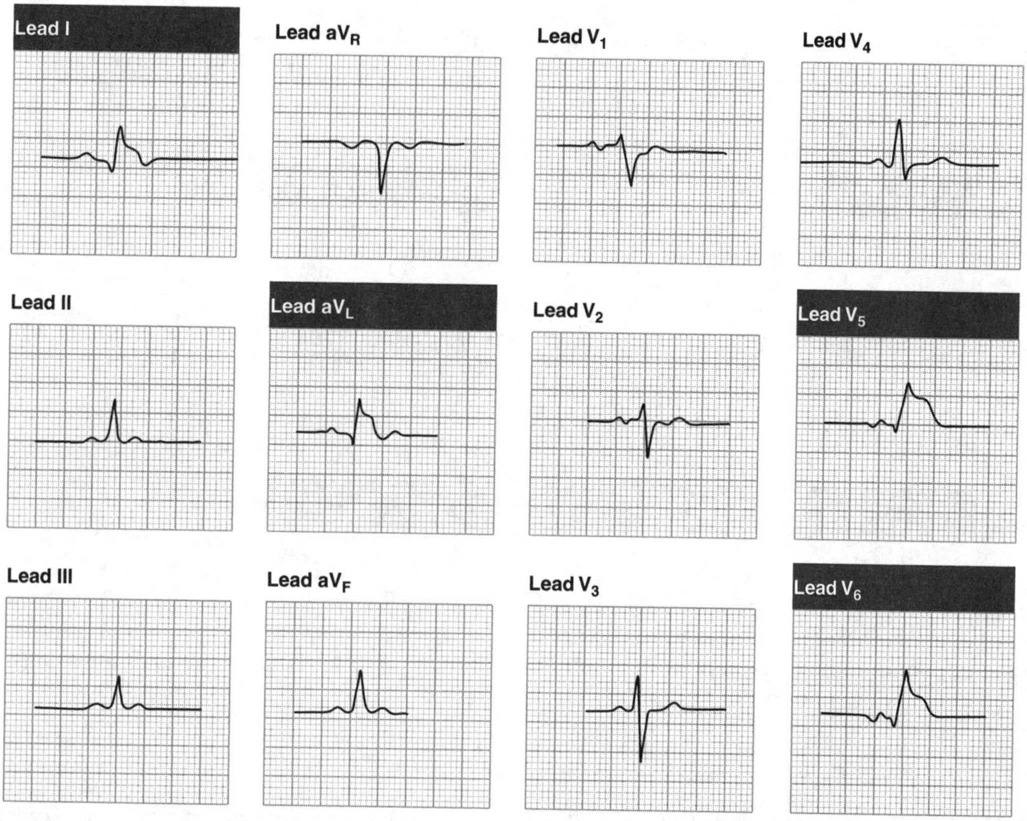

FIGURE 10–10 • **Lateral myocardial infarction.** Changes consistent with a lateral wall myocardial infarction are seen in leads I, aVL, V_5, and V_6. (*From ECG Interpretation Made Incredibly Easy 5e. Wolters Kluwer Lippincott Williams and Wilkins 2011.*)

Septal Myocardial Infarction

Leads to locate a septal MI in are V_1 and V_2 (Fig. 10–11). R waves can disappear when lack of oxygenated blood is delivered to the areas that are replenished by the left anterior descending artery. This area of infarction may accompany an anterior MI. The bundle of His and the bundle branch blocks are located in this area of delivery as well. This is commonly seen with an anterior myocardial infarction. Dysrhythmias that are commonly seen with this type of myocardial infarction are AV blocks, especially second degree type II and complete (third degree).

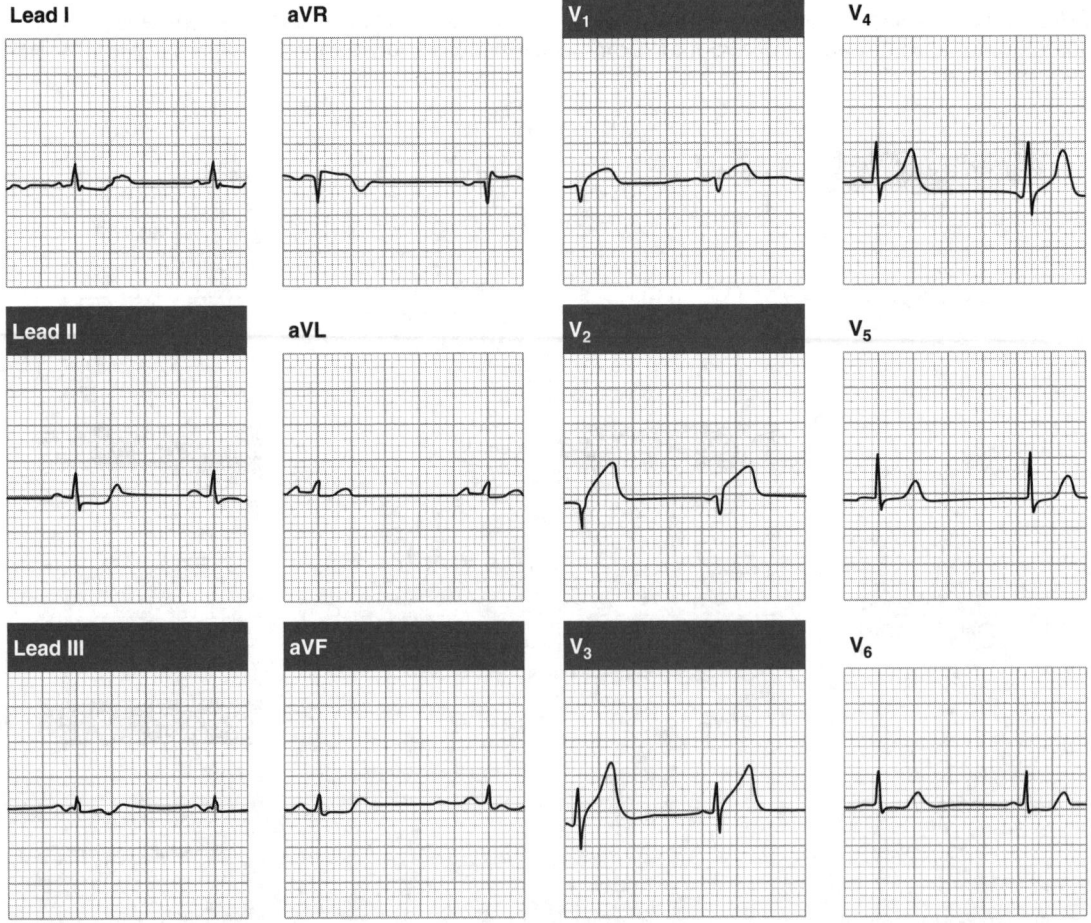

FIGURE 10–11 • **Septal myocardial infarction.** The septal wall is part of the anterior aspect of the heart. Leads to view for this aspect include leads V_1 and V_2. In this example, V_3 is also implicated. The inferior leads II, III, and aVF show reciprocal changes. (*From ECG Interpretation Made Incredibly Easy 5e. Wolters Kluwer Lippincott Williams and Wilkins 2011.*)

Inferior Myocardial Infarction

The right coronary artery feeds the area concerned with an inferior myocardial infarction through the posterior descending branch. Leads which view the inferior aspect of the left ventricle are II, III, and aVF (Fig. 10–12). Dysrhythmias that are usually seen with this type of MI are bradycardias (from increased parasympathetic activity) such as sinus bradycardia and sinus arrest and AV conduction delays such as first- and second-degree block (type I). PVCs can also occur. In these patients, the Q wave that is usually present throughout life may disappear after a period of time. Reciprocal changes would be seen in the leads representing the lateral aspect of the heart, I, aVL.

CLINICAL ALERT

Another aspect of the heart that can be involved is the right ventricle. While most infarctions concern the left ventricle due to the location and branching of the LCA, the right ventricle can be associated with an inferior MI. This occurs when the marginal branch which is derived from the RCA is occluded. If only the right marginal branch is occluded, the infarction site can be isolated to the right ventricle. When it occurs proximal to this branch, symptoms from both the right ventricle and inferior aspect of the heart can occur. A decrease in cardiac output can be realized with the right ventricular infarct because the right ventricle does not pump well diminishing the amount of blood that is returning to the left side of the heart. Another problem with the right ventricular infarct is that blood volume builds up in the right ventricle due to the reduced function of this chamber. These pathophysiologic responses lead the patient to the triad of "classic" symptoms that are associated with this disease process. These are: hypotension (from the decreased cardiac output), jugular venous distention (from the build up of blood in the right ventricle and thus the venous system), and clear lung sounds (left ventricular failure causes pulmonary edema). This triad is not always present in all patients with this problem, however, it is considered to be the characteristic symptoms for right ventricular infarct. A right-sided EKG is necessary to see the ST segment elevation for this type of myocardial infarction. V_4R to V_6R are the leads that are obtained when this infarct is suspected. Left-sided chest leads are transferred to the right side of the chest for these leads.

Posterior Myocardial Infarction

The posterior aspect of the heart is fed by the RCA and the circumflex. The leads that are noted to be different in this MI are leads V_1 and V_2. Leads V_3, and

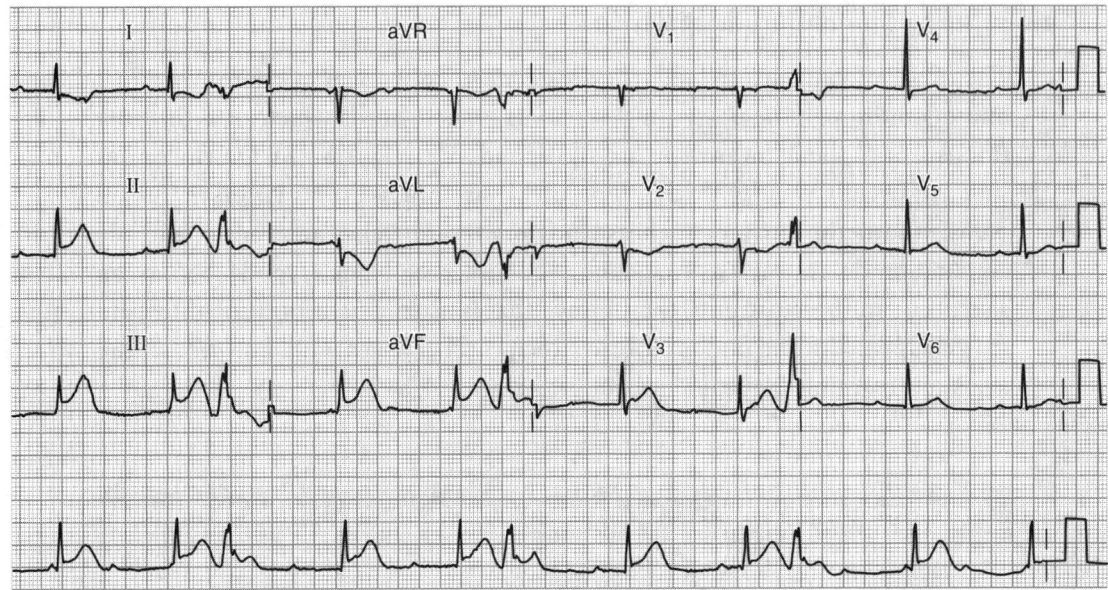

FIGURE 10−12 • **Inferior myocardial infarction.** ST segment elevation is seen in II, III, and aVF. This EKG also demonstrates a third-degree (complete) heart block associated with this infarction. This is best noted in the rhythm strip at the bottom of the EKG. Premature ventricular contractions are also seen as escape beats due to the slow rate. Reciprocal changes are seen in I and aVL.

V_4 can also be included in this diagnosis (Fig. 10–13). However, these leads show reciprocal changes, ST segment depression, since these leads reflect the mirror image of the posterior aspect, the anterior part of the heart. Other EKG changes to be seen in these anterior leads are tall R waves. In order to see the ST segment elevation expected with a posterior wall MI, a posterior EKG must be done. This includes leads V_7, V_8, and V_9. These leads are placed on the left side of the back in the following positions: V_7—left posterior axillary line, V_8—under the tip of the scapula, V_9—at the left vertebral column.

Another way to look at an EKG to determine if it is a posterior MI is to use the "mirror" test. In this test, turn the EKG upside down and hold it toward a mirror. Look at the EKG in the mirror. This will show the ST segments as being elevated, similar to what would be seen with the posterior leads. Another way is called *reversed transillumination*. Turn the EKG upside down and backwards to the health care practitioner (so that the back of the EKG is toward the practitioner). Hold it up to a light. The ST "elevation" should now show on leads V_1 and V_2 (Fig. 10–14).

CLINICAL ALERT

When special EKGs are needed to assist in determining the type of myocardial infarction the patient is experiencing, they may be labeled differently in each institution. The terms, "15-lead" and "18-lead" EKGs, can thus mean distinct ideas. Sometimes the terms right-sided EKG (V_4R, V_5R, V_6R) and posterior EKG (V_7, V_8, V_9) are used. Be sure to determine which of these are used in the institution in which the health care professional has chosen to work.

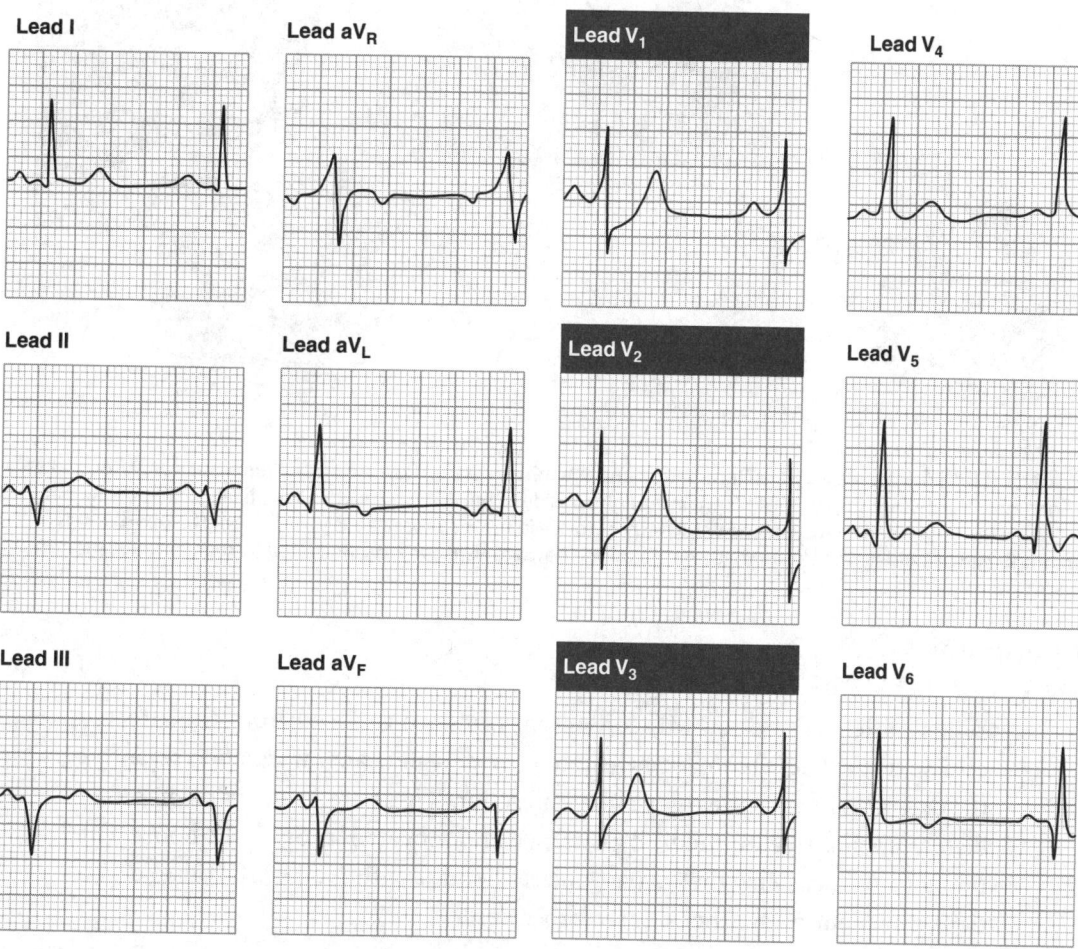

FIGURE 10–13 • **Posterior myocardial infarction.** In a posterior MI, leads V_1 and V_2 will demonstrate reciprocal changes. These reciprocal changes are also seen in V_3 in this EKG. Leads V_7, V_8, and V_9 are necessary to see the ST segment elevation that correlates with a posterior MI. (*Modified from ECG Interpretation Made Incredibly Easy 5e. Wolters Kluwer Lippincott Williams and Wilkins 2011.*)

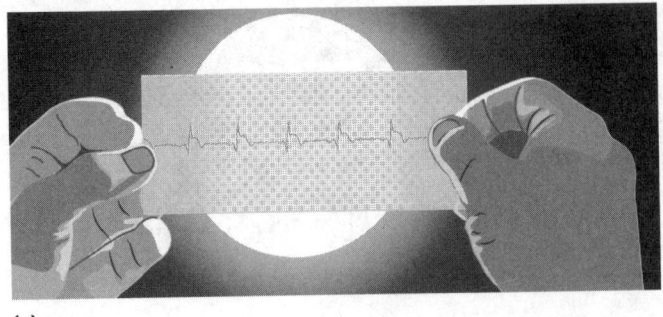

(a)

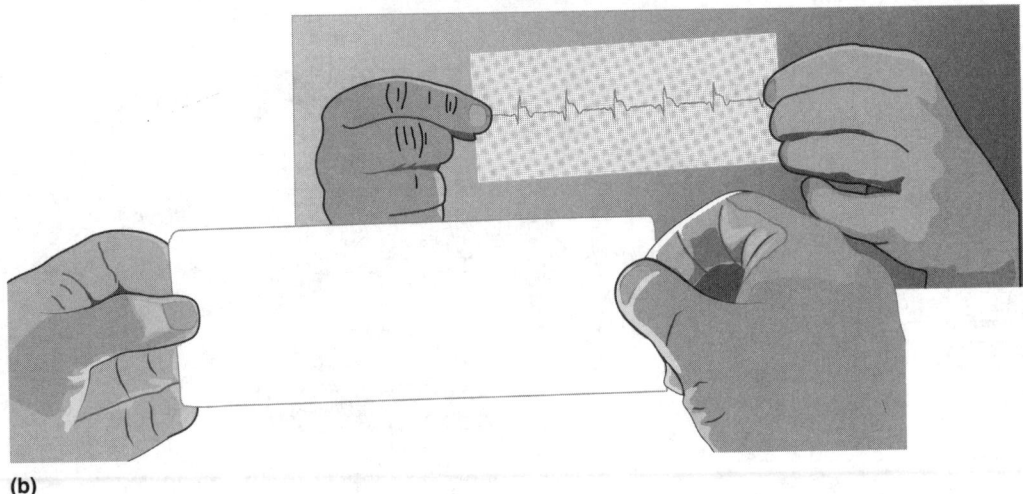

(b)

FIGURE 10–14 • **Reversed transillumination and the mirror test.** (a) Reversed transillumination is performed using a light. Hold the rhythm strip or the EKG against a light, upside down and backwards to the health care practitioner. This will show the ST segment elevation one would expect to see in the reciprocal leads V_1 and V_2. (b) The mirror test is accomplished by holding the EKG or rhythm strip upside down toward a mirror. "Read" the ST segment "elevation" in leads V_1 and V_2.

Biomarkers

When patients suffer an MI, certain enzymes are released from the affected cardiac tissue. These biomarkers help to provide significant information regarding the diagnosis of an acute myocardial infarction. These are usually drawn immediately upon arrival to medical assistance and repeated in 6 and 12 hours. The presence of these enzymes is particularly helpful with NSTEMI. "False" elevations can occur with other disease processes.

- **Troponin**: Released quickly and stays elevated for longer period of time (up to 5 days).
- **CK-MB**: An isoenzyme of creatinine kinase—released within 3 to12 hours with a peak in 24 hours. Returns to normal within 48 to 72 hours.

- **Myoglobin:** Released rapidly and may be found in urine soon after initial chest pain.

Symptoms

Patients presenting with angina or an AMI will typically complain of chest pain. It is important to help the patient to understand that "pressure" and "tightness" are "pain." Always ask the patient if these sensations are present because they may be quick to state that no pain is present. Also, certain populations, especially diabetic patients and the elderly may not experience pain at all. Others may have atypical pain such as sharp, stabbing pains. The pain of an acute MI is present for longer periods of time and more intense than angina.

> ## CLINICAL ALERT
>
> Not every patient with an AMI will portray typical symptoms such as clutching their chest. Everyone responds to pain, crisis, and fear in their own ways. Always be alert to the non-typical patient as well and ask pertinent questions in a quick, effective manner.

Other manifestations that may accompany an AMI are shortness of breath, diaphoresis, dizziness, lightheadedness, palpitations, fatigue, malaise, syncope or near syncope, a feeling of "indigestion," upper mid epigastric pain, a feeling of "fullness," radiation of pain to the left arm or shoulder area, jaw or neck pain, or numbness to the left arm or hand. When patients faint due to a bradycardic rhythm, this is known as a **"Stokes-Adams"** attack.

The patient may appear pale and feel cool or clammy to the touch, and have vital sign changes such as hypotension, tachycardia, bradycardia, increased respiratory rate, and a slight increase in temperature.

Treatment

Treatment for patients with an AMI includes prompt recognition of the problem. Every minute that passes without appropriate treatment allows for additional heart muscle to die. Health care professionals must be alert to symptoms, both specific and vague. Treat dysrhythmias that arise with proper interventions. Be sure to attach monitor patches and obtain an EKG immediately upon arrival. Oxygen should be supplied as per institution policy. Utilize a cardiology consult and transfer the patient if necessary depending on the needs of the patient and the services supplied by the institution.

CLINICAL ALERT

The use of nitroglycerin for chest pain is standard procedure. Always have intravenous access before administering nitroglycerin. Patients can respond to the vasodilatory effects of this medication with negative effects such as hypotension. It is not unusual for blood pressures to drop significantly after either sublingual or spray nitroglycerin. If this occurs, be prepared to administer a small bolus of normal saline to counter the vasodilatory effects. Other side effects include headache and the more uncommon reflex tachycardia. These effects are usually short lived due to the short half-life (2-3 minutes) of this medication. Also ask patients about the use of medications for erectile dysfunction since the combination of these can cause very strong episodes of hypotension. Some of these medications are also now being used or explored for their positive outcomes for females.

Other treatment options for these patients includes the use aspirin or clopidogrel (Plavix), glycoprotein IIb-IIIa inhibitors, beta-blockers, calcium channel blockers, angiotensin-converting enzyme inhibitors, thrombolytic medications, percutaneous angiography with stent placement, angioplasty, or atherectomy, coronary artery bypass graft, or the use of a balloon pump.

Conclusion

AMI are a major cause of death and disability in the United States. The most common reason for this event in the adult population is atherosclerotic coronary artery disease. Major points from this chapter include the following:

- Plaques develop below the intimal layer of coronary arteries and then break through the layer to cause narrowed passages for blood flow.
- Two major arteries supply blood to the heart—the right and left coronary arteries.
- Branches from the two main arteries encircle the heart.
- A "left dominant" individual will have the PDA arise from the circumflex branch of the left coronary artery.

- A "right dominant" individual will have the PDA arise from the right coronary artery.

- The usual etiology for a myocardial infarction is atherosclerotic heart disease; however there are other reasons for patients to have an MI.

- Acute coronary syndrome is divided into unstable angina, NSTEMI, and STEMI.

- Stable angina occurs with activity and is relieved by rest or the use of nitroglycerin.

- Unstable angina occurs after very slight exertion or at rest.

- Prinzmetal's angina is another form of angina that occurs due to coronary artery spasm and is not associated with activity.

- NSTEMI is diagnosed initially based on increased levels of biomarkers.

- STEMI will carry the injury pattern of ST elevation in the affected areas of the heart.

- An inverted T wave is an indicator of ischemia.

- In early stages of an AMI, the T wave can be hyperacute.

- There are three areas of infarcted tissue—the zone of ischemia, the zone of injury, and the zone of infarction.

- Elevated ST segments do not show actual damage.

- Reciprocal changes occur in areas opposite of where the actual injury is occurring.

- Pathologic Q waves indicate infarcted myocardium.

- A pathologic Q wave is greater than 0.04 seconds in width or one third the overall QRS height.

- Lead aVR is not used to determine changes associated with myocardial infarctions.

- Contiguous leads mean that leads look at similar parts of the heart.

- When determining the site of the infarction, both the arteries involved and the leads that "look" at the area are involved.

- An anterior MI will show changes in V_1, V_2, V_3, and V_4 and involves the left coronary artery (LCA) and the left anterior descending artery (LAD).

- An infarction of the left coronary artery is called "the widow maker."

- A lateral MI involves the circumflex artery and is shown as changes in leads I, aVL, V_5, and V_6.

- A septal MI is seen in leads V_1 and V_2 and involves the LAD.

- An inferior MI is seen in leads II, III, and aVF and the artery blocked is the posterior descending branch of the right coronary artery.
- A right ventricular infarct can accompany an inferior MI.
- A right-sided EKG must be done to see the ST elevation in a right ventricular infarct.
- The triad of symptoms with a right ventricular infarct is: hypotension, increased jugular venous distention (JVD), and clear lungs.
- A posterior MI is seen with reciprocal changes in leads V_1 and V_2.
- Posterior leads—V_7, V_8, and V_9—must be done to visualize the ST segment elevation in a posterior MI.
- Biomarkers are enzymes that are released from infarcted tissue and help to make the diagnosis of an acute myocardial infarction.
- The three biomarkers used in AMI are: troponin, CK-MB, and myoglobin.
- Patients will usually present with chest pain when an MI is present, but not every patient will actually have chest pain or recognize it as such.
- Other symptoms that are associated with an MI are: shortness of breath, lightheadedness, dizziness, sweating, syncope or near syncope, "indigestion," and arm, neck, and jaw pain.
- Stokes—Adams attack occurs when a patient has a syncopal event due to a slow heart rate.
- Treatment options for patients with an AMI include: oxygen, nitroglycerin, aspirin, or clopidogrel (Plavix), treating dysrhythmias, beta-blockers, calcium channel blockers, angiotensin-converting enzyme inhibitors, thrombolytics, angiography, stents, angioplasty, atherectomy, coronary artery bypass grafting, and balloon pump.

PRACTICE QUESTIONS

1. In atherosclerotic heart disease, plaque builds up under which of the following?
    A. Medial layer of the vessel
    B. Intimal layer of the vessel
    C. Ostial openings
    D. Aortic valve

2. **A person who is said to be "right dominant" would have which of the following present on the coronary arteries?**

   A. The circumflex artery would arise from the right coronary artery

   B. The right coronary artery is larger and longer than the left coronary artery

   C. The posterior descending artery would branch off of the right coronary artery

   D. The right coronary artery makes a complete circle around the apex of the heart

3. **Acute coronary syndrome includes all the following EXCEPT:**

   A. unstable angina.

   B. non-ST segment elevation myocardial infarction.

   C. ST segment elevation myocardial infarction.

   D. stable angina.

4. **Prinzmetal's angina occurs during:**

   A. emotional stress.

   B. rest or sleep.

   C. strong physical exertion.

   D. minimal exercise.

5. **Non-ST segment elevation MI is diagnosed via:**

   A. cardiac enzymes.

   B. clinical picture.

   C. electrolyte imbalances.

   D. 12-lead EKG.

6. **ST segment elevation indicates:**

   A. ischemia.

   B. injury.

   C. infarction.

   D. necrosis.

7. **Reciprocal changes will be seen in which leads with an anterior myocardial infarction?**

   A. Inferior

   B. Posterior

   C. Septal

   D. Lateral

8. Which of the following leads should not be used to interpret an acute myocardial infarction in a 12-lead EKG?

A. II

B. V_6

C. aVR

D. V_7

9. Which of the following populations of patients may have normal Q waves?

A. Geriatric

B. Diabetic

C. Pediatric

D. Autistic

10. Which of the following would be considered to be "contiguous" leads?

A. II and aVF

B. V_1 and V_5

C. I and aVR

D. V_2 and V_6

11. A lateral myocardial infarction would be seen in which of the following leads?

A. II and III

B. I and aVL

C. V_2 and V_3

D. V_1 and V_2

12. Which of the following leads would be examined closely for the presence of a right ventricular infarct?

A. V_4

B. V_1

C. V_4R

D. V_8R

13. Injury and ischemia changes are noted in leads V_1 and V_2. Which of the following areas of the myocardium are involved?

A. Lateral

B. Inferior

C. Septal

D. Posterior

14. In which of the following leads would a posterior myocardial infarction be manifested best?

   A. V_6
   B. II
   C. V_8
   D. V_4R

15. Which of the following is a true statement regarding the cardiac enzyme, troponin?

   A. It is found easily in urine.
   B. It returns to normal within 72 hours.
   C. It can stay elevated for up to 5 days.
   D. It is an isoenzyme of creatinine kinase.

ANSWER KEY

1. **B.** Atherosclerotic plaques develop under the intima or the innermost layer of vessels. They then rupture through into the vessel.

2. **C.** A "right dominant" individual has the posterior descending artery (PDA) arising from the right coronary artery. In a "left dominant" person the PDA arises from the circumflex artery.

3. **D.** Acute coronary syndrome includes unstable angina, NSTEMI, and STEMI.

4. **B.** Prinzmetal's angina typically occurs during sleep or rest. It is not usually associated with emotional or physical stress.

5. **A.** Cardiac enzymes or biomarkers are used to help with the diagnosis of myocardial infarction in the absence of ST segment elevation on the 12-lead EKG.

6. **B.** ST segment elevation indicates an injury pattern. T wave inversion shows ischemia and a pathologic Q wave designates necrosis or infarction.

7. **A.** An anterior myocardial infarction will show reciprocal or "mirror image" changes in the inferior leads.

8. **C.** Lead aVR normally has a deep and negatively deflected Q wave and should not be used in the diagnosis of an acute myocardial infarction.

9. **C.** Pediatric patients can have normal Q waves present in II, III, aVF, V_5, and V_6.

10. **A.** Contiguous leads look at the same area of the heart. Leads II and aVF both look at the inferior aspect of the heart.

11. **B.** A lateral myocardial infarction is noted in leads I, aVL, V_5, and V_6.

12. **C.** V_4R is part of the right-sided EKG that would need to be performed for the diagnosis of a right ventricular infarction.

13. **C.** V_1 and V_2 look at the septal portion of the heart. These leads would help to diagnose this type of myocardial infarction. A lateral MI would be seen in I, aVL, V_5 and V_6. An inferior MI would show changes in II, III, and aVF. An anterior MI would be indicated with changes in V_1, V_2, V_3, or V_4.

14. **C.** A posterior MI would need a posterior EKG to visualize ST segment elevations. The leads to be used in this type of EKG are V_7, V_8, and V_9. Recipricol changes would be seen in V_1 and V_2.

15. **C.** Troponin is very useful in that it rises early and stays elevated for longer periods of time—up to 5 days. CK-MB is an isoenzyme of creatinine kinase and returns to normal at about 72 hours. Myoglobin is excreted in the urine.

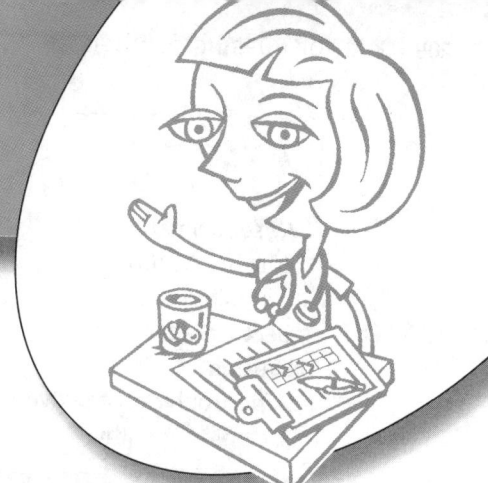

chapter 11

EKG Changes Other Than Myocardial Infarction

At the end of this chapter, the student will be able to:

1. Identify EKG changes occurring with disease processes other than myocardial infarction (MI).

2. Understand the causes of EKG changes occurring with disease processes other than MI.

3. List common dysrhythmias associated with disease processes other than MI.

4. Describe pacemaker spikes and common complications associated with pacemaker malfunctions.

5. List some medications that can create EKG changes.

6. Identify the EKG changes that occur with some medications.

KEY WORDS

AV sequential
Brugada syndrome
Cor pulmonale
Electrical alternans
Effusion
Hypertrophic obstructive
  cardiomyopathy

Idiopathic hypertrophic subaortic stenosis
J wave
Osborne wave
Pericarditis
Pulmonary embolus
Subarachnoid hemorrhage
Wellens syndrome

Overview

Patients can display a variety of EKG changes for reasons other than acute myocardial infarctions (AMI). Many of these have been mentioned in previous chapters. This chapter will look at some of these deviations from normal as they relate to EKG tracing and cardiac monitor irregularities. When examining these changes, always do so with the patient in mind. Patient past history, symptoms, vital sign assessment, and events surrounding the presentation should be considered when making definitive decisions about EKG changes. Also, comparing the patient's EKG with a prior EKG is an important facet of interpretation. Correlate lab studies and put the entire picture into perspective before arriving at a final decision.

CLINICAL ALERT

Today's cardiac monitors have the capacity to recognize many changes to waveforms, including ST segment elevations, QTc intervals, etc. One of the problems that health care personnel must be aware of is called alarm fatigue. Technology affords the medical world in many ingenious ways to "watch" the patient and with this comes more noises, bells, and alarms to bring changes to the attention of those who are caring for the ill or injured individual. Guard against becoming lax regarding responding to alarms. Always check the patient. Make sure that there is clear understanding about what the alarms mean. Be familiar with the mechanics of the monitoring equipment including retrieving important information and creating a hard copy of events. Never assume that alarms are simply patient movement or the loss of a lead wire.

Table 11–1 lists the EKG changes that occur with factors other than an AMI.

TABLE 11–1 EKG Changes Associated with Processes Other Than Myocardial Infarction

Process	EKG Changes	Common Dysrhythmias
Hyperkalemia	• Diffuse, high, peaked T waves • Broad QRS complexes • Prolonged PR interval • Loss of P wave	• PVC • Ventricular fibrillation
Hypokalemia	• Depressed T wave • Depressed ST segments • Presence of U wave	• Torsades de pointes
Hypercalcemia	• Shortened QT interval	
Hypocalcemia	• Prolonged QT interval	• Torsades de pointes
Hypermagnesemia	• Prolonged PR • Wide QRS • Elevated T wave	• Complete heart block
Hypomagnesemia	• Presence of U waves • Prolonged QT interval	• PVCs • Ventricular tachycardia • Ventricular fibrillation • Torsades de pointes
Hypothermia	• J wave (Osborne wave)	• Bradycardia • Atrial fibrillation (slow)
Subarachnoid hemorrhage	• Deeply inverted T waves • Presence of U waves	• Bradycardia
Pulmonary embolus	• Large S wave in lead I • Deep Q wave in lead III • Inverted T wave in lead III • Right bundle branch block • Right ventricular hypertrophy	• Sinus tachycardia • Atrial fibrillation • PVCs • Ventricular tachycardia • Ventricular fibrillation
Emphysema	• Low voltage • Right axis deviation • Poor R wave progression	• Atrial fibrillation • Atrial flutter • Multifocal atrial tachycardia
Pericarditis	• Diffuse ST segment elevation • T wave inversion • T wave flattening • Depressed PR interval	
Idiopathic hypertrophic subaortic stenosis (IHSS)	• Left ventricular hypertrophy • Left axis deviation • Q waves in lateral and inferior leads	• Sudden death
Brugada syndrome	• Right bundle branch block • ST segment elevation in V_1, V_2, V_3	• Polymorphic ventricular tachycardia • Ventricular fibrillation
Wellens syndrome	• T wave inversion in V_2 and V_3	

Electrolyte Imbalances

Potassium

Both hypo and hyperkalemia can create changes in EKG morphology. Hypokalemia will be noted as a depressed or flattened T wave, depressed ST segments, and/or the presence of a U wave. A U wave is an extra waveform after the T wave. It can be present in other processes as well. Dysrhythmias which can occur with low potassium are ventricular in nature and include the development of torsades de pointes (Fig. 11–1).

Hyperkalemia is noted to have diffuse, high, peaked T waves and broad QRS complexes. These T waves are not restricted to certain areas of the heart. The P wave is also important in high potassium situations as the PR interval will prolong and then flatten and sometimes disappear. The cardiotoxic effects of hyperkalemia which creates the wide QRS complexes can predispose the patient to PVCs and subsequent ventricular fibrillation (Fig. 11–2).

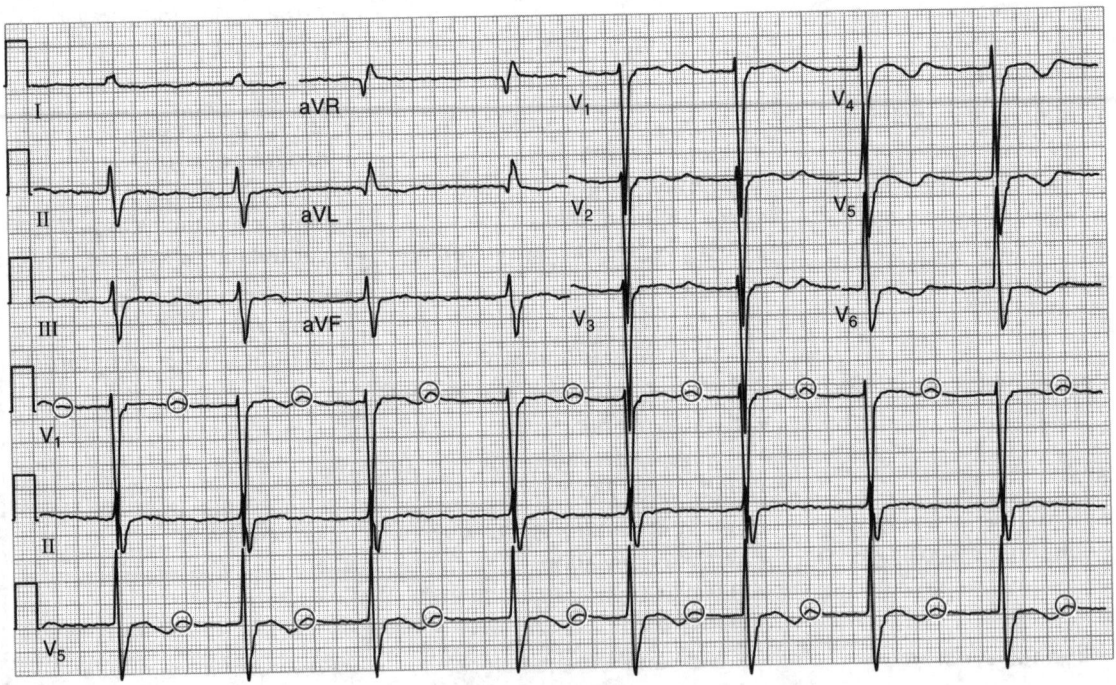

FIGURE 11–1 • EKG changes associated with hypokalemia. Notice the flattened T waves and the presence of U waves in this EKG tracing from a patient with a K level of 2.1 mmol/L.

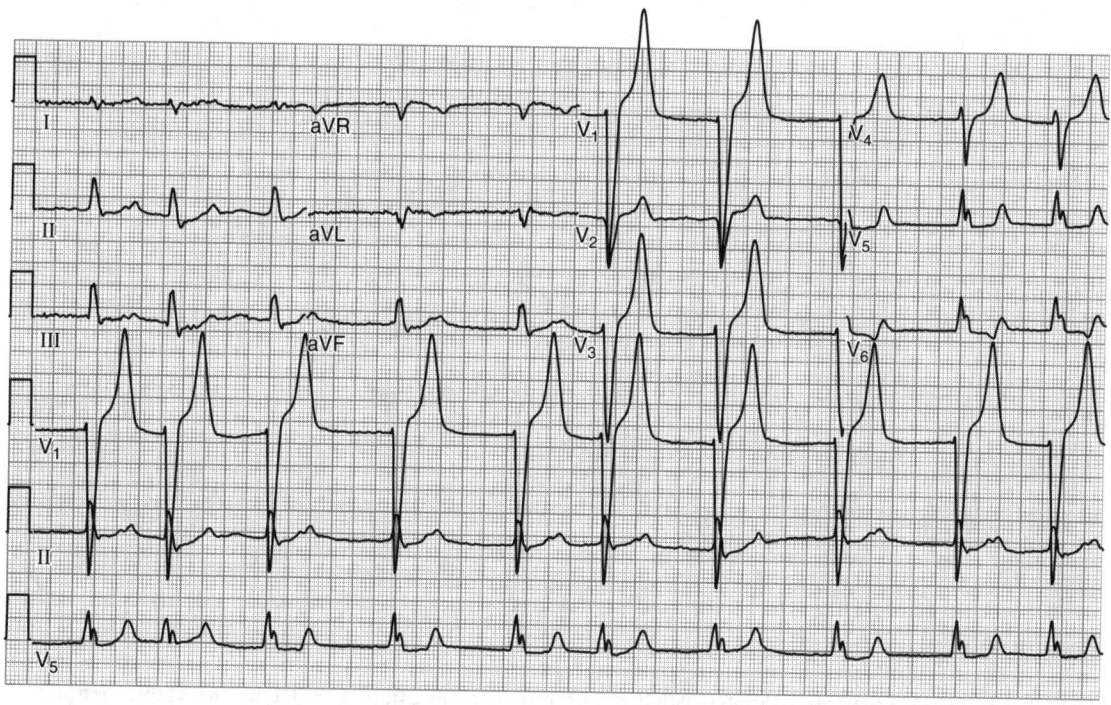

FIGURE 11–2 • EKG changes associated with hyperkalemia. Notice the high peaked T waves, the loss of P waves, and the widened QRS complex from a patient with a K level of 8.2 mmol/L.

Calcium

As has been noted in previous chapters, calcium is a necessary electrolyte for the normal functioning of the heart. Hypocalcemia can be a dangerous electrolyte imbalance. This causes the QT interval to lengthen which can be a precursor of torsades de pointes. The QT interval should be less than half the entire length of the cardiac cycle. Some causes of hypocalcemia are pancreatitis, hydrogen fluoride burns, and the administration of multiple units of blood. The ST segment can also be flattened. Hypercalcemia can cause the QT interval to shorten (Fig. 11–3).

Magnesium

Hypomagnesemia can present with similar changes to the EKG as hypokalemia with the presence of U waves and nonspecific T wave changes as well as the prolongation of the QT interval. This places the patient at high risk for torsades de pointes and other ventricular dysrhythmias such as PVCs, ventricular

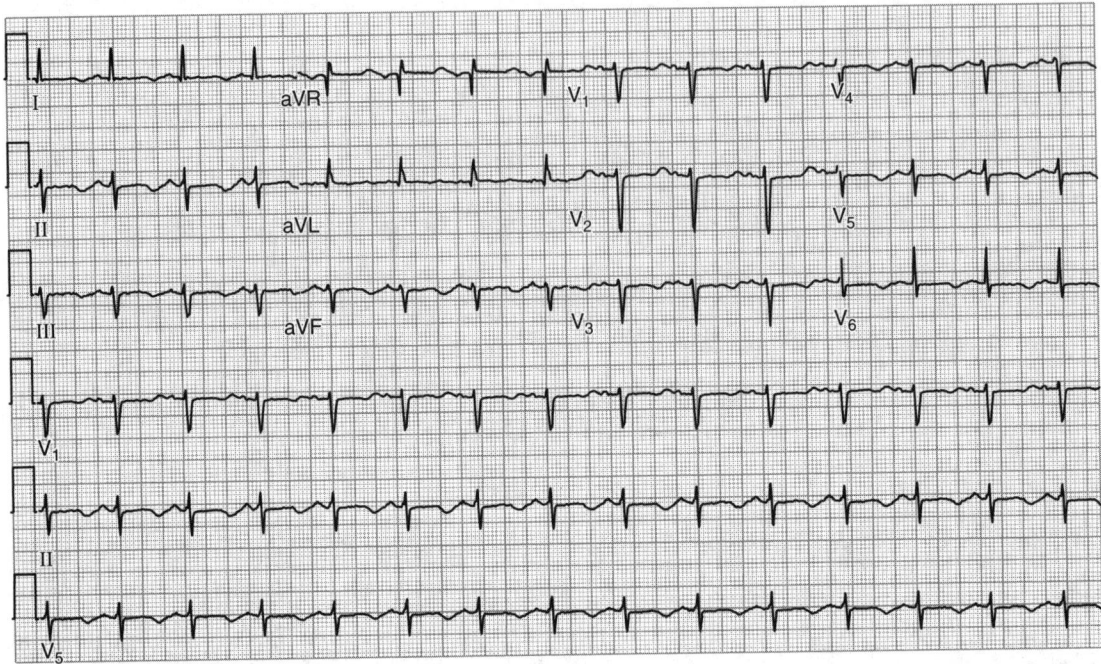

FIGURE 11–3 • EKG changes associated with hypocalcemia. In this EKG tracing, the QT interval is prolonged and the ST segment is flattened in a patient with known hypocalcemia.

tachycardia, and ventricular fibrillation. Some causes of low magnesium are diuresis, increased calcium, increased ingestion of vitamin D, administration of steroids, chemotherapy, and the development of sepsis.

Hypermagnesemia can cause a prolonged PR interval, a widened QRS, and elevated T waves. Complete heart block can occur with this electrolyte disturbance. Etiologies of high magnesium include renal failure, administration of magnesium, and use of antacids.

Environmental

Hypothermia

The biggest issue with environmental problems is that of hypothermia. Bradycardia is the most common dysrhythmia, including a slow atrial fibrillation. All intervals have a tendency to prolong. The **J wave** or **Osborne wave** is the most distinguishing characteristic for this environmentally related concern. This is an extra "hump" or positive deflection in the EKG tracing between the ST segment and the T wave at the "J point" (Fig. 11–4).

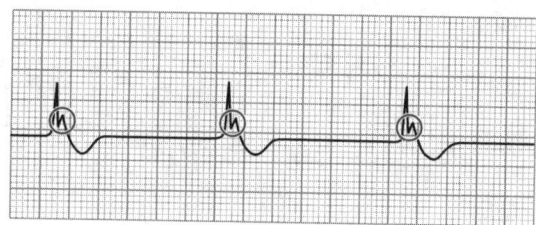

FIGURE 11–4 • J wave. The J wave, also known as the Osborne wave, is an extra positive deflection after the QRS.

> ### CLINICAL ALERT
>
> Be aware that when individuals are presenting with hypothermia, they may be shivering or trembling. When this happens, artifact on the EKG can cause misinterpretations. Be sure to distinguish between artifact and what might appear to be atrial flutter, atrial fibrillation, or ventricular fibrillation.

Central Nervous System

Subarachnoid Hemorrhage

Patients with central nervous system disturbances such as a **subarachnoid hemorrhage**, an intracranial bleeding problem, can present with EKG changes. These will be demonstrated by deeply inverted T waves. Bradycardia and U waves can also be present as well as prolongation of the QT interval (Fig. 11–5).

Pulmonary System

Pulmonary Embolus

A major **pulmonary embolus**, a blood clot in the lungs, can present with significant EKG changes. One of these is the S1Q3 pattern. In this abnormality, lead I demonstrates a significant S wave and lead III reveals a deep Q wave (Fig. 11–6). Another aspect of this may be the inclusion of an inverted T wave in lead III (S1Q3T3). The Q wave is differentiated from that of an AMI since it is found in only one lead and not contiguous leads associated with different parts of the cardiac anatomy. Other changes that might be present include indications of a right bundle branch block and right ventricular hypertrophy.

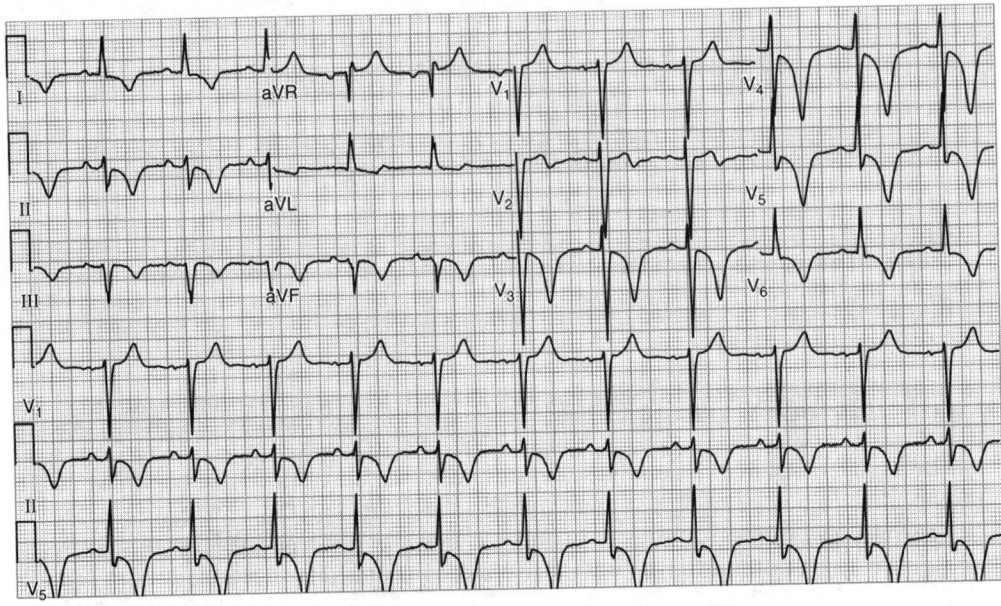

FIGURE 11–5 • EKG changes associated with a subarachnoid hemorrhage. The deeply inverted T waves associated with a subarachnoid hemorrhage are clearly seen in leads I, II, III, V_3, V_4, V_5, and V_6.

CLINICAL ALERT

Several different dysrhythmias can be present in a pulmonary embolus. The more common ones are sinus tachycardia and atrial fibrillation; though it is not uncommon for patients with large pulmonary emboli to have PVCs which will then progress to ventricular tachycardia or fibrillation. Patients who have smaller pulmonary emboli may only present with sinus tachycardia and this is a significant factor when people present with sudden onset of shortness of breath and chest or back pain that is sharp or pleuritic in nature. This tachycardia is not always extremely rapid. Rates of 110 to 120 should also be suspect.

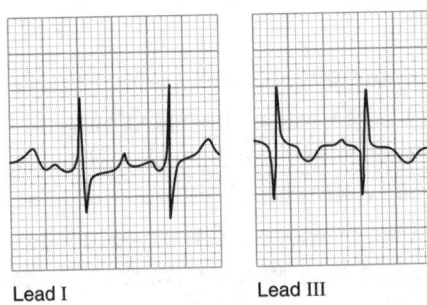

Lead I   Lead III

FIGURE 11–6 • EKG changes associated with pulmonary embolus. A massive pulmonary embolus can have an S1Q3 pattern in which there is a large S wave present in lead I and a deep Q wave in lead III. (*From Thaler, M. The Only EKG Book You'll Ever Need, 6e. 2011.*)

Chronic Obstructive Pulmonary Disease

Patients with long standing chronic obstructive pulmonary disease (COPD) can have changes to their EKG tracing. COPD is divided into chronic obstructive bronchitis and emphysema. Changes within the thoracic cavity due to increases in the volume of the lung from alveolar air trapping, the change in the position of the diaphragm, and the subsequent change in orientation of the heart within the chest cavity can create the following changes in the emphysemic patient (Fig. 11–7):

- Low voltage
- Right axis deviation
- Poor R wave progression

Dysrhythmias that occur include both atrial and ventricular, but atrial fibrillation and flutter are common as well as multifocal atrial tachycardia. These dysrhythmias may occur due to the disease process or medications that are used to treat the patient.

CLINICAL ALERT

When patients experience right-sided heart failure as a consequence of pulmonary disease, it is known as **cor pulmonale**. P pulmonale is an EKG change associated with this disease process. This is an indication of right atrial enlargement and is expressed as an increase in the amplitude of the first upswing of the P wave in the inferior leads II, III, aVF.

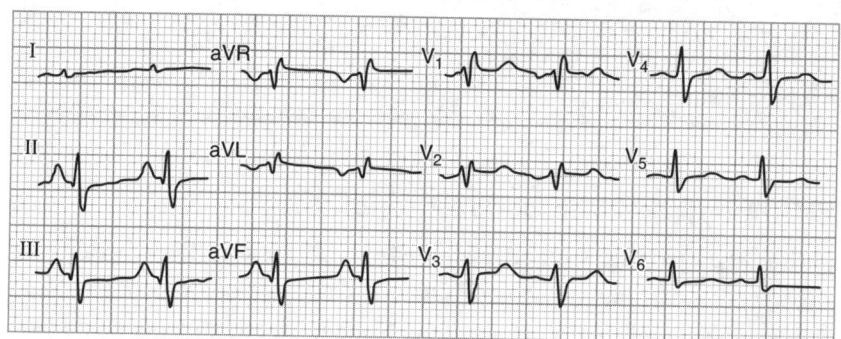

FIGURE 11–7 • **EKG changes associated with chronic obstructive pulmonary disease.** Chronic obstructive pulmonary disease can present with poor R wave progression, low voltage QRS complexes, and P pulmonale. (*Reproduced from ABC of clinical electrocardiography: conditions affecting the right side of the heart, Harrigan RA and Jones K, Vol. 324, Page 1202, © 2002. With permission from BMJ Publishing Group Ltd.*)

Cardiac System

Pericarditis

Pericarditis is an inflammatory disease process of the heart. When this occurs, several EKG changes can be seen. These occur in the large majority of cases, but the early signs may not be seen if the patient has had the problem for several days (Fig. 11–8). These changes are:

- Diffuse ST segment elevation
- T wave inversion (after ST segments have returned to the isoelectric line)
- T wave flattening and then return to normal
- Depressed PR interval

If an **effusion** (a collection of fluid) is present in the pericardial sac, low voltage would be seen in all leads. **Electrical alternans**, a change in the amplitude of successive QRS complexes, can be exhibited due to a rotation of the heart as fluid continues to fill the pericardial sac with the effusion.

CLINICAL ALERT

These patients often appear to have large, extended infarctions on their EKG tracings due to the diffuse pattern of the ST segment elevation. Although it is imperative to prove that infarction has not occurred, the following changes can also provide clarity for the health care provider:

- More leads than would be associated with a localized area of infarction demonstrate the ST segment elevation.
- If a patient is in the process of myocardial infarction, the T wave inversion, indicating ischemia, would most likely lead the changes on the EKG rather than appear after the ST segment elevation.
- No Q waves occur with pericarditis.

Idiopathic Hypertrophic Subaortic Stenosis

Idiopathic hypertrophic subaortic stenosis (IHSS) is also known as **hypertrophic obstructive cardiomyopathy** (HOCM). This is a disease process seen very often in young people who are athletic. Sudden death can occur due to the enlargement and stiffness of heart muscle that does not allow for good filling and causes problems with ventricular outflow. Patients may also complain of lightheadedness, chest pain, or syncopal episodes. EKG changes that will be found on the 12-lead EKG are (Fig. 11–9):

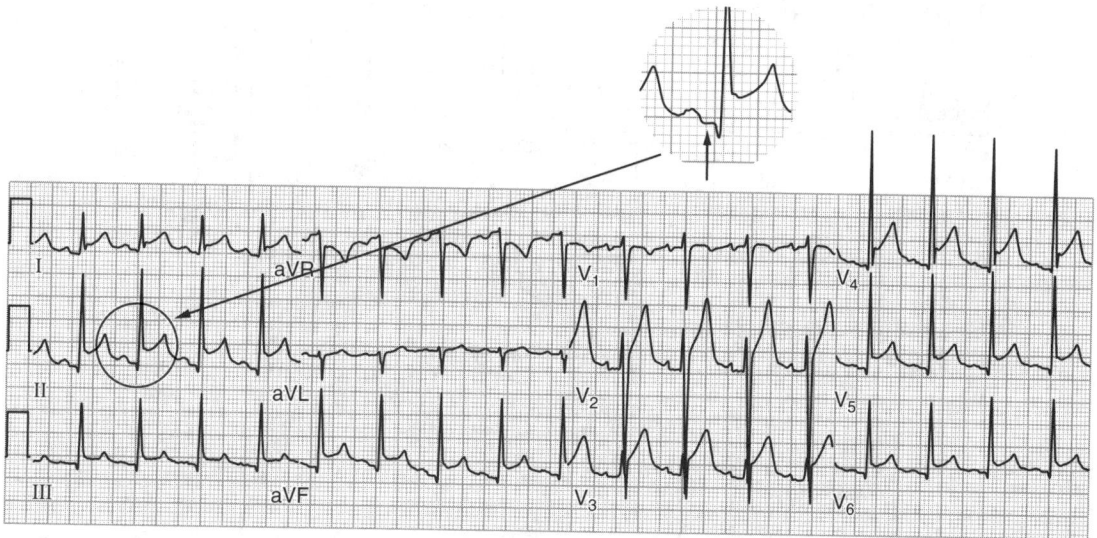

FIGURE 11–8 • EKG Tracing in pericarditis. Diffuse ST segment elevation and the presence of PR segment depression as demonstrated in lead II can indicate pericarditis. (*From Ferry D., ECG in 10 Days, 2e. McGraw Hill, 2007.*)

- Left ventricular hypertrophy (larger R waves in leads that look at the left ventricle—V_5 and V_6—with V_6 being greater than V_5)
- Left axis deviation (lead I QRS positive with a negative QRS in aVF)
- Lateral and inferior Q waves (not associated with infarction)

CLINICAL ALERT

Some individuals who are athletic can have changes to their EKG simply due to the fact that they have been in training and their heart has made alterations that will maximize their efforts. This is especially true for runners. Some of these changes include dysrhythmias such as profound bradycardia, junctional rhythms, first-degree AV block, second-degree AV block (Wenckebach), or wandering atrial pacemaker. Other changes that might be seen are: ST segment elevations, T wave inversions, right and left ventricular hypertrophy, and right bundle branch block.

Brugada Syndrome

Brugada syndrome is an inherited autosomal dominant disease process that causes sudden death in otherwise healthy, younger male patients (age 30-50). Females can have this syndrome, but it is more common in men. It is also more common in Asian populations. Patients with this syndrome develop

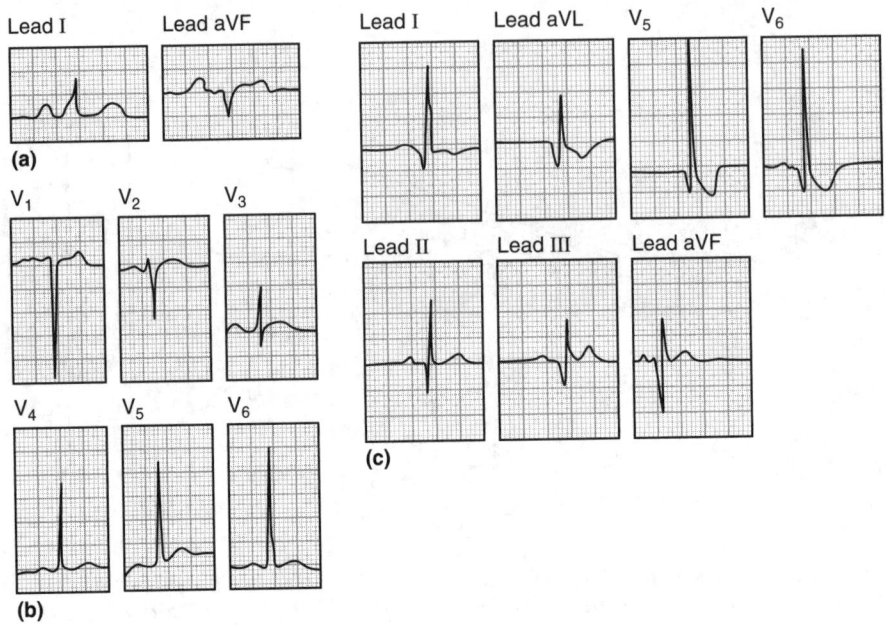

FIGURE 11–9 • EKG changes associated with IHSS. Possible changes which can occur with this disease process are: (a) Left Axis Deviation - depicted by a positive R wave in Lead I and a negative R wave in Lead aVF. (b) Left Ventricular Hypertrophy - depicted by a large S wave in V_1, large R wave in V_6 (greater than 18 mm), greater R wave height in V_6 than V_5, and combined height of S wave in V_1 and R wave in V_6 greater than 35 mm. (c) Deep/narrow Q waves (less than 40 ms) in lateral and inferior leads (not associated with acute myocardial infarction Q waves - usually greater than 40 ms). (Every disease process will not always depict "picture perfect" signatory EKG changes.) (*Modified from Thaler, M. The Only EKG Book You'll Ever Need, 6e. 2011.*)

polymorphic ventricular tachycardia and subsequent ventricular fibrillation. EKG changes that are associated with this cardiac disturbance are right bundle branch block and ST segment elevation in precordial leads, V_1, V_2, and V_3 not associated with an injury pattern (Fig. 11–10). The insertion of an automatic

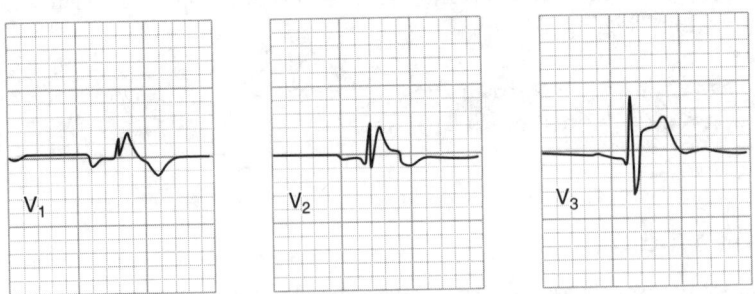

FIGURE 11–10 • EKG changes associated with Brugada syndrome. Leads V_1, V_2, and V_3 carry the indicative changes for Brugada syndrome of right bundle branch block and ST segment elevation that is not consistent with injury pattern in an acute myocardial infarction. (*From Thaler, M. The Only EKG Book You'll Ever Need, 6e. 2011.*)

implantable cardioversion defibrillator is the treatment of choice at this time. Identifying these changes in the routine EKG can be life saving for these individuals.

Wellens Syndrome

Wellens syndrome is another disease process that can cause sudden death in patients. In this abnormality, the left anterior descending artery (LAD) is stenosed and can be treated with angioplasty and placement of coronary stents. The EKG findings in this preinfarction disease state are T wave inversion in leads V_2 and V_3. Without treatment, these patients will progress to an anterior myocardial infarction. Patients will have chest pain with these specific EKG changes and no ST segment elevation or Q waves (Fig. 11–11).

Pacemakers

In general pacemakers are placed when heart rates are too slow such as bradycardia and AV blocks. When the patient's heart does not generate an impulse, the pacemaker will take over to perform this function. Other reasons for pacemakers are tachydysrhythmias or sick sinus syndrome.

Electrodes are positioned within the heart and attached to a generator. In emergency situations a temporary pacemaker is placed. The leads that are used for pacemakers can be unipolar (a negative pole) or bipolar (both a negative and a positive pole). There are different kinds of pacemakers and each is programmed to assist the heart in the best manner available.

When patients have pacemakers, the EKG or cardiac monitor tracing will show a pacer spike or "blip." On many cardiac monitors, this spike can be marked so that it shows up in a different color for easy recognition. Depending on the type of pacemaker placed, the spike or "blip" will appear prior to the P wave or the QRS. Atrial pacing will produce a pacer spike before the P wave and ventricular pacing will demonstrate a pacer spike before the QRS complex. Some pacemakers are called "**AV sequential.**" In this instance, there will be two

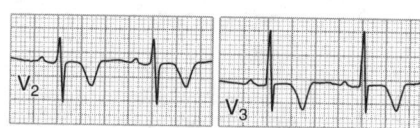

FIGURE 11–11 • EKG changes associated with Wellens syndrome. Deep T wave inversion seen in leads V_2 and V_3 can be Wellen syndrome.

pacer spikes for each complex—one before the P wave and one before the QRS. There are a variety of pacemakers and a number of ways in which they can be set specific for the patient's underlying disease process. They are based on the chamber that is paced, the chamber that is sensing the stimulus, and the activity that occurs from that generated impulse. The ones listed above are the most common (Fig. 11–12).

When pacemakers are in place, watch for failure to pace or failure to capture. Failure to pace is indicated when no pacing spikes are noted on the EKG tracing or cardiac monitor. This could mean that the battery needs to be changed or that there is some type of failure of the circuitry. This could be caused by a lead that has broken, has become disconnected, or that the amperage has been set too low. If this happens with a temporary pacemaker, the voltage or mA can be set higher until the pacer blip or spike is noted on the tracing or monitor.

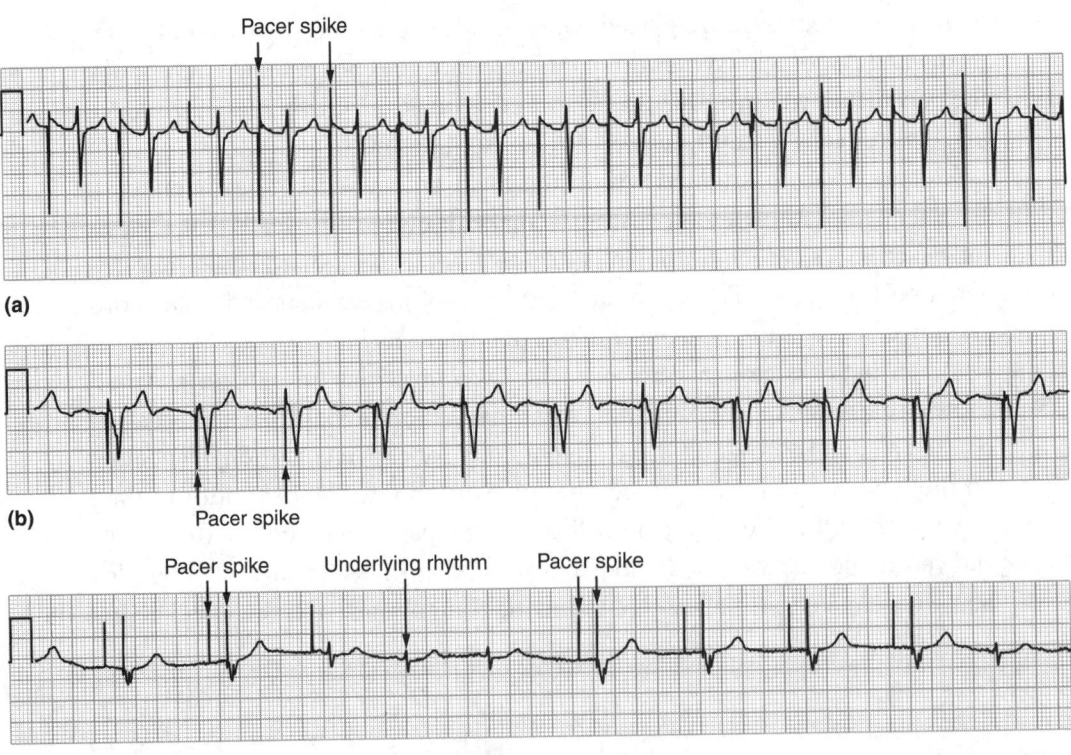

FIGURE 11–12 • **Pacer spikes.** Pacer spikes or "blips" are noted one each of these rhythm strips. (a) Atrial pacing will show a spike before the P wave. (b) Ventricular pacing is seen in this rhythm strip. The spike occurs before the QRS complex. (c) AV sequential pacing shows two pacer spikes before each complex. One is stimulating the atria and the other, the ventricles. The beats without pacer spikes are the patient's own underlying rhythm and contractions.

Pacer failure to capture is identified when the pacer spike is seen but no atrial or ventricular waveforms are noted. Etiologies for this problem include incorrect lead positioning, deficient battery, faulty lead wires, a lead wire that has actually perforated through the myocardium, or disease processes such as electrolyte imbalances or hypoxia leading to acidotic conditions.

Pacemakers can also undersense and oversense. Undersensing causes the production of pacer spikes when they are not necessary, that is, the patient's underlying rhythm is already producing a heart rate that is perfusing the body. These spikes can cause problems if they occur on the vulnerable portion of the T wave which can then cause ventricular fibrillation. Oversensing picks up other activity that is not cardiac in nature such as tremors or other muscular movements. At this point, the pacemaker will not fire in an attempt to correct the heart rate for the patient and the patient can become asystolic (Fig. 11–13).

CLINICAL ALERT

Some patients have a special pacemaker that is called a "Biventricular Pacemaker." This was developed to assist patients who have heart failure. This is also known as *cardiac resynchronization therapy* and causes the ventricles to contract in a more synchronous fashion. There are three leads for this pacemaker—one that is placed in the right atrium, one in the right ventricle, and the last in the left ventricle.

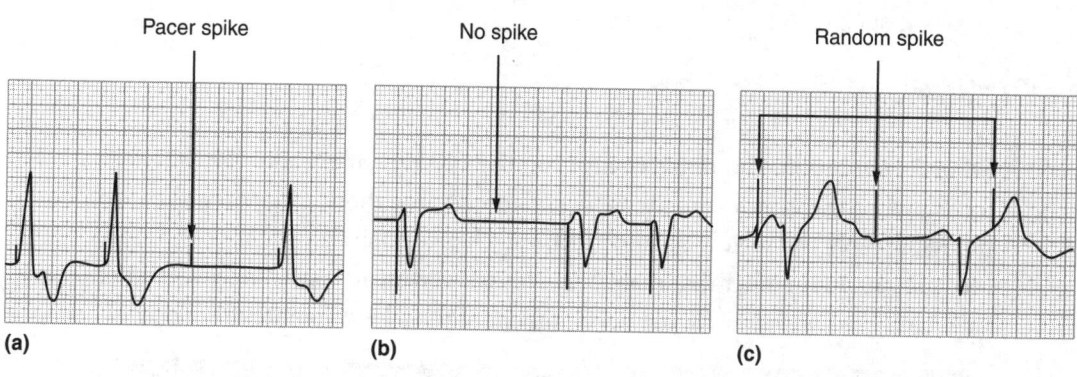

FIGURE 11–13 • Pacemaker malfunctions. (a) In failure to capture, pacemaker spikes are seen without a concurrent QRS complex. **(b)** In failure to pace, the pacer spike is not present where it would be expected to generate an impulse. The area between the 1st and the 2nd QRS complex (generated by the pacemaker) is lacking a pacer spike and the QRS complex. **(c)** When pacer spikes occur randomly throughout the rhythm, there is a failure to sense which may be due to over or undersensing.

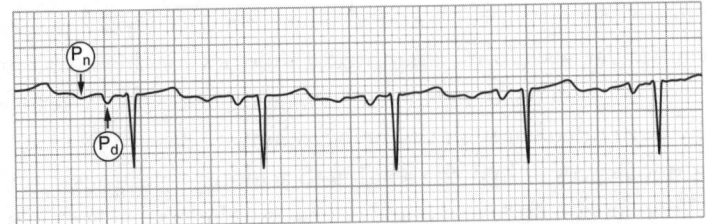

FIGURE 11–14 • **Native and donor P waves.** The first P wave comes from the patient's native SA node. The second P wave is derived from the donor's SA nodal tissue. (*Modified from Dubin D, Rapid Interpretation of EKG's, 6e., Cover Publishing Company, 2010.*)

Heart Transplant

Heart transplant patients can have changes on their EKG tracing and cardiac monitor. The most interesting of these is the presence of two P waves. Due to the manner in which the heart is attached to the existing piece of right atrium and thus maintains their own SA node, the patient will have both a "native P wave" and a "donor P wave" (Fig. 11–14). The native P wave, denoted as P_n, is not able to conduct the impulse beyond the sutured area. The donor P wave, denoted as P_d, becomes the dominant area of generated impulses and conducts the impulse through the myocardium. Other changes that may be seen with transplanted hearts are:

- An increase in the sinus rate
- Rotation of the axis
- A right bundle branch block
- Nonspecific ST-T wave changes

Medications

Several medications can make changes on the EKG tracing or the cardiac monitor. Some of these have already been discussed throughout other chapters. The following table is a review of some of these changes that can occur with certain medications. Remember that many medications can create a prolonged QT interval which can then allow for the development of torsades de pointes (Table 11–2).

> **CLINICAL ALERT**
>
> Many medications can cause cardiac changes for the patient. Sometimes these changes occur due to the combined effects of two or more medications that the patient may be taking. Always take this into consideration when diagnosing and treating patients for EKG changes or dysrhythmias that are taking place.

TABLE 11–2 Some Medications Implicated in EKG Changes		
Medication	**EKG Changes**	**Dysrhythmias**

Digitalis (Digoxin)	Depression of the ST segment / flattened or depressed T wave ("digitalis effect")
	
	(this is a gradual downward sloping)
		• PACs
		• PJCs
		• PVCs
		• Blocks
		  • PAT with block
		  • Sinus block
		  • AV blocks
		• Atrial tachydysrhythmia
		• Junctional tachydysrhythmia
		• Ventricular bigeminy
		• Ventricular fibrillation

Quinidine (Quinaglute)	Prolonged QRS Prolonged QT	• Torsades de pointes
Sotalol (Betapace)	Prolonged PR Prolonged QRS Prolonged QT	• Bradycardia • Torsades de pointes
Amiodarone (Cordarone)	Prolonged PR Prolonged QRS Prolonged QT	• Torsades de pointes
Verapamil (Calan)	Prolonged PR	• Sinus bradycardia • AV Blocks
Diltiazem (Cardizem)	Prolonged QRS	• Sinus bradycardia • AV Blocks
Tricyclic Antidepressants	Prolonged PR Prolonged QT Widened QRS ST Depression	• Sinus Tachycardia • PVCs • Supraventricular tachycardia • Ventricular tachycardia

Conclusion

Many processes can cause cardiac abnormalities for patients. These can be derived from a variety of sources and can impact the cardiac health of individuals in many unique ways. Body systems intertwine and it is important for the health care professional to understand the various adjustments that these systems make when disease processes or medication related events occur.

Some of the highlights from this chapter are:

- Hypokalemia is noted on the EKG by a flattened T wave, depressed ST segments, and the presence of U waves.

- Torsades de pointes can be caused by hypokalemia.

- Hyperkalemia will present with tall, peaked T waves.

- Ventricular fibrillation can be caused by hyperkalemia.

- Hypocalcemia causes a prolongation of the QT interval which can be a precursor to torsades de pointes.

- Hypercalcemia can cause the QT interval to shorten.

- Hypomagnesemia can look very similar to hypokalemia.

- Ventricular dysrhythmias can be caused by hypomagnesemia including torsades de pointes.

- Complete heart block can be caused by hypermagnesemia.

- The J wave (Osborne wave) is present with hypothermia.

- Intracranial events such as subarachnoid hemorrhage can produce deeply inverted T waves as well as bradycardia and prolongation of the QT interval.

- A pulmonary embolus has a special S1Q3 pattern. This can also include an inverted T wave in lead III (S1Q3T3).

- Tachycardia is a common dysrhythmia with pulmonary embolus.

- Patients with COPD will have low voltage, right axis deviation, and poor R wave progression on their EKG.

- Cor pulmonale is right-sided heart failure caused by an underlying pulmonary disease process.

- P pulmonale is the EKG change associated with cor pulmonale.

- Pericarditis appears with diffuse ST segment elevation across the EKG.

- T wave changes will also occur with pericarditis, but this will happen after the ST segment elevation, rather than before as with an acute myocardial infarction.

- An effusion can cause electrical alternans, a change in the amplitude of successive QRS complexes.

- Idiopathic hypertrophic subaortic stenosis (IHSS) can cause sudden death in young people, especially athletes.

- IHSS changes to the heart include left ventricular hypertrophy, left axis deviation, and Q waves in the inferior and lateral leads.

- Some athletic individuals can have some changes on their EKG and dysrhythmias which are considered to be "normal" for them.
- Many athletes will have a severe or profound bradycardia.
- Brugada syndrome is most common in Asian males and causes sudden death.
- The characteristic changes on the EKG for Brugada syndrome is a right bundle branch block and ST segment elevation in the precordial leads.
- Wellens syndrome is caused by a stenosed LAD.
- Wellens syndrome can be picked up on the 12-lead EKG as T wave inversion in V_2 and V_3.
- Patients with pacemakers will have a pacer spike or "blip" before captured QRS complexes.
- Pacemakers are usually used for bradycardias and AV blocks.
- Pacemakers can be atrial, ventricular, or AV sequential.
- Failure to pace, failure to capture, oversensing, and undersensing are complications that can occur with pacemakers.
- Undersensing can cause pacer spikes to appear throughout the EKG and these can fall on the vulnerable portion of the T wave causing ventricular fibrillation.
- Oversensing causes the pacemaker to fail to fire and the patient can become asystolic.
- Biventricular pacemakers are used to keep patients out of heart failure.
- Heart transplant patients will have two P waves—a native P wave (Pn) and a donor P wave (Pd).
- Many different medications can cause a variety of EKG changes including prolonged PR, QRS, or QT.

PRACTICE QUESTIONS

1. **Hyperkalemia will cause which of the following EKG changes?**
   A. Depressed ST segment
   B. Peaked T wave
   C. Shortened QRS complex
   D. Presence of U wave

2. Hypocalcemia can cause which of the following EKG changes?

   A. Prolonged QT interval
   B. Elevated ST segment
   C. Increased PR interval
   D. Depressed T wave

3. Which of the following dysrhythmias would most likely be caused by hypermagnesemia?

   A. Premature ventricular contractions
   B. Ventricular tachycardia
   C. Torsades de pointes
   D. Complete heart block

4. A J wave (Osborn wave) is associated with which of the following processes?

   A. Subarachnoid hemorrhage
   B. Hyperkalemia
   C. Hypothermia
   D. Heart transplant

5. Which of the following will cause deeply inverted T waves?

   A. Subarachnoid hemorrhage
   B. Hyperkalemia
   C. Hypothermia
   D. Heart transplant

6. Which of the following would NOT be a sign of a pulmonary embolus?

   A. Large S wave in lead I
   B. Prolonged PR interval in lead II
   C. Deep Q wave in lead III
   D. Inverted T wave in lead III

7. Which of the following dysrhythmias would be a significant indicator for a pulmonary embolus?

   A. Sinus tachycardia
   B. Complete heart block
   C. Ventricular tachycardia
   D. Wenckebach

8. Emphysema causes several changes on the EKG due to which of the following?

   A. Increased mucous production
   B. Loss of defense mechanisms
   C. Change in position of the diaphragm
   D. Increased number of alveoli

9. **Which of the following is a true statement regarding cor pulmonale?**

   A. Cor pulmonale is a form of left-sided heart failure.

   B. Cor pulmonale is caused by gastric disease processes.

   C. Cor pulmonale causes pulmonary edema.

   D. Cor pulmonale is a consequence of pulmonary disease.

10. **Pericarditis will mimic signs of which of the following on the 12-lead EKG?**

    A. Massive pulmonary embolus

    B. Extended myocardial infarction

    C. Advanced subarachnoid hemorrhage

    D. Extreme hyperkalemia

11. **Which of the following is a known cause of sudden death in young athletes?**

    A. Brugada syndrome

    B. Wellens syndrome

    C. Pericarditis

    D. Idiopathic hypertrophic subaortic stenosis

12. **Which of the following is the cause of pacer spikes being seen without a QRS complex?**

    A. Pacer failure to pace

    B. Pacer failure to capture

    C. Pacer oversensing

    D. Pacer undersensing

13. **A biventricular pacemaker is used to treat which of the following?**

    A. Heart failure

    B. Ventricular tachycardia

    C. Torsades de pointes

    D. Pulmonary hypertension

14. **A patient with a heart transplant will have two:**

    A. S waves

    B. T waves

    C. R waves

    D. P waves

15. **Digitalis toxicity will cause:**

    A. peaked T waves.

    B. depressed ST segment.

    C. biphasic P wave.

    D. prolonged PR interval.

ANSWER KEY

1. **B.** Hyperkalemia is indicated on the EKG or cardiac monitor by high peaked T waves. ST depression can be seen with hypokalemia and a U wave is seen with hypomagnesemia.

2. **A.** Hypocalcemia can cause prolonged QT intervals which can be a precursor to torsades de pointes. Elevated ST segments and depressed T waves can be seen with pericarditis and increased PR interval may be present in hypermagnesiemia and several medications. Depressed T waves can be seen with hypokalemia as well.

3. **D.** Hypermagnesemia can produce complete heart block. Causes of hypermagnesemia include renal failure, the administration of magnesium, or the overuse of antacids.

4. **C.** Hypothermia causes the presence of a J wave, also known as an Osborne wave on the EKG. This is an extra positive deflection between the ST segment and the T wave. A subarachnoid hemorrhage can have deeply inverted T waves, hyperkalemia may be demonstrated with high peaked T waves, and heart transplants will have an extra P wave.

5. **A.** Intracranial events such as a subarachnoid hemorrhage can affect the EKG or cardiac monitor by producing deeply inverted T waves.

6. **B.** A massive pulmonary embolus can be demonstrated on the 12-lead EKG with a particular pattern known as S1Q3T3. This is represented by a significant S wave in lead I, and a deep Q wave and inverted T wave in lead III.

7. **A.** Sinus tachycardia is often the dysrhythmia when patients are experiencing a pulmonary embolus. This does not have to be at extremely high rates. Even rates as high as 110 to 120 beats per minute can be significant for a pulmonary embolus.

8. **C.** Patients with emphysema, a type of chronic obstructive pulmonary disease, can have low voltage, right axis deviation, and poor R wave progression due to changes within the thoracic cavity. These changes include increases in the volume of the lung due to alveolar air trapping, diaphragm positioning, and a change in the orientation of the heart.

9. **D.** Cor pulmonale is a consequence of pulmonary disease that causes right sided heart failure.

10. **B.** Pericarditis can appear with diffuse ST segment elevation. This can appear as a massive myocardial infarction. After the ST segments return to the isoelectric line, T wave inversion will occur. This is different than with an MI, but, the myocardial infarction must be ruled out.

11. **D.** IHSS, idiopathic hypertrophic subaortic stenosis, can cause sudden death in young people, especially athletes. This causes enlargement and stiffness of the heart muscle which then prevents proper filling and disorders of the outflow. Brugada does cause sudden death but the individuals are usually young Asian males, ages 30 to 50, and the cause of death is polymorphic ventricular tachycardia and

ventricular fibrillation. Wellens syndrome is caused by a stenotic LAD causing an acute anterior myocardial infarction. Pericarditis is an inflammatory disease process of the heart.

12. **B.** Failure to capture is seen on the EKG as pacer spikes that do not have subsequent QRS complexes. Failure to pace would be seen as no pacer spikes appearing on the EKG strip. Oversensing picks up activity that is not cardiac in nature such as tremors or other muscular movements such as seizures and therefore the pacemaker does not fire since it "thinks" that the patient is having QRS complexes. Undersensing causes the production of pacer spikes when they are not necessary. This can cause a major problem if the spike falls on the vulnerable portion of the T wave.

13. **A.** A biventricular pacemaker causes the ventricles to work more synchronously and keeps patients out of heart failure.

14. **D.** Heart transplant patients will have two P waves. These are known as the native P wave, P_n, and the donor P wave, P_d.

15. **B.** The "digitalis effect" is a gradual downward sloping of the ST segment.

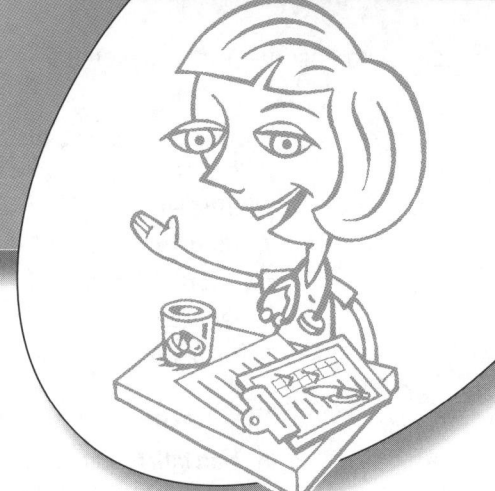

Final Exam

1. **Which of the following is a correct definition of a rhythm strip?**

   A. A special test that involves 12 views of the heart's electrical activity

   B. A tool that can be used to definitively diagnose a myocardial infarction

   C. A designated view of the heart that is used to monitor rate and rhythm

   D. A translation of the contraction of each of the chambers of the heart

2. **Einthoven assigned which of the following letters to denote each of the waveforms found on an EKG tracing?**

   A. A, B, C, D, E

   B. L, M, N, O, P

   C. U, V, W, X, Y

   D. P, Q, R, S, T

3. **An abnormal heart rhythm is known as a/an:**

   A. dysrhythmia.

   B. monorhythmia.

   C. transrhythmia.

   D. polyrhythmia.

4. **Tachycardia is a term that means:**

   A. a slow heart rate.

   B. extra beats that occur.

   C. a fast heart rate.

   D. the loss of beats.

5. A patient is seeing his physician for multiple complaints. For which of the following symptoms would the physician feel that an EKG would assist in his diagnosis?

   A. Ringing in the ears
   B. Shortness of breath
   C. One leg swelling
   D. Increased salivation

6. The term pericarditis would mean that the patient's heart:

   A. had inflammation to the sac surrounding it.
   B. had a lack of blood flow to the arteries feeding it.
   C. was not pumping effectively to produce good cardiac output.
   D. was too thick or enlarged to beat efficiently.

7. Which of the following would most likely be able to legally interpret an EKG tracing for diagnostic purposes?

   A. EKG technician
   B. Registered Nurse
   C. Physician
   D. Paramedic

8. The apex of the heart is located on the:

   A. top of the heart.
   B. left side of the heart.
   C. bottom of the heart.
   D. right side of the heart.

9. Which of the following is a true statement regarding the myocardial layer of the heart?

   A. It is the innermost layer made up of endothelium and connective tissue.
   B. The main coronary arteries are located in this area.
   C. It is continuous with the interior layer of the vessels.
   D. It is the thick, muscular layer consisting of cardiac muscle fiber.

10. The tricuspid valve lies between the:

    A. right atrium and right ventricle.
    B. left atrium and left ventricle.
    C. pulmonary artery and right ventricle.
    D. left ventricle and the aorta.

11. **When blood flows backward due to a dysfunctional heart valve, this is known as:**

    A. valvular stenosis.

    B. valvular prolapse.

    C. valvular regurgitation.

    D. valvular inversion.

12. **An S3 heart sound is:**

    A. considered to be normal in older people.

    B. the normal first heart sound in the cycle.

    C. occurs due to closure of the aortic valve.

    D. can be associated with heart failure.

13. **Which of the following would be considered to be a positive chronotropic response?**

    A. Heart rate of 42

    B. Blood pressure of 140/54

    C. Heart rate of 120

    D. Blood pressure of 182/112

14. **The parasympathetic nervous system would exert which of the following responses in the heart?**

    A. Heart rate of 42

    B. Blood pressure of 140/54

    C. Heart rate of 120

    D. Blood pressure of 182/112

15. **Carotid sinus massage might be utilized in which of the following circumstances?**

    A. Slow heart rates

    B. Rapid heart rates

    C. Increased blood pressure

    D. Decreased blood pressure

16. **Which of the following is the correct sequence of the cardiac cycle?**

    A. Isovolumetric ventricular contraction, ventricular ejection, ventricular filling, isovolumetric relaxation

    B. Isovolumetric relaxation, ventricular filling, ventricular ejection, isovolumetric ventricular contraction

    C. Ventricular ejection, isovolumetric relaxation, ventricular filling, isovolumetric ventricular contraction

    D. Ventricular filling, isovolumetric ventricular contraction, ventricular ejection, isovolumetric relaxation

17. Which of the following would indicate a normal ejection fraction?

 A. 60%

 B. 45%

 C. 30%

 D. 20%

18. Which of the following is the correct formula utilized for cardiac output?

 A. Cardiac output = stroke volume × ejection fraction

 B. Cardiac output = heart rate × blood pressure

 C. Cardiac output = stroke volume × heart rate

 D. Cardiac output = blood pressure × ejection fraction

19. Which of the following is the correct definition for the term "automaticity"?

 A. Ability of the pacemaker cells to create an electrical impulse without nerve stimulation

 B. Ability of the cardiac muscle cells to respond to chemical, mechanical, and electrical stimulation

 C. Ability to receive an electrical impulse and transmit it to another cardiac cell

 D. Ability of the cardiac muscle to contract after receiving an electrical impulse

20. When the movement of electrolytes across cell membranes causes the inside of the cell to become more positive, this translates to:

 A. an isoelectric line on the EKG.

 B. a spike or positive wave on the EKG.

 C. a negative deflection on the EKG.

 D. a biphasic waveform on the EKG.

21. PEA or Pulseless Electrical Activity is seen on the EKG recording when:

 A. only mechanical activity is occurring within the heart muscle.

 B. only electrical activity occurs within the heart muscle.

 C. extra contractions are occurring within the heart muscle.

 D. fewer contractions are occurring within the heart muscle.

22. The term "refractoriness" relates to the cardiac cycle in which of the following ways?

 A. This is the same as contractility.

 B. This coincides with conductivity.

 C. This is related to unresponsiveness to stimuli.

 D. This is the ability to create an impulse.

23. **Which of the following presents the correct normal electrical pathway of an electrical impulse?**

    A. AV node, bundle of His, SA node, bundle branches, Purkinje fibers
    B. SA node, bundle of His, bundle branches, AV node, Purkinje fibers
    C. Purkinje fibers, bundle branches, bundle of His, AV node, SA node
    D. SA node, AV node, bundle of His, bundle branches, Purkinje fibers

24. **Which of the following parts of the electrical pathway is considered to be a protective device during rapid atrial rates such as atrial fibrillation?**

    A. SA node
    B. AV node
    C. Bundle of His
    D. Purkinje fibers

25. **Wolff-Parkinson-White (WPW) syndrome occurs due to which of the following abnormal cardiac impulses?**

    A. Enhanced automaticity
    B. Retrograde conduction
    C. Escape rhythms
    D. Reentry rhythms

26. **Which of the following would be an example of triggered activity?**

    A. Ventricular fibrillation
    B. Supraventricular tachycardia
    C. Premature atrial contractions
    D. Atrioventricular blocks

27. **Which of the following best describes a 12-lead EKG?**

    A. It is displayed on a cardiac monitor.
    B. It uses only the bipolar leads.
    C. Electrodes are placed on the chest only.
    D. It provides a complete picture of the electrical activity.

28. **The EASI system is a:**

    A. way to remember how to attach three leads for monitoring.
    B. form of the five electrode system so that 12 leads can be monitored.
    C. particular form of color coding of the electrodes.
    D. system that can be used in place of a conventional 12-lead EKG.

29. If a patient is exhibiting premature ventricular contractions on the EKG, which of the following would be an important clinical aspect of assessing the patient?

    A. Auscultating the lungs
    B. Visualizing the neck area
    C. Palpating the pulse
    D. Percussing the back

30. Which of the following actions should be taken when baseline issues are seen on the EKG?

    A. Reposition the electrodes
    B. Check for electrical interference
    C. Connect electrodes wires to appropriate electrodes
    D. Reapply disconnected electrode wires

31. Which of the following electrolyte abnormalities might create a false alarm reading?

    A. Hyperkalemia
    B. Hypermagnesemia
    C. Hypernatremia
    D. Hyperchloremia

32. Each large box on the special EKG paper is equal to:

    A. 0.04 seconds.
    B. 0.20 seconds.
    C. 0.30 seconds.
    D. 0.60 seconds.

33. Which of the following is a true statement regarding a bipolar lead?

    A. A bipolar lead has both a negative and a positive electrode.
    B. Lead aVR is an example of a bipolar lead.
    C. Lead augmented vector foot is an example of a bipolar lead.
    D. A bipolar lead uses the heart as a relative negative electrode.

34. Einthoven's triangle is created by the:

    A. unipolar leads.
    B. horizontal leads.
    C. vertical leads.
    D. bipolar leads.

35. **Lead II would be created by placing the electrodes in which of the following locations?**

    A. Positive electrode to the right leg and negative electrode to the right arm
    B. Positive electrode to the left leg and negative electrode to the left arm
    C. Positive electrode to the right leg and negative electrode to the left arm
    D. Positive electrode to the left leg and negative electrode to the right arm

36. **For Lead V_2, the positive electrode is placed at the:**

    A. fourth intercostal space to the right of the sternum.
    B. fourth intercostal space to the left of the sternum.
    C. fifth intercostal space at the midclavicular line.
    D. fifth intercostal space at the anterior axillary line.

37. **Proper placement of the positive electrode in order to view Lead V_4R is:**

    A. fourth intercostal space to the right of the sternum.
    B. fifth intercostal space to the right of the sternum.
    C. fourth intercostal space to the left of the sternum.
    D. fifth intercostal space at the right midclavicular line.

38. **Lead V_8 would be placed correctly on the fifth intercostal space:**

    A. midaxillary line.
    B. posterior axillary line.
    C. posterior scapular area.
    D. border of the spine.

39. **Which of the following might be used to assist in the detection of bundle branch blocks?**

    A. Right chest leads
    B. Posterior leads
    C. Modified chest leads
    D. Horizontal leads

40. **Depolarization of the atria is seen with which of the following?**

    A. P wave
    B. Q wave
    C. R wave
    D. T wave

41. **Which of the following is a true statement regarding the QRS complex?**
    A. All three wave forms are always present in the QRS complex.
    B. A Q, R, or S wave that has an amplitude below 5 mm is denoted with a small case letter.
    C. A notched R wave is known as an R prime and is noted as a change in direction.
    D. The highest amplitude for the R wave should be in lead V_1.

42. **Which of the following might be a cause of poor R wave progression?**
    A. Cholecystitis
    B. Fibromyalgia
    C. Dextrocardia
    D. Atrial fibrillation

43. **T wave inversion might be associated with which of the following disease processes?**
    A. Hyperkalemia
    B. Myocardial injury
    C. Pacemakers
    D. Cerebral hemorrhage

44. **The normal PR interval is:**
    A. 0.02 to 0.06 seconds.
    B. 0.04 to 0.20 seconds.
    C. 0.12 to 0.20 seconds.
    D. 0.36 to 0.44 seconds.

45. **A prolonged QT interval can place the patient at risk for which of the following?**
    A. Torsades de pointes
    B. First-degree AV block
    C. Atrial fibrillation
    D. Supraventricular tachycardia

46. **Calipers would be used to assist in determining which of the following?**
    A. Heart rate
    B. Rhythm regularity
    C. PR interval
    D. QRS width

47. Using the small box method, what would the heart rate be if there were 15 small squares in between each R wave?

    A. 20 beats per minute
    B. 60 beats per minute
    C. 80 beats per minute
    D. 100 beats per minute

48. Which of the following would be indicative of a normal sinus rhythm?

    A. Heart rate of 104
    B. PR interval of 0.24 seconds
    C. QRS interval of 0.40 seconds
    D. Presence of ectopic beats

49. Which of the following is a true statement regarding axis?

    A. The mean electrical axis is the opposite direction in which the electrical axis is traveling.
    B. In the hexaxial reference system, the upper segments represent negative degrees.
    C. Normally the mean electrical axis should fall within the scope of +180° to −90°.
    D. In right axis deviation the axis would correspond to −90° to 0°on the reference system.

50. Which of the following readings on the EKG would indicate a left axis deviation?

    A. Lead I positive, lead aVF positive
    B. Lead I negative, lead aVF positive
    C. Lead I negative, lead aVF negative
    D. Lead I positive, lead aVF negative

51. Which type of axis deviation might be most commonly associated with pregnancy?

    A. Left axis deviation
    B. Right axis deviation
    C. Extreme right axis deviation
    D. No axis deviation

52. Which of the following is a true statement regarding the difference between hypertrophy and enlargement?

    A. Enlargement reflects an expansion of actual muscle mass.
    B. Hypertrophy can be caused by hypertension.
    C. Aortic insufficiency could be a cause of hypertrophy.
    D. The term enlargement is most commonly used to describe the ventricles.

53. Right atrial enlargement would be seen in which parts of the following waveforms?

    A. Downstroke of the P wave
    B. Height of the QRS
    C. Upswing of the P wave
    D. Length of the QRS

54. A complete bundle branch block would have which of the following characteristics on the QRS complex?

    A. The Q wave will be deeper.
    B. The height will be increased.
    C. The width will be greater than 0.12 seconds.
    D. An S prime will occur.

55. In which of the following leads will a left bundle branch block be represented?

    A. Leads V_1 and V_2
    B. Leads II and III
    C. Leads I and aVR
    D. Leads V_5 and V_6

56. Which of the following disease processes is most difficult to determine when a patient presents with a left bundle branch block?

    A. Acute myocardial infarction
    B. Second-degree AV block
    C. Right ventricular hypertrophy
    D. Hypokalemia

57. The Valsalva maneuver would create which of the following actions?

    A. Increase the heart rate
    B. Slow the heart rate
    C. Create premature beats
    D. Decrease premature beats

58. Which of the following heart rates would be considered to be bradycardic in an infant?

    A. 140 beats per minute
    B. 120 beats per minute
    C. 110 beats per minute
    D. 80 beats per minute

59. When a child is in a situation that is taxing to the heart, which of the following will occur in order to attempt to increase cardiac output?

    A. Increase stroke volume
    B. Decrease heart rate
    C. Increase heart rate
    D. Decrease stroke volume

60. Which patient population would normally exhibit sinus arrhythmia associated with respiratory rate?

    A. Pregnant patients
    B. Children
    C. Senior adults
    D. Middle aged adults

61. When escape beats occur due to a bradycardia, which of the following is the best treatment?

    A. Provide treatment to speed up the heart rate
    B. Administer medication to eradicate the extra beats
    C. No treatment is necessary at this time
    D. Stabilize the patient with beta blockers

62. Another term for sick sinus syndrome is:

    A. sinus arrest.
    B. AV nodal dysfunction.
    C. brady-tachy syndrome.
    D. sinus arrhythmia.

63. Which of the following would be characteristic on the EKG for a premature atrial contraction (PAC)?

    A. No P waves present
    B. Noncompensatory pause
    C. Regular rhythm
    D. Wide QRS

64. What is the term that is used when a premature ventricular contraction occurs on every third beat?

    A. Bigeminy
    B. Trigeminy
    C. Quadrigeminy
    D. Coupling

65. Which of the following is the determining characteristic for multifocal atrial tachycardia?

A. Changing configurations of the P wave

B. Prolonged PR interval

C. Widened QRS complex

D. Rate greater than 100 beats per minute

66. The bundle of Kent is significant in which of the following types of tachydys-rhythmias?

A. Wolff-Parkinson-White (WPW) syndrome

B. Multifocal atrial tachycardia

C. Wandering atrial pacemaker

D. Sinus tachycardia

67. Which of the following are important aspects of care with the administration of adenosine (Adenocard)?

A. Initiate intravenous access in the right antecubital space.

B. Administer this medication slowly over at least 5 minutes.

C. Patients with Wolff-Parkinson-White (WPW) syndrome can receive this medication.

D. Watch for the development of rapid atrial fibrillation or atrial flutter.

68. Which of the following is a correct statement when administering synchro-nized cardioversion?

A. Synchronized cardioversion is utilized for the treatment of unstable ventricu-lar tachycardia.

B. When using synchronized cardioversion, press the "shock" buttons quickly.

C. Medication patches on the patient's chest are a problem with this procedure.

D. The patient should be on the main cardiac monitor only for this procedure.

69. Which of the following is the best explanation for the loss of cardiac output for the patient with atrial fibrillation?

A. Increase in stroke volume

B. Loss of atrial kick

C. Lengthened depolarization

D. Prolonged T wave

70. Which of the following is usually seen on the EKG for a patient with atrial fibrillation?

A. Sawtooth pattern

B. Lengthened PR interval

C. Widened QRS

D. Loss of P waves

71. The normal rate for a junctional rhythm would most likely be:
    A. 60 to 100 beats per minute.
    B. 20 to 40 beats per minute.
    C. 40 to 60 beats per minute.
    D. 100 to 150 beats per minute.

72. The term "multifocal PVCs" means that premature ventricular contractions:
    A. have differing configurations.
    B. are occurring from multiple sites.
    C. have a uniform appearance.
    D. are occurring from the same site.

73. Which of the following can occur with R on T phenomenon?
    A. Ventricular tachycardia
    B. Third-degree AV block
    C. Atrial fibrillation
    D. Sinus tachycardia

74. Which of the following provides the correct answer for the 5 H's associated with pulseless electrical activity (PEA)?
    A. Hypervolemia, Hypoxia, Hypothermia, Hypokalemia, Hydrogen ion (acidosis)
    B. Hypovolemia, Hypoxia, Hyperthermia, Hyperkalemia, Hydrogen ion (alkalosis)
    C. Hypovolemia, Hypoxia, Hyperthermia, Hyperkalemia, Hydrogen ion (acidosis)
    D. Hypervolemia, Hyperoxia, Hyperthermia, Hyperkalemia, Hydrogen ion (acidosis)

75. Which of the following would indicate mechanical capture of a pacemaker?
    A. Palpable pulse
    B. Pacer spike
    C. QRS complex
    D. P wave

76. Which of the following are associated with torsades de pointes (TdP)?
    A. Monomorphic morphology
    B. Prolonged QT interval
    C. QRS complexes with uniform height
    D. Widened QRS complexes

77. Which of the following would have a progressive lengthening of the PR interval with a subsequent dropped QRS complex?
    A. First-degree AV block
    B. Mobitz type I AV block
    C. Mobitz type II AV block
    D. Complete AV block

78. Patients with Prinzmetal's angina will usually have episodes:

    A. with extreme activity or emotional upset.
    B. from midnight to 8 o'clock in the morning.
    C. with depressed ST segments.
    D. from atherosclerotic heart disease.

79. Which of the following would indicate an injury pattern on an EKG?

    A. Depressed T wave
    B. Pathologic Q wave
    C. Presence of a J wave
    D. Elevated ST segment

80. Which of the following is a true statement regarding reciprocal changes?

    A. Reciprocal changes are a mirror image of the injury site.
    B. Reciprocal changes are seen as ST segment elevation.
    C. Reciprocal changes are present in leads that are next to the area of infarction.
    D. Reciprocal changes appear in the true area of infarction.

81. Which of the following leads would indicate damage to the lateral aspect of the heart?

    A. Leads II, III, aVF
    B. Leads I, II, III
    C. Leads V_1, V_2, V_3, V_4
    D. Leads I, aVL, V_5, V_6

82. The main portion of the right coronary artery supplies the:

    A. interventricular septum.
    B. SA node.
    C. right ventricle.
    D. left atrium.

83. Which of the following biomarkers will stay elevated for a longer period of time?

    A. CK-MB
    B. Myoglobin
    C. Troponin
    D. Creatinine kinase

84. Which of the following electrolyte depletions can cause a patient to be predisposed to torsades de pointes (TdP)?

    A. Phosphorus
    B. Sodium
    C. Chloride
    D. Magnesium

85. **A patient with a subarachnoid hemorrhage might be most likely to present with which of the following?**

    A. Deeply inverted T waves

    B. Prolonged PR interval

    C. Very wide QRS complexes

    D. Biphasic P wave

Identify the following dysrhythmias.

86.

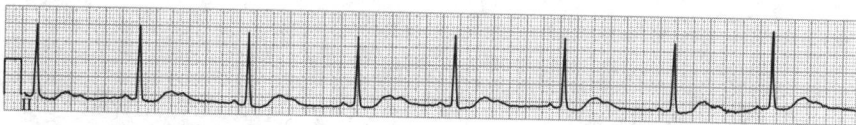

    A. Normal sinus rhythm

    B. Sinus bradycardia

    C. Sinus tachycardia

    D. First-degree AV block

87. Lead II

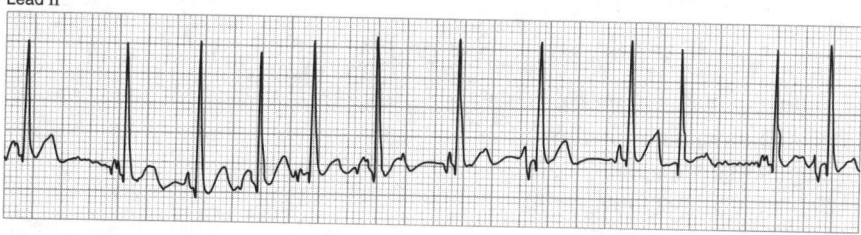

    A. Wandering atrial pacemaker

    B. Multifocal atrial tachycardia

    C. Sinus tachycardia

    D. Atrial fibrillation

88.

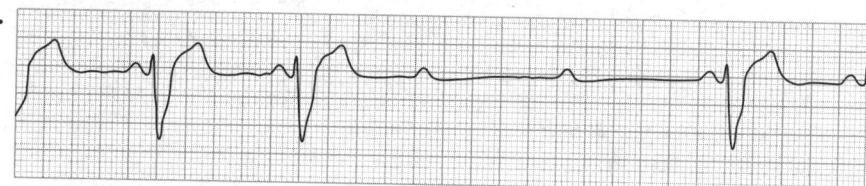

    A. First-degree AV block

    B. Mobitz type I

    C. Mobitz type II

    D. Third-degree AV block

89. Lead II

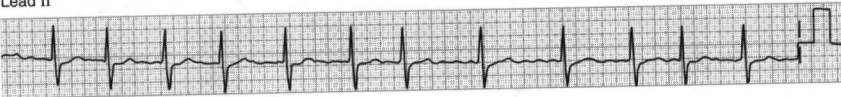

    A. Polymorphic ventricular tachycardia

    B. Ventricular fibrillation

    C. Asystole

    D. Monomorphic ventricular tachycardia

90. Lead II

    A. Ventricular fibrillation

    B. Atrial fibrillation

    C. Atrial tachycardia

    D. Atrial flutter

91.

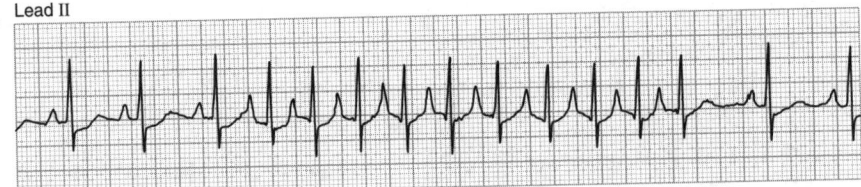

    A. Normal sinus rhythm

    B. Atrial fibrillation

    C. Sinus tachycardia

    D. Ventricular tachycardia

92. Lead II

    A. Paroxysmal supraventricular tachycardia

    B. Atrial fibrillation

    C. Atrial flutter

    D. Multifocal atrial tachycardia

93.

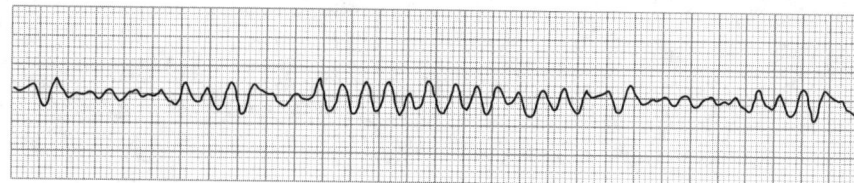

    A. Polymorphic ventricular tachycardia
    B. Coarse ventricular fibrillation
    C. Monomorphic ventricular tachycardia
    D. Atrial fibrillation

94. Lead II

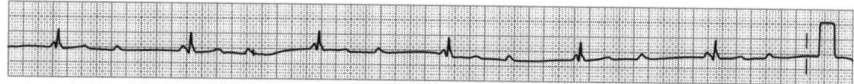

    A. First-degree AV block
    B. Mobitz type II
    C. Sinus bradycardia
    D. Third-degree AV block

95.

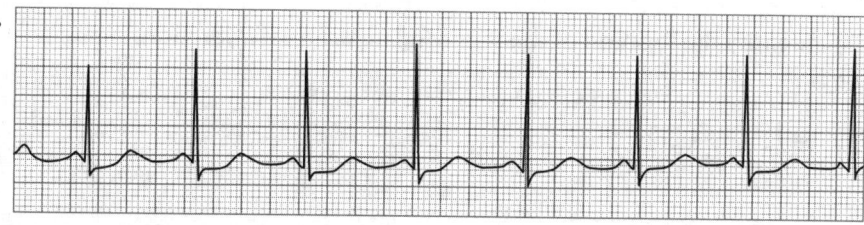

    A. Sinus bradycardia
    B. Normal sinus rhythm
    C. Sinus tachycardia
    D. Wandering atrial pacemaker

96. Lead II

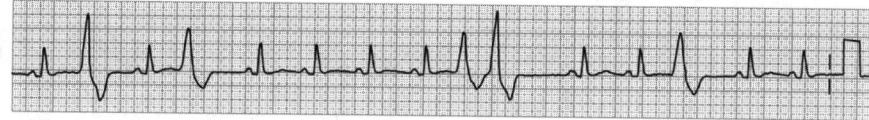

    A. Normal sinus rhythm with premature ventricular coupling
    B. Normal sinus rhythm with premature atrial coupling
    C. Normal sinus rhythm with premature junctional coupling
    D. Normal sinus rhythm with premature sinus coupling

97.

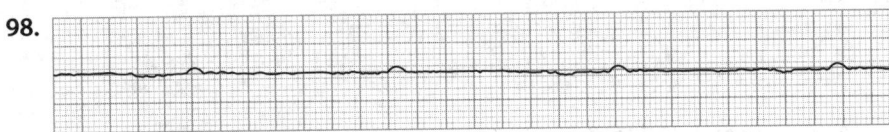

A. Sinus bradycardia
B. Idioventricular rhythm
C. Mobitz type II
D. Third-degree AV block

98.

A. Asystole
B. Ventricular fibrillation
C. Ventricular standstill
D. Ventricular tachycardia

Identify the location of the following myocardial infarction.

99.

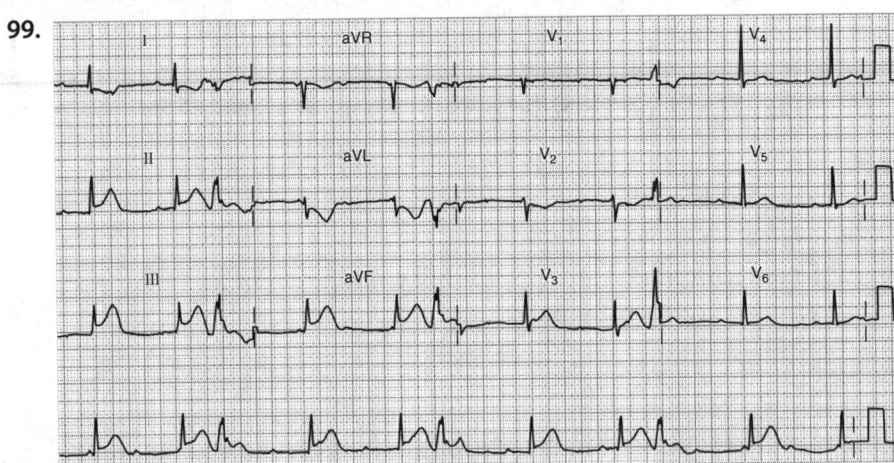

A. Posterior
B. Anterior
C. Lateral
D. Inferior

Identify the most likely diagnosis for the following EKG.

100.

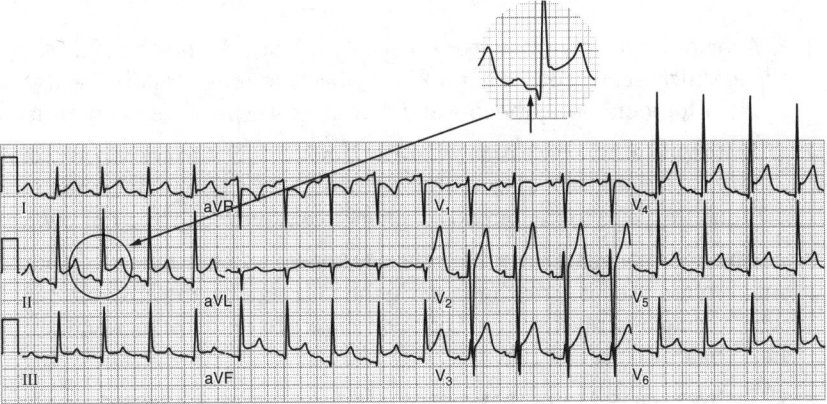

A. Hypothermia

B. Pericarditis

C. Hyperkalemia

D. Subarachnoid hemorrhage

Final Exam Answers and Rationales

1. **C.** A rhythm strip only looks at one view of the heart. A 12-lead or full EKG involves the electrical activity of the entire heart which requires 12 leads. The rhythm strip is useful for monitoring the rate and rhythm of the patient's heart during care.

2. **D.** Einthoven arbitrarily assigned the letters P, Q, R, S, T to the waveforms to designate each complete electrical heart beat. Other letters have been assigned through the years to denote other adjunctive waves such as a J or U wave.

3. **A.** An abnormal heart rhythm is officially known as a dysrhythmia. Another term that is often used is arrhythmia. Arrhythmia is actually the absence of a rhythm, which could describe asystole. Dysrhythmia is a better term to describe abnormal heart beats that can occur.

4. **C.** Tachycardia is a term that means a fast heart rate. Bradycardia is the correct term for slow heart rates. Extra beats within the heart cycle are called premature or escape beats. Lost beats can occur with heart blocks.

5. **B.** Shortness of breath can be a symptom of cardiac problems. In some patients, this can be the only symptom of a myocardial infarction. Not all patients have classic chest pain associated with an acute cardiac event. The other symptoms are not usually associated with cardiac problems.

6. **A.** Pericarditis is a term meaning that the pericardial sac surrounding the heart has become inflamed. A lack of blood flow would involve coronary heart disease. Heart failure causes the heart to not pump effectively and cardiomyopathy occurs when the heart muscle is too thick or too big to function correctly.

7. **C.** In most states the only person who can legally interpret an EKG for diagnostic purposes is the physician. Other health care professionals utilize their skill in EKG reading and rhythm identification to properly care for their patients.

8. **C.** The apex of the heart is the lower portion and is made of up of the left ventricle. The top of the heart is the broader portion and is known as the base and is comprised mostly of the left atrium.

9. **D.** The myocardium is the thick, muscular layer of the heart wall which consists of cardiac muscle fibers. It is responsible for the pumping action of the heart. The endocardium is the innermost layer made up of endothelial cells and connective tissue and is continuous with the interior layer of the arteries and veins. The epicardium is the outermost layer and is the location of the coronary arteries.

10. **A.** The tricuspid valve has three leaflets and controls the flow of blood between the right atrium and right ventricle. The mitral valve (bicuspid) lies between the left atrium and left ventricle. The valve between the pulmonary artery and the right ventricle is the pulmonic valve and the aortic valve is the one that lies between the left ventricle and the aorta.

11. **C.** Valvular regurgitation, also known as incompetence and insufficiency, occurs when blood flows back into heart chambers because the valve is not closing properly. Valvular stenosis involves a rigid or thickened valve, causing the heart to work harder to attempt to push blood through the less flexible valve. A valvular prolapse is when one of the cusps inverts.

12. **D.** An S$_3$ heart sound is an abnormal sound that can be associated with heart failure or a mitral valve regurgitation. It can be normal in young people. S$_1$ is the normal first heart sound and the closure of the aortic and pulmonic valves is the normal S$_2$ sound.

13. **C.** A positive chronotropic response is an increase in heart rate.

14. **A.** The parasympathetic nervous system slows the heart rate. The heart is innervated by the vagus nerve, the largest parasympathetic nerve in the body. When it is stimulated the heart rate decreases.

15. **B.** Rapid heart rates are often reduced by the performance of carotid sinus massage. This is done by the physician or provider. This causes stimulation of the baroreceptors which in turn activates the vagus nerve and slows the heart.

16. **D.** The four stages of the cardiac cycle start with ventricular filling. It then goes through isovolumetric ventricular contraction. Ventricular ejection is the third stage. This is when the semilunar valves open and blood is ejected. After this occurs, it is followed by isovolumetric relaxation in which all valves are closed and blood begins to fill the atria again.

17. **A.** The ejection fraction, which can be measured by an echocardiogram, assesses contractile function. The normal range is 55% to 80%.

18. **C.** Cardiac output is measured by multiplying the stroke volume (the amount of blood ejected from a ventricle) times the heart rate. Normal cardiac output in most adults is 4 to 8 L/minute.

19. **A.** Automaticity is the ability of the cardiac pacemaker cells to create an electrical impulse without stimulation by a nerve. Excitability is the ability of the cardiac cells to respond chemical, electrical, or mechanical stimuli. Conductivity is the cell's ability to receive an electrical impulse and then transmit it to another cell. Contractility is the ability to actually create a contraction after receiving an electrical impulse.

20. **B.** When the inside of the cell becomes more positive due to the movement of electrolytes across the cell membrane, a spike or positive wave appears on the EKG recording.

21. **B.** Pulseless electrical activity (PEA) occurs when only electrical activity is seen on the EKG recording. No contractions are occurring at this time. The patient will have no blood pressure or pulse.

22. **C.** Refractoriness is the ability to remain unresponsive to a stimulus or to reject an impulse. There are three refractory periods—absolute, relative, and supernormal. During the relative refractory period, a very strong stimulus can cause depolarization. This is a very vulnerable period. During the supernormal period, weaker stimuli can cause responses and is also a vulnerable period of time for the development of dysrhythmias.

23. **D.** The normal electrical pathway in the heart starts in the SA node, traveling then through the AV node, the bundle of His, the bundle branches, and finally the Purkinje fibers.

24. **B.** The AV node is a protective section of the whole impulse generating system. If it is not functioning correctly, increased rates of impulses from the atria such as with atrial fibrillation would be able to be conducted through to the ventricles.

25. **D.** Wolff-Parkinson-White (WPW) syndrome, is caused by a reentry mechanism in which an impulse spreads through the conduction system and then reenters the system again. Several factors can be present when a reentry pathway occurs.

26. **C.** In triggered activity, one of the abnormal heart impulses that can occur to create dysrhythmias, electrical impulses are conducted during the normal resting period of repolarization. An example of this is a premature atrial or junctional beat. Ventricular fibrillation and supraventricular tachycardia are caused by enhanced automaticity. Atrioventricular blocks are the result of conduction disturbances.

27. **D.** A 12-lead EKG provides for a complete picture of the electrical activity of the heart. It provides for 12 different views. A rhythm strip looks at one lead obtained by placing electrodes on the chest, is displayed on the cardiac monitor and utilizes the bipolar leads to continuously monitor the heart's activity.

28. **B.** The EASI system is a way to place a five-lead system of monitoring that can be correlated to the 12-lead EKG. The monitor that it is attached to must be able to conduct special calculations in order to provide a three dimensional view and a total of 12 views. It should not be used as a replacement for the 12-lead EKG.

29. **C.** When premature ventricular contractions are noted on the EKG, it is important to palpate the radial pulse to determine if these beats are perfusing the patient. Often, the recorder on the monitor will count these beats as part of the "heart rate", but if they are not providing mechanical contraction and perfusing the patient's body, they are not really part of the heart rate.

30. **B.** Baseline issues with the EKG recording are usually associated with patient movement or electrical interference in the room (60-cycle interference) from items such as razors, hair dryers, or radios. Replacing electrodes may help, but the positioning of the electrodes should not cause baseline issues. Repositioning the electrodes and reapplying the electrodes would help with the lack of a waveform. Checking to make sure that the correct electrode is connected to the correct wire would assist with waveform abnormalities.

31. **A.** Hyperkalemia can cause high, peaked T waves which can then be incorrectly read by the cardiac monitor to be a QRS complex. This would double the actual heart rate on the monitor and cause the high alarm to activate.

32. **B.** Each large box on the special EKG paper is made up of five of the small boxes. Each small box is equal to 0.04 seconds. Therefore, each large box is equal to 0.20 seconds.

33. **A.** A bipolar lead utilizes both a positive and a negative electrode. The standard limb leads, leads I, II, III are the bipolar leads. The augmented leads, aVR, aVL, and aVF, are unipolar leads which uses the heart as a relative negative "electrode."

34. **D.** Einthoven's triangle is an imaginary triangle that is formed by the three bipolar leads. This shows the frontal plane views of the heart.

35. **D.** Lead II is accomplished by placing the positive electrode on the patient's left leg and the negative electrode on the right arm. For lead I, positive electrode is on the left arm and the negative electrode is on the right arm. For lead III, the

positive electrode is placed on the left leg and the negative electrode is on the left arm.

36. **B.** Lead V_2 is correctly placed at the fourth intercostal space to the left of the sternum. The fourth intercostal space to the right of the sternum is the correct placement for lead V_1. Lead V_4 is placed at the fifth intercostal space at the midclavicular line and lead V_5 is at the fifth intercostal space at the anterior axillary line. Lead V_3 is placed between lead V_2 and V_4 and lead V_6 is at the fifth intercostal space at the midaxillary line.

37. **D.** Lead V_4R looks at the right side of the heart. Its proper placement would be the fifth intercostal space at the right midclavicular line.

38. **C.** Lead V_8, which would be accomplished to view changes for a posterior wall infarct, is placed correctly at the fifth intercostal space in the area of the posterior scapular area. Lead V_7 is placed at the posterior axillary line in the fifth intercostal space. Lead V_9 is placed at the fifth intercostal space at the border of the spine on the left side.

39. **C.** Modified chest leads can be used to help in distinguishing bundle branch blocks, premature beats, and supraventricular rhythms. These bipolar leads are MCL_1 and MCL_6.

40. **A.** The P wave designates depolarization of the atria. The Q and R waves are part of the QRS complex and is related to ventricular depolarization. The T wave displays ventricular repolarization.

41. **B.** Any part of the QRS complex that is 5 mm or more below the isoelectric line is denoted with a lower case letter. All three parts of this complex can be present or there may only be a QS, RS, qS, etc. An R (or S) prime occurs when there is an extra R (or S) wave and it actually touches and crosses the baseline. When it simply changes directions, it is called a notch. The lowest amplitude for the R wave occurs in V_1 and then progressively increases in size, with the greatest amplitude being in V_6.

42. **C.** Poor R wave progression can be caused by many etiologies including dextrocardia, bundle branch blocks, hypertrophy, acute myocardial infarction, pacing rhythms, Wolff-Parkinson-White (WPW) syndrome, tension pneumothorax, emphysema, and precordial lead displacement.

43. **D.** Inverted or depressed T waves can be seen with cerebral bleeding such as a subarachnoid hemorrhage. It can also be manifested with myocardial ischemia, hypokalemia, and hypomagnesemia. High or peaked T waves are seen with hyperkalemia, pacemakers, and myocardial injury.

44. **C.** The normal PR interval falls between 0.12 and 0.20 seconds. The pediatric patient usually reaches the normal adult PR interval by age 12 to 16 years of age. At birth the PR interval is very short, 0.07 to 0.14 seconds, due to the faster heart rate and the smaller ventricles. The normal QT interval is 0.36 to 0.44 seconds.

45. **A.** A prolonged QT interval can predispose patients to a life-threatening tachydysrhythmia known as torsades de pointes. Many different situations can cause this increased threat.

46. **B.** Calipers can assist in determining and verifying regularity of a rhythm. Another way to do this is to use an index card or other piece of paper to mark out each R wave. Heart rate, PR interval, and QRS width is established by using the small and large boxes to measure.

47. **D.** Using the small box method to determine the heart rate is the most precise. Count the number of small boxes between two R waves and divide that number into 1500. With 15 small boxes counted, the heart rate would then be 100. In the large box method, the number to use to divide into is 300.

48. **C.** For normal sinus rhythm to be truly present, the QRS width should fall between 0.36 and 0.44 seconds. Normal sinus rhythm (NSR) should have a heart rate between 60 to 100 beats per minute, have a PR interval between 0.12 to 0.20 seconds, and have no ectopic beats.

49. **B.** In the hexaxial reference system, the upper segments represent negative degrees and the lower or bottom sections carry positive degrees. The mean electrical axis is defined as the direction that the mean vector is taking when it is viewed from a circle of degrees on the frontal plane. The normal mean electrical axis should fall within the scope of 0° to +90°. Right axis deviation is represented by a range of +180° to +90°. Left axis deviation corresponds to −90° to 0° on the hexaxial reference system.

50. **D.** A left axis deviation is noted when lead I is positive and aVF is negative. Right axis deviation is occurring when lead I is negative and aVF is positive. Extreme right axis deviation is shown with a negative lead I and a negative aVF. The normal axis is for both leads I and aVF to have positive deflections.

51. **A.** Pregnancy, along with other processes in which the diaphragm is pushed upwards (ascites, abdominal distention, and obesity) can cause a left axis deviation. Other causes of left axis deviation might be an inferior myocardial infarction, a left bundle branch block, left ventricular hypertrophy, or a pacemaker.

52. **B.** Hypertrophy, caused by an increase in the muscle mass itself, occurs because of an increase in pressure rather than volume. Hypertension and aortic insufficiency are two possible causes of hypertrophy. Enlargement, an expansion or dilation of a chamber from an increase in volume, is usually used to describe the atria and hypertrophy usually relates to the ventricles.

53. **C.** Right atrial enlargement would be recognized on the upswing of the P wave. This part of the P wave denotes right atrial activity. When this portion of the P wave is tall and peaked, it is known as P pulmonale. The left atrium is seen through the downstroke, or second portion, of the P wave. When it is prominent and deep, it can represent left atrial enlargement. P mitrale, seen with a notched P wave, is indicative of left atrial enlargement.

54. **C.** For a bundle branch block to be considered to be complete, the width of the QRS complex must be greater than 0.12 seconds. A bundle branch block, noted with an R prime (R'), that is incomplete will have a shorter width.

55. **D.** A left bundle branch block will distinguish itself in leads V_5 and V_6. A right bundle branch block will be represented in leads V_1 and V_2.

56. **A.** When a patient presents with a left bundle branch block, it is difficult to note the changes that are consistent with an acute myocardial infarction.

57. **B.** The Valsalva maneuver is a process in which the vagus nerve is stimulated in an effort to slow the heart rate. It is performed by having the patient cough, hold their breath and push down as if having a bowel movement, or by placing their face in ice cold water. This is used to treat some tachydysrhythmias.

58. **D.** Infants normally have a higher heart rate. Any rate below 90 to 100 would be considered to be bradycardic for this age group.

59. **C.** Infants and young children are not able to change their stroke volume. In order to increase cardiac output, which is the outcome of stroke volume times heart rate, they can only increase their heart rate. This is the way that their body attempts to compensate for a low cardiac output.

60. **B.** Sinus arrhythmia can be a normal phenomenon in children. This is associated with respirations and is seen as a fluctuating increase and decrease in heart rate. A non-respiratory sinus arrhythmia can be seen in older adults due to the aging process.

61. **A.** Bradycardic heart rhythms associated with escape beats should be given medications to speed up the heart. The escape beats are there in an attempt to "rescue" the patient. Do not give medications to eradicate the extra beats or medication, such as beta blockers, that would work to slow the heart rate further.

62. **C.** Sick sinus syndrome is also known as Brady-tachy syndrome. This is a dysrhythmia that is caused by problems in both the conductivity and automaticity of the heart. It is most common in older adults and in children who have had open heart procedures.

63. **B.** Premature atrial contractions (PACs) will have a noncompensatory pause after each one. A premature ventricular contraction (PVC) will have a compensatory pause. PACs will have P waves and will have an irregular rhythm. The QRS is not wide with a PAC.

64. **B.** Trigeminy is the correct term for premature beats when they occur after two normal beats, that is, every third beat is a premature beat. Bigeminy occurs when every other beat is premature. Quadrigeminy is when every fourth beat is premature. The term coupling is used when two premature beats occur together.

65. **D.** When wandering atrial pacemaker rates increase over 100 beats per minute, it is known as multifocal atrial tachycardia. The majority of the other characteristics remain the same for both of these dysrhythmias.

66. **A.** Wolff-Parkinson-White (WPW) syndrome, a type of reentry supraventricular tachycardia, occurs due to a congenital bridge of tissue called the bundle of Kent.

67. **A.** When administering adenosine (Adenocard), the best intravenous access is the right antecubital space. A larger catheter is recommended and the medication must be administered very quickly due to the half-life of this drug being extremely short. It should be administered with a rapid infusion of normal saline and the rhythm to watch for would be a short period of asystole immediately after injection. Patients with Wolff-Parkinson-White (WPW) syndrome should not receive this medication.

68. **C.** When administering synchronized cardioversion for stable ventricular tachy-cardia, medication patches on the patient's chest should be removed. The patient should be on the monitor that is being used to administer the shocks and "blips" should be marking each QRS complex. The buttons or paddles must be held down until the shock is delivered.

69. **B.** When atrial fibrillation occurs, there is a loss of atrial kick, which normally increases cardiac output. The atria are not providing good quality contractions during this time.

70. **D.** In atrial fibrillation, the P waves are undetectable. The atrial rate is so fast, 400 to 600 beats per minute, that they cannot be seen. The sawtooth pattern is seen with atrial flutter. There is not PR interval to measure and the QRS is not normally widened.

71. **C.** The inherent rate for a junctional rhythm is 40 to 60 beats per minute. A tachycardic version of a junctional rhythm can occur, but the normal rate would be as stated.

72. **A.** Premature ventricular contractions that are "multiform" or "multifocal" have dif-ferent configurations. It can signify diverse ectopic sites however, a single ectopic site can actually produce multiform PVCs.

73. **A.** R on T phenomenon can occur with a single premature ventricular contraction (PVC). When this PVC falls on the T wave of the preceding complex, the repolariza-tion process is unable to complete and ventricular tachycardia or ventricular fibrillation can occur.

74. **C.** The 5 H's of pulseless electrical activity (PEA) are: Hypovolemia, Hypoxia, Hypo/ Hyperthermia, Hypo/Hyperkalemia, Hydrogen Ion (acidosis).

75. **A.** Mechanical capture of a pacemaker would be indicated by the presence of a palpable pulse. A pacer blip or spike would designate electrical activity of the pacemaker and the QRS after each blip or spike would indicate electrical capture.

76. **B.** Torsades de pointes (TdP) is associated with a prolonged QT interval that can occur for a variety of reasons. This is a term that means "twisting of the points" and is seen on the EKG as QRS complexes that are of varying shapes, sizes, and amplitude.

77. **B.** Mobitz type I AV block is also known as Wenckebach. This occurs when the PR interval lengthens progressively until a complete QRS complex is dropped. The process then starts again for the next dropped beat. Mobitz type II (type II AV block) has constant PR intervals and the dropped beats occur throughout the rhythm strip. First-degree AV block has a prolonged PR interval and in third-degree or complete AV block there is no correlation between the P waves and the QRS complexes.

78. **B.** Prinzmetal or variant angina usually occurs during rest and peaks between midnight and 8 o'clock in the morning. During the time of coronary artery spasm, ST segments are elevated on the EKG. Atherosclerotic heart disease can occur with this type of angina, but is not always present.

79. **D.** An injury pattern on the EKG is seen through an elevation of the ST segment. T wave depression is indicative of ischemia. The pathologic Q wave indicates infarction.

80. **A.** Reciprocal changes, ST segment depression, is seen as a mirror image of the site of the injury. They occur opposite of the area in which the actual injury is occurring.

81. **D.** A lateral myocardial infarction would be indicated with changes occurring in leads I, aVL, V_5 and V_6. Leads II, III, and aVF will look at the inferior portion of the heart. Leads V_1, V_2, V_3, and V_4 are indicative of changes in the anterior portion of the heart. Leads I, II and III do not look at the same aspect of the heart.

82. **B.** The major right coronary artery supplies the right atrium, the SA node and AV node. The interventricular septum is nourished by the left anterior descending (LAD) artery and the posterior interventricular branch of the right coronary artery. The right ventricle is supplied by the LAD and the right marginal and posterior interventricular branches of the right coronary artery. The circumflex (CX) branch of the left coronary artery supplies the left atrium.

83. **C.** Troponin is the biomarker that remains elevated for the longest period of time (up to 5 days). CK-MB, an isoenzyme of creatinine kinase, usually returns to normal within 48 to 72 hours. Myoglobin, is released rapidly but does not stay elevated for a lengthy time.

84. **D.** Hypomagnesemia can be a precursor to torsades de pointes (TdP).

85. **A.** Subarachnoid hemorrhage might present with deeply inverted or depressed T waves. Other EKG changes that might accompany this central nervous system disease process are bradycardia, the presence of u waves and prolongation of the QT interval.

86. **B.** The PR interval is normal and the rate is less than 60 beats per minute.

87. **B.** The P waves vary in morphology and the rate is greater than 100 beats per minute. The rhythm is regular.

88. **C.** There is no lengthened PR interval and no progressive "dropped" beats. The P waves and QRS complexes do have a coordination. The PR intervals are constant.

89. **D.** The rhythm is regular and the QRS complexes are of the same shape and height. There is a pattern to the rhythm.

90. **B.** The rhythm is irregularly irregular. The PR is not measurable as no P waves are detectable. No sawtooth pattern is seen. There are distinct QRS complexes.

91. **C.** The rate is faster than 100 beats per minute. The P waves and QRS complexes are distinct.

92. **A.** The rhythm is regular and rapid (>150-250 beats per minute). The P waves are indistinguishable due to the fast rate. No sawtooth pattern is seen.

93. **B.** The rhythm is chaotic and irregular. No rate, waves or complexes are discernible.

94. **D.** The atrial and ventricular rates are regular but are independent of each other. There is no correlation between each P wave and QRS complex. The ventricular rate is slower.

95. **B.** The rate is between 60 to 100 beats per minute. The P waves and QRS complexes are discernible and have correlation between each other. The P wave is consistent.

96. **A.** Premature ventricular contractions are wide and bizarre. Premature atrial and junctional complexes look like their counterparts within the rhythm and are not wide. A premature atrial contraction will have a P wave and a premature junctional contraction may have no P wave, a depressed P wave, or a P wave occurring within the QRS complex.

97. **B.** The rhythm is regular and the rate is between 20 to 40 beats per minute. The QRS complex is wide and bizarre and no P waves are noted.

98. **C.** P waves are present but no ventricular activity is discernible.

99. **D.** ST segment inferior myocardial infarctions (STEMI) are seen in leads II, III, and aVF.

100. **B.** Pericarditis can present with diffuse ST segment elevation across multiple leads on the EKG in the early stages. Hypothermia can have a distinguishing J wave or Osborne wave. Hyperkalemia would have high peaked T waves. A subarachnoid hemorrhage would have EKG changes that would present as deeply inverted T waves, bradycardia, and the presence of U waves.

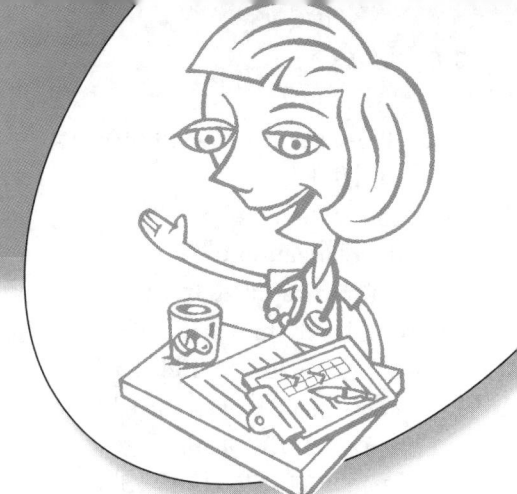

Index

A